Barbara Vincent

Adaptation

See Mrs. Diles about Achievement Test

2- -66

# Basic
# Medical-Surgical
# Nursing

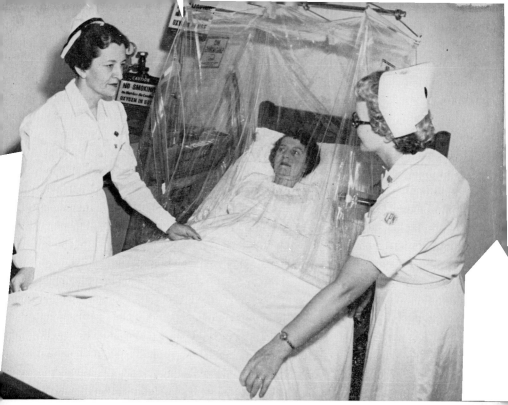

The registered professional nurse and the licensed practical nurse working as a team in caring for the patient. (Long's Photo Service, Norfolk,
Virginia.)

# Basic
# Medical-Surgical
# Nursing

MILDRED A. MASON, R.N., B.S.

SUPERVISOR, PRACTICAL NURSE EDUCATION
NORFOLK CITY SCHOOLS

New York
The Macmillan Company

DEDICATED TO

MRS. MILDRED LAWRENCE BRADSHAW, R.N
A *Pioneer in Practical Nurse Education*

# *Preface*

Along with the rapid growth of practical nursing schools, following World War II, the licensed practical or licensed vocational nurse has become an integral part of nursing. Her responsibilities have been increased in scope, especially in the care of patients with the more common diseases. *Basic Medical-Surgical Nursing* was written to help meet the need for a textbook which deals with these responsibilities.

Throughout the textbook, emphasis is placed on the individual who is affected by disease. When either medical or surgical treatment or a combination of both is frequently used for an individual with a specific disease, all methods of treatment have been discussed.

Part I contains background information. A special feature of this section is a chapter dealing with the common symptoms of illness. Knowledge of these symptoms makes more effective the practical nurse's ability to nurse the patients entrusted to her care.

Part II discusses the responsibilities of the practical nurse in caring for a patient with a general disease condition, such as an inflammation or cancer.

Parts III through XI deal with the role of the practical nurse in caring for the patient with one of the more common diseases of a system of his body.

Each part is interrelated with preceding and subsequent discussions. For example, knowledge of the common symptoms of illness (Part I, Chapter 4) and the body's reaction to an inflammation (Part II, Chapter 6) is essential for the practical nurse's understanding of an infection such as pneumonia (Part IV, Chapter 13) and appendicitis (Part V, Chapter 15). The practical nurse must have such knowledge and understanding if she is to give effective nursing care.

Effort has been made to correlate such areas of knowledge without undue repetition. In teaching courses commonly known as "Introduction to Conditions of Illness" and "Medical and Surgical Nursing" or "Common Diseases," the instructor of practical nurses should find this correlation a decided asset when using *Basic Medical-Surgical Nursing* as a student textbook.

Helpful adjuncts to the text discussion include "Suggestions for Study" and "References" at the end of each of the twenty-four chapters, as well as a "Glossary" containing approximately five hundred entries.

Although this text has been prepared primarily for the student practical nurse, it also serves as a source of information for the licensed practical nurse who is already engaged in nursing.

                                                   M.A.M.

Norfolk, Virginia

March 10, 1959

# *Acknowledgments*

Many persons have made the preparation of this text possible. The author is especially grateful to Mrs. Mildred L. Bradshaw, R.N., director of nurses at the Leigh Memorial Hospital in Norfolk, Virginia, for giving her the opportunity to enter into practical nursing over ten years ago when it was in its infancy. Her wise counsel has been a constant source of help in the teaching of practical nurses as well as in the preparation of this book. A special debt of gratitude is owed Mrs. Jean L. Miller, R.N., for her consistent encouragement, cooperation, and material help to the author.

Grateful appreciation is extended to Mrs. Nettie B. Spence, L.P.N., and Mrs. Sallie H. Parrish, L.P.N., editor of *Practical Nurses Digest*, who have made innumerable suggestions regarding the content which they believed would be of value to the practical nurse student as well as the licensed practical nurse.

Acknowledgment is made to Robert W. Alfriend, M.D., and Elliott D. Floyd, M.D., for reading the major portion of the manuscript and making many excellent recommendations. Gratitude is also expressed to Milton H. Bland, M.D.; Miss Hazel Dunaway, B.S.; R. J. Faulconer, M.D.; W. C. Salley, M.D., Ph.D.; D. C. Whitehead, M.D.; and F. G. Woodson, M.D., for reviewing parts of the book and giving suggestions.

The author wishes to express her appreciation to the following: Kathlyn Y. Egan, R.N., consultant, Oxygen Therapy Department, Linde Company, Division of the Union Carbide Corporation, New York City, for helping to prepare the information regarding oxygen therapy; Misses Elizabeth Boggs and Janice Bland for editing the original manuscript; Miss Lillian Hooper for helping to prepare the illustrations; and Mrs. Beulah P. Griffin, L.P.N., for typing the manuscript. Also, sincere thanks are extended to the staff of The Macmillan Company for their constant and invaluable assistance in making this textbook possible.

M.A.M.

# Contents

Contents                                    xi

# xii Contents

Contagiosa, Nursing Care. Breast Conditions: Structure and Function, Mastitis, Chronic Cystic Mastitis, Benign Tumor, Cancer. Burn. Cancer

*Introduction
to the
Practical Nurse's
Role in Caring
for the Medical
and Surgical Patient*

PART I

Chapter 1              *HISTORICAL DEVELOPMENT OF PRACTICAL NURSING*

| Chapter Outline | MEDICINE SURGERY PRACTICAL NURSING | HEALTH TEAM NURSING TEAM |
|---|---|---|

The roots of practical nursing grow deeply into the past history of man, especially in the fields of medicine and surgery. If the practical nurse of today is to fulfill her responsibility in caring for the medical and surgical patient, it is necessary for her to be aware of and to appreciate the rapid advances being made in medical science. In order to do this, a brief review of past progress is essential.

## MEDICINE

Primitive man based his care of the sick on instinct and superstitions. He believed that evil spirits caused illness. Therefore, magic was used in an attempt to appease the evil spirits or to frighten them away. This is still the belief of some primitive tribes today.

Man has made gradual progress through the centuries in discovering and using scientific knowledge for the improvement of health. Several thousand years before the birth of Christ the early Egyptians and Babylonians practiced surgery and were skillful in mixing drugs. Approximately seven hundred years before Christ was born, the Hebrews believed that disease was the result of Jehovah's anger. An appeal to Jehovah was necessary for the person to be cured. The teachings of Moses stressed cleanliness, sanitation, and the separation of ill people from the healthy in order to prevent the spread of disease.

Several hundred years before the birth of Christ, the people of ancient Greece placed great importance on health and beauty. Hippocrates, known as the father of medicine, appeared on the scene

3

during this period. He emphasized the study of the patient rather than the seeking of magic formulas for treating disease. His writings contain descriptions of surgical conditions such as fractured vertebrae and clubfoot.

Just before the birth of Christ and following His death, the Romans made great progress in public sanitation. The streets were clean; the water, pure; and the houses, well ventilated. Following the fall of the Roman Empire, medicine, as well as other sciences, was enveloped in the darkness of the Middle Ages. Living conditions lapsed into an unsanitary state. The bubonic plague, or the Black Death, swept over Europe, causing many deaths in 1348. This dread disease occurred at intervals until the end of the seventeenth century. Ships and people were quarantined in an effort to prevent the spread of bubonic plague. Hospitals were first organized during the early Middle Ages.

During the sixteenth and seventeenth centuries there was a re-birth of the sciences. Surgery had become a separate branch of medicine. Anatomy was established as a science, the circulation of the blood discovered, and the microscope was developed and used.

In the eighteenth century, hospitals were overcrowded and noted for their uncleanliness. A movement to improve living and working conditions was begun. Vaccination against smallpox was introduced during this century.

The nineteenth century was a period of rapid advance in medicine. The fact that communicable diseases are caused by germs entering the body was established. Hospitals were improved; new laws of sanitation were passed; public health departments were organized; and x-ray, radium, and vaccines to prevent diseases such as diphtheria and typhoid fever were discovered.

During the present century the progress which has already been made by man in his fight against disease is amazing. Blood trans-fusions are a daily occurrence in hospitals as a result of the discovery of blood groups. Insulin to treat diabetes, liver extract to treat pernicious anemia, drugs to relieve allergies, a vaccine to prevent poliomyelitis, and drugs to cure syphilis have been discovered. Na-tional, state, and local health services have been developed. Advances have been made in mother and baby care. Patients with mental ill-ness are now treated kindly and scientifically. The modern science of nutrition has been founded. The sulfonamides and antibiotics used in fighting infection have been discovered. These are some of the outstanding developments of the twentieth century. At present, research is being done on cancer, heart disease, and many other diseases.

## SURGERY

Surgery is a branch of medicine which deals with the treatment of disease by manual or instrumental operations. Prior to the nineteenth century, surgery usually resulted in infection, gangrene, and often death. Antiseptics and sterilization were not used then. After studying Pasteur's work with microorganisms, Joseph Lister used carbolic acid for disinfection in the operating room in 1865. The horrible infections associated with surgery began to decrease as he improved his method of antisepsis. The surgeon of today uses the aseptic technique in which no microorganisms are allowed to come in contact with the operative area.

The use of anesthesia was started in the middle of the nineteenth century. As a result, the patient could have surgery without feeling the surgeon's knife.

The greatest progress has been made in surgery since the beginning of the twentieth century. Research has made it possible for the surgeon to increase his knowledge. Early ambulation, getting the patient out of bed within 24 to 48 hours after surgery, has reduced postoperative complications such as pneumonia and the formation of blood clots. New anesthetics, antibiotics, and new drugs to relieve pain have been introduced. Advances have been made in improving the actual techniques of operation. Remarkable progress is being made in brain, heart, and lung surgery.

## PRACTICAL NURSING

In glancing over the brief historical background of medicine and surgery, the practical nurse will realize that she is entering the health field at an exciting time, since man is making amazing progress in the conquest of disease. She is one of many important members who contribute to the health and welfare of our people.

Although practical nursing is as old as mankind, planned teaching of practical nurses is relatively new. The first practical nurses were people who cared for the sick in their homes. There was usually someone in the family or village who liked to care for the sick. This kind person used her knowledge of homemaking to comfort and to care for the ill.

As civilization progressed, the need for especially prepared nurses grew. Modern nursing was born of this need. In 1860 Florence Nightingale established the first modern school for nurses in England. The movement of training nurses spread, and in **1873 a training** school was started in the United States. The practical nurse continued to care for the sick in their homes, while the trained nurse cared for hospitalized patients. It was not until the early 1900's that the practical nurse was replaced to a great extent by the trained nurse. A critical shortage of professional nurses to care for hospitalized patients occurred during World War II. This shortage resulted from a transfer of graduate nurses from civilian hospitals to the armed forces, and a marked increase in the number of people who went to hospitals. Other changes in our society which influenced the development of practical nurse education were: (1) emphasis on preventive medicine and public health, (2) rapid construction of hospitals, and (3) increase of specialties in medicine and surgery. With these changes the duties of the professional nurse increased. Also, the need for nurses outgrew the supply of nurses. The medical and nursing professions realized the necessity for providing nursing care to supplement that given by the professional nurse. The hospitals began to employ practical nurses. Because the number of practical nurses with training was small, farsighted professional nurses began to plan courses for practical nurses.

The growth of practical nursing schools has been rapid. Approximately 12 schools were functioning before World War II. By the end of the war in 1945 the number of approved schools of practical nursing had increased to 46. The number has increased to over 500 at the present time.

The registered or professional nurse acts as the team leader. She is responsible for planning, supervising, and giving nursing care. The registered nurse determines the needs of the individual patient. She then assigns the members of the nursing team most capable of meeting those needs to care for him. For example, the team leader may assume the responsibility for teaching the patient to give himself insulin. She may assign the licensed practical nurse to change his dressing, and the nurse's aide to make his bed. The team members are responsible to each other for the care of all patients assigned to them and to the team leader. Each member can contribute information about the patient or his condition to others on the team to improve the patient's care.

Although the assignment of certain patients to a specific nursing team is not used in all hospitals, teamwork can still be practiced. *Teamwork* means sharing and working together for a common goal. All individuals responsible for the nursing care of a patient must work together for the patient's welfare.

## HEALTH TEAM

The health team is composed of individuals who work together to meet the health needs of an individual. Members of the health team often include a physician, a nurse, a social worker, a pharmacist, a dietitian, a dentist, a sanitation engineer, an occupational therapist, a spiritual adviser, a psychologist, and a physical therapist. Usually the doctor is the leader, who calls upon the services of other members for help. Each member of the health team makes a contribution, but its smooth functioning depends upon how well each cooperates.

## NURSING TEAM

The nursing team is an important part of the over-all health team. Members of the team responsible for nursing include the registered or professional nurse, the licensed practical nurse, the student nurse, the nurse's aide, and the orderly. Their aim is to give the patient the best care possible.

The physician is responsible for diagnosis and treatment. He outlines the plan to be followed when he writes orders for the patient. The nursing team follows his decisions in caring for the patient.

## SUGGESTIONS FOR STUDY

1. Talk with an older member of your community about the changes that he has seen in medicine and surgery.
2. Discuss superstitions regarding health which you have heard.
3. When was surgery first practiced?

4. Who was Hippocrates? When did he live?
5. Make a brief outline showing when the following were discovered: circulation of the blood, microscope, smallpox vaccination, germs, x-ray, disinfection, anesthesia, typhoid vaccine, insulin, and liver extract.
6. Who were the first practical nurses?
7. When was the first training school for nurses established in England? In the United States?
8. List some of the changes in our society which influenced the growth of practical nurse education.
9. How many schools of practical nursing were in this country before World War II? After World War II? What is the approximate number now?
10. How many members of the health team do you know? What are their duties?
11. Discuss the meaning of *teamwork*.

REFERENCES FOR CHAPTER 1

Dakin, Florence; Thompson, Ella M.; and Le Baron, Margaret: *Simplified Nursing*, 6th ed. J. B. Lippincott Co., Philadelphia, 1956, pp. 3-15.
Deming, Dorothy: "Practical Nursing and the Changing Professional Attitude," *Am. J. Nursing*, 46:366-70, (June) 1946.
———: *The Practical Nurse*. Commonwealth Fund, New York, 1947.
———: "Practical Nursing Then and Now," *Am. J. Nursing*, 50:621-23, (Oct.) 1950.
Eliason, Eldridge; Ferguson, L. Kraeer; and Sholtis, Lillian A.: *Surgical Nursing*, 10th ed. J. B. Lippincott Co., Philadelphia, 1955, pp. 1-11 and 32-33.
Emerson, Charles P., Jr., and Bragdon, Jane S.: *Essentials of Medicine*, 17th ed. J. B. Lippincott Co., Philadelphia, 1955, pp. 3-13.
Field, Minna: "The Nurse and the Social Worker on the Hospital Team," *Am. J. Nursing*, 55:694-96, (June) 1955.
Fuerst, Elinor V., and Wolff, LuVerne: *Fundamentals of Nursing*. J. B. Lippincott Co., Philadelphia, 1956, pp. 1-8.
Gill, Helen Z. (ed.): *Basic Nursing*, 4th ed. The Macmillan Company, New York, 1955, pp. 3-10.
Jamieson, Elizabeth, and Sewall, Mary: *Trends in Nursing History*, 4th ed. W. B. Saunders Co., Philadelphia, 1954.
Jensen, Julius, and Jensen, Deborah: *Nursing in Clinical Medicine*, 4th ed. The Macmillan Company, New York, 1954, pp. 6-11 and 19-24.
Knapp, Margaret F.: "Public Schools Train Practical Nurses," *Nursing World*, 216:37-39, (Jan.) 1952.

"Practical Nursing Programs in 1957," *Nursing Oultook,* 6:443-45, (Aug.) 1958.
Stafford, Edward S., and Diller, Doris: *Surgery and Surgical Nursing,* 3rd ed. W. B. Saunders Co., Philadelphia, 1958, pp. 1-4.
Todd, C. Edwina: "Teamwork in Practical Nursing," *Practical Nurses Digest,* 2:10-11, (July) 1955.
Torrop, Hilda M.: "Developments in the Field of Practical Nursing," *Am. J. Nursing,* 52:72-73, (Jan.) 1952.
Weddige, Dorothy: "The Work of Practical Nurses in New York City Municipal Hospitals," *Practical Nurses Digest,* 2:3-5, (Apr.) 1955.

# Chapter 2

# THE INDIVIDUAL AS A PATIENT

## INTRODUCTION

A *patient* is an *individual* who needs care. He is under the care of the physician and other members of the health team because of sickness or disease. Although the sick person is a patient, he retains his individuality. It is of vital importance for the practical nurse to understand that when a person is ill, the entire individual is affected and not only the appendix which is inflamed or the bone which is broken. Thus, the entire individual needs care.

*Psychosomatic medicine* is a special branch of medicine which is being developed as a result of the realization that illness must be considered and treated in relation to the whole individual. *"Psycho"* refers to the soul or mind and *"soma"* to the body. The term *psychosomatic* indicates the close relationship between the mind and the body. It implies that the mind cannot be sick without affecting the physical body, or the physical body without affecting the mind. A person's mind and body influence his health.

An individual may develop a psychosomatic illness as a result of stresses put on his body by unpleasant feelings, such as worry and fear. These feelings can disturb the functioning of an organ or a certain part of his body and cause physical symptoms. For example, fear can cause an individual to secrete more urine. The functioning of the urinary system is disturbed. Another example is seen in the person who is angry. His stomach may contract faster, and secrete more gastric juice during this time. The walls of his stomach can also become reddened. These functional changes may cause him to complain of indigestion and pain. If he continues to have this feeling of anger for a prolonged period of time, he may eventually develop a peptic ulcer. Thus, the person with a psychosomatic illness has symptoms of physical disease. He may not have a physical disease or he may have one.

## BEHAVIOR CHANGES

When a person is sick, he is confronted with problems such as discomfort, pain, disability, and loss of income or even the loss of life. It is understandable that an individual's behavior is affected by illness. The practical nurse should understand that a person usually acts differently when he is sick. For example, a patient may cry more easily, may be depressed, or may be overly critical of the hospital. Such a change in the individual's behavior may be a direct result of disease, or it may be associated with the frustrations of illness as illustrated in the following cases.

The case of Mr. Thompson is an example of a behavior change which was a direct result of disease. This patient was recuperating from a stroke (cerebral accident). On one occasion, after the practical nurse and the orderly had assisted him in walking to a chair, he cried. This middle-aged man had not wept since he was a boy. In a few minutes he was laughing and talking. The practical nurse had learned that sudden emotional outbursts, such as crying and laughing, are associated with a stroke. Since the nurse understood the relationship of emotional reactions to the physical condition of a patient with a stroke, she was not surprised by Mr. Thompson's behavior. The practical nurse can easily understand that the entire individual is affected and not only the diseased area of his brain.

Another example of disease affecting the entire individual is seen in the case of Mr. Adams, who was in a body cast because of three fractured vertebrae. He appeared depressed to the student practical nurse when she began his daily bath. Mr. Adams responded to the kindly attitude of the nurse by talking about his family and his job as a truck driver. The patient seemed most concerned about the welfare of his wife and four children while he was unable to earn a livelihood. It is evident that Mr. Adams' depressed mood was associated with his illness. He was suffering from depression as well as from fractured vertebrae.

The practical nurse needs to understand that the healthy individual has many channels into which he directs his efforts and interests. Many of these channels are closed when a person becomes ill. The physical confinement of the patient to a smaller unit of living, the loss of energy associated with disease, and the patient's concern over his welfare are important factors in the narrowing of his personal interests.

This may be illustrated by the illness of Mrs. East. She and her husband lived in a newly acquired brick home. Mrs. East had joined several of the local community clubs and was especially interested in the garden club. She spent many happy hours digging, planting, and caring for her flower garden. The night after she had planted several rose bushes she started having chills and fever. The next day she was admitted to the hospital for observation. During this period of observation, Mrs. East spent many long hours looking at the four walls of the hospital room. Her thoughts were centered on herself. She wondered what was causing her illness, when she would be feeling better, and whether she were going to get well. Prior to this Mrs. East had had many interests other than herself. Being sick caused her to focus her thoughts primarily on herself. She was temporarily egocentric, or self-centered. As Mrs. East improved, she became less self-centered, and her interest in outside activities returned.

Patients frequently lose interest in things which have previously been important to them. This loss may be slight in the case of one person and markedly greater in another. Factors which may seem unimportant to the well person frequently become extremely important to a patient. An example of this is seen in the patient's diet which often assumes greater importance than it assumed previously. Mealtime becomes one of the anticipated highlights of his day. The patient can usually depend on the diversion of having his tray served three times a day. The practical nurse needs to realize that patients look forward to mealtime as a break in an otherwise monotonous day, but often do not feel hungry. For this reason she can expect some patients to be overly critical of their food. This should be a challenge to the practical nurse to do whatever possible to make the meal more appetizing to the patient.

## LISTENING TO THE PATIENT

The practical nurse is able to understand either a well or a sick person only if she develops the art of listening. Listening can be considered as a golden key to understanding. The term *listening* is not used in this text to imply an entirely one-sided conversation from the patient to the nurse. It means that the nurse talks *with the* patient rather than *to* him. She frequently injects into the conversation interested remarks which show that she is really listening. The nurse who is a persistent chatterer is not able to understand the patient because she does not listen to him.

Geniune interest is a basic requirement for developing the art of listening and leads to understanding. All of us have had the experience of talking with someone who did not appear interested in what we were saying. That person was not listening to us because of lack of interest. The practical nurse must have a genuine interest in the patient as a person if she is to understand him. She should remember that words and gestures are indications of the patient's feelings. What the patient says and how he says it can be considered symptoms of his thoughts and emotions. For example, Mr. Branch, a preoperative patient asked the practical nurse several times if she knew the surgeon who was to operate on him that morning. Mr. Branch seemed to be anxious when he asked the question. Since the practical nurse was really listening to what the patient was saying, she was able to understand that his repeated question probably indicated apprehension. She reported her observation to the head nurse, who asked the surgeon to stop by and see the patient before surgery. Because of her interest in the patient, she was able to listen and to understand him. She contributed to his emotional as well as his physical well-being.

A good listener can lighten another person's burden. The commonly heard expression referring to the load lifted from one's shoulders expresses the relief obtained when an individual finds an interested and understanding listener. Although a person may not find a solution to his worries and problems, he often finds relief in talking about them because he has shared his burden. As the practical nurse spends a great deal of time in giving actual bedside care to the patient, she frequently has the opportunity to give this kind of help.

The practical nurse needs to realize that the art of listening does not always indicate agreement. It does mean that the good listener tries to understand what is being said. If the patient feels that the practical nurse is critical of what he is saying, he may try to defend his statements. He may also stop talking when he feels the listener is criticizing instead of understanding.

The nurse who is overly concerned with the actual procedure rather than with the patient receiving it is placing an obstacle in the way of understanding. Although technical skill is necessary in the care of a patient, it should not receive so much emphasis that the nurse loses sight of the human being who is involved. For example, the nurse who focuses all of her attention on making the bed skillfully and quickly may give the patient the impression that the bed is more important than he is. He may feel the nurse is too busy to be bothered with him. The practical nurse needs to master the skills involved in nursing so well that she can focus her attention on the patient himself. Thus, she can develop the art of listening, which will lead to understanding.

Realizing the influence that worries, fears, anxieties, and problems may have on the patient's recovery helps the practical nurse to remember the importance of reporting these to her team leader or head nurse. She, in turn, transmits them to the doctor and other appropriate team members, such as the spiritual adviser, the social worker, and other nurses. The communication of this information through the head nurse to other team members often makes it possible for the problem to be solved. An example of this is seen in the patient with diabetes who told the practical nurse that he was afraid to give himself insulin. This was reported to the head nurse. After she had discussed the patient's fear with the doctor, the head nurse made plans with the team leader to begin teaching the patient how to give himself insulin. This teaching was begun early in an effort to help the patient overcome his fear.

## REASSURING THE PATIENT

The practical nurse who understands the patient because she has developed the art of listening is in an important position to reassure the patient. When a nurse reassures a sick person, she helps him to develop or to regain confidence. Understanding can be considered as a basic requirement for reassurance. A patient is reassured when he feels that members of the health team understand him as an individual. Having a feeling of trust in those caring for him also helps to inspire the patient's confidence.

A false idea about reassurance is to tell a person not to worry or to tell him that everything will be all right. Telling an individual not to worry may be compared with trying to stop the flow of a stream. The tension produced by the worry cannot be reduced by telling it to stop just as the power of a flowing stream cannot be stopped by telling it to stop. Frequently the tension produced by a worry can be reduced or relieved by talking. The practical nurse should realize that this does not mean that she solves the problem necessarily. It does mean that by being a good listener she allows the patient to reduce his tension or "let off steam." This in turn helps to reassure the patient because he feels that the practical nurse does understand him. For example, Mr. Carter told the practical nurse that he was worried about his invalid wife at home. Since she was genuinely interested in him as an individual, she asked him who was caring for his wife. This simple question gave Mr. Carter an opportunity to talk about his worry which had caused him several sleepless nights. He told the nurse that he had taken care of her before his illness, but now his son and daughter-in-law are doing it. Although it might seem to the nurse that the patient had nothing to worry about, he felt that he did. Since he was not told by the nurse to stop worrying, he felt that she understood him. This gave him an opportunity to reduce some of his tension by talking about his concern over his wife. Mr. Carter seemed to feel reassured because the nurse understood and respected him as an individual. She listened to him.

There are innumerable ways in which the practical nurse can reassure the patient by her thoughtfulness. For example, if the practical nurse tells her patient where she will be and how he can reach her, she helps to reassure him. The anxious patient feels more confident if the thoughtful nurse tells him that she will stop by his room frequently to see that he is all right. The mere presence of a kindly and understanding person can be reassuring. Frequently the presence of the practical nurse makes the patient feel more confident. An example of this is seen in the patient who is being transferred to the operating room. He has a feeling of reassurance if the nurse who has been caring for him goes with him. These are only a few examples of how the understanding practical nurse can reassure the patient.

A person frequently feels greater need for spiritual help when he becomes ill. He often seeks reassurance, support, comfort, and courage from his religious faith during an illness. This may be especially true when medical science seems to be failing. The patient's priest, rabbi, or minister is an important member of the health team. Many large hospitals have chaplains of the various faiths who minister to the patient's spiritual needs. The pastor from the patient's church usually visits him when he is hospitalized in his community. The practical nurse should provide the patient and his spiritual adviser with privacy during the visit.

The patient may ask the practical nurse if the hospital has a chaplain. Such a question may indicate that the patient feels the need for spiritual support. The practical nurse should be well informed regarding the services available in that particular hospital so that she can answer such questions. The patient may ask her to tell the chaplain or the pastor from his church to stop by to see him. This request should be handled with as much consideration and promptness as the patient's request for something to relieve pain. In addition to understanding the importance of religion to the patient's welfare, the practical nurse must respect his beliefs.

## SUGGESTIONS FOR STUDY

1. Have you ever been a patient? If so, did you feel that those who were caring for you understood and respected you as an individual?
2. What changes in your behavior can you recall which were associated with a minor illness, such as a common cold?
3. Observe the behavior changes of a patient as he begins to improve.
4. Have you ever thought of one of your patients as a "ruptured appendix" or a "broken leg"? If so, compare your ideas with those presented in this chapter.
5. Select and read one of the articles listed at the end of this chapter which deal with the spiritual needs of a patient.
6. What is psychosomatic medicine?
7. Why is a person's diet likely to assume greater importance when he becomes sick?

8. What factor is discussed in this chapter as a basic requirement for becoming a good listener? Do you agree?

9. Discuss the ways in which the practical nurse can reassure the patient.

## REFERENCES FOR CHAPTER 2

Ashbrook, James B.: "Not by Bread Alone," *Am. J. Nursing,* **55:**164-68, (Feb.) 1955.

Cabot, Richard C., and Dicks, Russell L.: *The Art of Ministering to the Sick.* The Macmillan Company, New York, 1945.

Faddis, Margene O., and Hayman, Joseph M.: *Care of the Medical Patient.* McGraw-Hill Book Co., New York, 1952, pp. 22-27.

Fuerst, Elinor V., and Wolff, LuVerne: *Fundamentals of Nursing.* J. B. Lippincott Co., Philadelphia, 1956, pp. 271-88.

Gregg, Dorothy: "Reassurance," *Am. J. Nursing,* **55:**171-74, (Feb.) 1955.

Jackson, Joan K.: "Communication Is Important," *Am. J. Nursing,* **59:**90-93, (Jan.) 1959.

Madigan, Marian E.: *Psychology Principles and Applications,* 2nd ed. C. V. Mosby Co., St. Louis, 1957.

Pearce, Evelyn C.: *Nurse and Patient.* J. B. Lippincott Co., Philadelphia, 1953.

Westberg, Granger E.: *Nurse, Pastor, and Patient.* Augustana Press, Rock Island, Ill., 1955.

Westberg, Granger E.; Flanagan John J.; and Silver, Samuel M.: "The Spiritual Needs of the Patient," *Practical Nurses Digest,* **2:**16-17, 28, and 30, (Sept.) 1955.

# Chapter 3

# CAUSES
# AND METHODS OF
# TREATING DISEASE

| Chapter | INTRODUCTION | METHODS OF TREATMENT |
|---------|--------------|----------------------|
| Outline | CAUSES OF DISEASE | |

## INTRODUCTION

An individual under the care of a physician because of *disease* has a disturbance in either the structure or the function of some part of his body. Disease may be classified according to its etiology (cause), the symptoms which it produces, and the system of the body which it affects. Some of the major causes of disease—infections, tumors, and allergies—are discussed in a general manner in Part II. The more common symptoms of disease are presented in Chapter 4. Parts III-XI of this book deal with the diseases which commonly affect the various body systems. The responsibilities of the practical nurse in caring for the individual patient are discussed throughout the entire text. It is hoped that the early discussion of major causes and common symptoms aids the practical nurse in understanding these major causes and common symptoms in relation to a specific system when they are discussed later. For instance, the common symptoms included in Chapter 4 and the basic knowledge of inflammation given in Chapter 6 should be valuable to the practical nurse when she studies pneumonia (inflammation of the lungs) in Chapter 13 as well as appendicitis (inflammation of the appendix) in Chapter 15.

## CAUSES OF DISEASE

What causes a person to become sick or to be affected by disease? Infection, neoplasm, allergy, injury, congenital defect, degeneration, emotions, and metabolic disorders are some of the main factors known to cause disease. An individual develops an *infection* when

18

living microorganisms enter his body, overpower his natural resistance, and cause an inflammatory process to develop. This is discussed in detail in Chapter 6. A *neoplasm*, which is also known as
tumor, is a new growth or an abnormal growth of cells. As a rule
these cells grow faster than normal. A neoplasm may be either benign
or malignant. Diseases caused by an abnormal growth of cells are
known as *neoplastic diseases,* and are discussed in Chapter 7. The
patient with an *allergy* has an abnormal reaction to certain substances which ordinarily have no effect on other individuals. A discussion of this condition is included in Chapter 8.

*Injury* or *trauma* from mechanical violence causes disease. For example, a person's leg may be broken as a result of an automobile
accident. Injury can also be caused by physical agents, such as electricity, extreme heat, and excessive cold. Some chemicals injure the
body when they come into contact with it; for example, undiluted
phenol burns the body's tissues.

A person may have a disease because of a *congenital defect,* which
is an abnormal condition present at birth. An example of this is seen
in a baby who is born with a clubfoot, a cleft lip, or with a defective
heart.

*Degeneration* occurs in every person as he becomes older. The normal structure of the body's cells breaks down slowly as one ages. This
group of disease processes develops earlier in some than in others.
Frequently these changes develop in the blood vessels and joints.
Thus, arteriosclerosis (hardening of the arteries) and arthritis are
more common in older people.

*Emotions* are defined as one's feelings, such as love, hate, fear,
anxiety, worry, anger, jealousy, disgust, depression, and joy. The practical nurse can readily understand how emotions may cause disease if
she recalls some of the bodily changes she has experienced as a result
of an emotional reaction. For example, a student practical nurse may
be anxious about or even afraid of a final examination in one of her
courses. She may notice that her heart is pounding and that her
hands are cold and perspiring. A classmate may tell her that she has
a tight feeling in the pit of her stomach. It may be noticed that
another student goes to the bathroom more often before the examination. These symptoms or changes develop as a result of emotion.
The students became tense because of their emotion regarding the

examination. Usually these bodily symptoms disappear after they have finished the examination, and, if controlled, are of no lasting significance.

Realizing that bodily changes are caused by an emotional reaction enables the practical nurse to understand better how strong and persistent emotional conflict over a period of time can disturb the functioning of various organs. A person is said to have a *functional disease* when there is no change in either the organ or the system to account for his symptoms. The practical nurse needs to know that the patient with a functional disorder can suffer as much as the patient with an organic disease in which there is an actual change in the organ. Frequently emotional tension plays an important role in certain organic diseases, especially of the circulatory system and the digestive system. For example, emotional tension may be considered as a causative factor in some patients with high blood pressure or a peptic ulcer.

*Metabolism* is the process by which foodstuffs are used to produce energy, changed into tissue elements, and stored in the cells of the body. It includes the changes which occur to food from the time it is digested until it is eliminated. Metabolism also includes the complex chemical activities which take place within the cells. A disease caused by a change of metabolism is known as a metabolic disorder. An example of this is seen in a person who is unable to use carbohydrates because of an insufficient amount of insulin. He has a metabolic disease known as *diabetes mellitus*. Nutritional deficiencies are closely related to this group of diseases. A person will become sick if his diet lacks the essential substances. For example, rickets will develop in an individual whose diet is deficient in vitamin D.

## METHODS OF TREATMENT

The *treatment* or *therapy* of a patient includes measures used to aid in his recovery. It also includes measures to make the sick person comfortable and to keep him in the best possible condition. As the leader of the health team, the physician plans the treatment for the individual patient. He then depends upon other members of the health team to carry out their responsibilities. For example, he might prescribe a special diet which would be arranged by the dietitian. Another example is seen in the doctor's order for a certain drug to be given by mouth. The pharmacist would dispense the proper drug to the nurse who would administer it to the patient. As an important member of the health team, the practical nurse needs an understanding of special types of therapy which may be prescribed by the doctor. Diet therapy, drug therapy, physical therapy, psychotherapy, surgery, and rehabilitation are special methods of treatment commonly used.

### Diet Therapy

Diet therapy is the treatment of a patient by food. The normal diet is changed to meet the requirements of an individual during illness. The physician prescribes the diet, and the dietition arranges for it in the hospital. The *dietitian* is a person specially prepared in the scientific regulation of diet for healthful nutrition as well as for therapeutic reasons. Patients having certain diseases are treated primarily by diet. For example, one of the main treatments of a person with diabetes mellitus is diet.

The practical nurse is frequently responsible for some phase of diet therapy, such as preparing and serving food to the patient. For example, the practical nurse on duty with a diabetic patient in the home would have the responsibility for either preparing the special diet or supervising its preparation. She would also serve it and encourage the patient to eat. The practical nurse caring for a hospitalized diabetic patient might be responsible for serving the tray and feeding the patient. She should then report the amount eaten to her team leader or head nurse. In order to assist properly in diet therapy, the practical nurse needs to remember that the doctor's plan of treatment may fail in some cases if the dietary regimen is not followed accurately.

### Drug Therapy

Drug therapy is the treatment of a person by the use of a substance which prevents, cures, or treats disease. The use of substances to relieve pain and suffering is included also in drug therapy. *Pharmacology* is the study of these substances which are known as *drugs* or *medicines*. The scientific knowledge of drugs, such as the source, name, characteristics, and actions, is included in pharmacology.

The physician prescribes the drug. The *pharmacist prepares, compounds, and dispenses the medicine*. The nursing team usually is responsible for its proper administration to the patient. However, in some cases the doctor does this with the nurse's assistance. For instance, the nurse would assist him in injecting medication into the spinal canal. Members of the nursing team would then observe and report the effects of the drug.

In general, qualified members of the nursing team administer drugs orally (by mouth), subcutaneously (beneath the skin), intramuscularly (into the muscle), rectally, and vaginally. Nurses also give medicine by instillation, by local application, and by inhalation. Oxygen is an example of a substance given by inhalation for its therapeutic effect. The nursing care of a patient receiving oxygen is discussed on pages 122 to 134.

The responsibility of the practical nurse in regards to drug therapy varies in different hospitals and in different localities of the United States. She should be fully aware of what is expected of her by her employer in relation to the administration of medicines. After learning the policy of that particular institution, she should follow it conscientiously.

### Physical Therapy

Physical therapy is the use of physical agents and special procedures, such as massage and exercise. Heat, cold, electricity, water, and rays, such as infrared and ultraviolet, are examples of physical agents. These agents may involve the use of very simple methods or the use of highly technical machines. Physical therapy is used in the treatment of a patient with a motor disability. That is, he has a disease affecting the muscles, joints, or nerves responsible for movement. The *physical therapist* is a person specially prepared in the use of these physical agents and special procedures.

The doctor prescribes physical therapy. He works with the physical therapist in determining the amount of disability and in planning the course of treatment. Members of the nursing team frequently are asked to assist in physical therapy. For example, the physical therapist may be helping the patient to do self-help activities, such as combing his hair or feeding himself. The physical therapist would ask the nursing team to assist in this by allowing the patient to do these for himself instead of having the nurse do them for him.

## Psychotherapy

Psychotherapy means treatment of the mind. The *psychiatrist* is a physician specializing in this type of therapy. His aim is to find out what caused the illness, to relieve the patient of his symptoms, and to help him in overcoming his illness.

## Surgery

Surgery is a branch of medicine which deals with the treatment of disease by operation and by manipulation, which means skillful use of the hands. For example, the physician would treat the patient with a dislocated shoulder by manipulation. In other words, he would replace the bone which had slipped out of joint by skillful use of his hands. The *surgeon* is a physician who has specialized in this type of therapy. The responsibilities of the practical nurse in caring for a patient treated with surgery are discussed in Chapter 5.

## Rehabilitation

Rehabilitation may be defined as helping the patient to regain the greatest amount of usefulness and the maximum degree of health which are possible within the limitations of his handicap. A full re-habilitation program includes aspects other than physical ones. The mental, social, vocational, and economic factors must be considered in relation to that particular individual. A plan for rehabilitation is outlined after a careful study of the person has been made. The physician calls upon various members of the health team to assist in the plan. For example, a *speech therapist* may be needed to teach the person to talk. An *occupational therapist* is responsible for teaching the patient how to earn his living in a new way, how to return to his former job, or simply how to do things for diversion while he is under treatment. The physical therapist may be asked to use measures, such as heat and exercise. Members of the nursing team need to know what the other members of the health team are doing for the patient. This makes continuity of care possible. For example, the physical therapist may instruct the patient to take certain exercises during the day. It may be the responsibility of the nursing team to help the patient with these at given times throughout the day. The speech therapist may want the patient to practice a certain sound or word during the day. Members of the nursing team can encourage the patient with his homework.

## SUGGESTIONS FOR STUDY

1. What is disease?
2. What bodily symptoms have you experienced because of emotions?
3. Discuss the factors known to cause an individual to develop a disease.
4. Discuss the difference between a functional disorder and an organic disorder.
5. What rehabilitation facilities are available in your community?
6. Is there a physical therapy department in your hospital? If so, make arrangements with the physical therapist for a visit.
7. What responsibilities do the licensed practical nurses assume in your hospital in regard to diet therapy and drug therapy?

## REFERENCES FOR CHAPTER 3

Brown, Amy F.: *Medical Nursing*, 3rd ed. W. B. Saunders Co., Philadelphia, 1957, pp. 44-59.
Emerson, Charles P., Jr., and Bragdon, Jane S.: *Essentials of Medicine*, 17th ed. J. B. Lippincott Co., Philadelphia, 1955, pp. 3-13.
Harmer, Bertha, and Henderson, Virginia: *Textbook of the Principles and Practice of Nursing*, 5th ed. The Macmillan Company, New York, 1955, pp. 508-31.
Hull, Edgar, and Perrodin, Cecilia: *Medical Nursing*, 5th ed. F. A. Davis Co., Philadelphia, 1954, pp. 3-30.
Jensen, Julius, and Jensen, Deborah: *Nursing in Clinical Medicine*, 4th ed. The Macmillan Company, New York, 1954, pp. 12-18 and 82-109.
Muller, Gulli L., and Dawes, Dorothy E.: *Introduction to Medical*

*Science*, 4th ed. W. B. Saunders Co., Philadelphia, 1958, pp. 38-105 and 384-401.

Musser, Ruth D., and Bird, Joseph G.: *Modern Pharmacology and Therapeutics*. The Macmillan Company, New York, 1958, pp. 5-6 and 84-97.

Proudfit, Fairfax T., and Robinson, Corinne H.: *Nutrition and Diet Therapy*, 11th ed. The Macmillan Company, New York, 1955, pp. 3-224, 285-309, and 530-39.

Rapier, Dorothy K.; Koch, Marianna J.; Moran, Lois P.; Fleming, Viola L.; Cady, Elwyn L.; and Jensen, Deborah: *Practical Nursing, A Textbook for Students and Graduates*. C. V. Mosby Co., St. Louis, 1958, pp. 449-69.

Terry, Florence J.; Benz, Gladys S.; Mereness, Dorothy; and Kleffner, Frank R.: *Principles and Technics of Rehabilitation Nursing*. C. V. Mosby Co., St. Louis, 1957, pp. 32-56.

Chapter 4     # THE PATIENT WITH
# COMMON SYMPTOMS
# OF ILLNESS

## INTRODUCTION

A *symptom* is any change in the body or functioning of the body which indicates disease or a change in the disease. Symptoms may be referred to as either subjective or objective. Subjective symptoms are changes felt by the patient, such as pain, itching, burning, and nausea. Objective symptoms are changes which are seen, felt, heard, or smelled by others. For example, the practical nurse can see cyanosis (blueness of skin), feel a swollen area, hear difficult breathing, and smell the sweetish odor of a diabetic patient's breath.

The term *physical sign* may be used in referring to either subjective or objective symptoms. The more correct usage of this phrase is in reference to objective symptoms which are found by special methods of examination, such as measuring the body temperature with a thermometer and determining blood pressure with a sphygmoma-nometer. As there is usually no sharp distinction between a sign and a symptom in the field of medicine, no sharp distinction is made in this text.

It is essential for the practical nurse to develop the ability to observe the patient's symptoms. Since she spends much of her time with the patient, other members of the health team depend upon her

25

to report matters of importance. Observations made by the practical nurse and other members of the nursing team guide the team leader in planning and changing the nursing care for an individual patient. Also, observations made by the nurse guide the physician in his diagnosis, treatment, and prognosis. The term *prognosis* means the prediction of the length, course, and outcome of the disease.

In addition to developing the ability to observe a patient's symptoms, the practical nurse needs to know what should be reported, to understand the common causes of a symptom, and to know her role in its relief. The practical nurse who understands the common causes of a patient's symptom is able to give more intelligent nursing care. For example, the practical nurse who knows that diarrhea is caused by an irritation in the bowel understands the importance of a non-irritating diet ordered by the doctor. Both the treatment and nursing care of many patients are *symptomatic,* which means that they are directed toward relieving symptoms. For this reason the practical nurse needs to know her role in relieving the patient of his symptom.

## ANOREXIA

The patient with anorexia has a loss of appetite. This symptom may be associated with a disease of the digestive system, such as an ulcer, or a disease in another part of the body, such as an infection, and emotional tension.

Although the patient should not be forced to eat, he should be encouraged to eat the type of food prescribed by his doctor. The practical nurse is in a key position for helping this patient. Surroundings which are clean, neat, orderly, and free from odor help to improve the patient's desire for food. Such objects as a half-filled emesis basin or an empty transfusion bottle can ruin a patient's meal. The patient should also be made as comfortable as possible. The sight and smell of tempting food served as attractively as possible aid in stimulating the appetite. The diet should be served in small portions at regular times. If at all possible, the patient's desire for a special food should be fulfilled. Placing a bloom in a small bud vase or other simple favors on the tray add to its attractiveness. After the patient has finished with his tray, the practical nurse should report the type and amount of food which the patient ate.

## NAUSEA AND VOMITING

### Definition

The patient with nausea has a feeling of discomfort in the region of his stomach, anorexia, and a tendency to vomit. When vomiting occurs, he ejects or throws out the contents of his stomach through his mouth. The ejected contents are referred to as *vomitus*. The actual act of vomiting results from a sudden and strong contraction of the diaphragm and stomach muscles.

### Cause

Nausea and vomiting are commonly caused by excessive fatigue, strong emotional reactions, drugs such as opium, the intake of poisons, and many diseases. A peptic ulcer, appendicitis, gallstones, and a brain tumor are only a few examples of diseases producing nausea and vomiting.

### Nursing Care

The patient who is vomiting needs understanding care from the practical nurse. After placing the emesis basin in a convenient place, the nurse should hold the patient's head on the side so that he cannot aspirate (breathe in) vomitus. This gives both physical and moral support. When the patient seems to have finished vomiting, the basin should be removed, cleaned thoroughly, and put in a convenient place for use again if necessary. It is not wise to keep the emesis basin in plain view of the patient as the sight of it may cause more vomiting.

The bad taste in the patient's mouth should be relieved according to his choice. Some individuals may want to rinse their mouth with clear water, some with mouthwash, and some may want to brush their teeth. The practical nurse should wash the patient's face. Clothing and linen, which have been soiled with vomitus, should be changed. Encouraging the patient to lie quietly and to take deep breaths through his mouth often helps to relieve the feeling of nausea and to prevent the return of vomiting.

The practical nurse should observe and report the time of vomiting, its nature, odor, amount, and color. She should notice whether or not *contents* it is associated with a spell of coughing, or with the intake of food *ejected* and drugs. It is also important to report projectile vomiting. In this *will force* case the contents of the stomach are expelled with great force. In noting the nature of the vomitus the nurse can ask herself these questions: Is it clear? Does it appear to contain partially digested food? Does it seem to contain blood or mucus? When the blood has been acted upon by gastric juice, it has the appearance of coffee grounds.

The presence of either a foul or a fecal odor should be reported. It is important to report the approximate amount and color of vomitus. For example, it may be observed that the fluid is colorless, green, yellow, or red. Bright red vomitus usually indicates recent hemorrhage. *Hematemesis* is the term used in referring to the vomiting of blood. If the vomitus appears unusual or if it is a kind of vomitus which has not been seen in this patient before, it should be saved for either the team leader or the doctor to see.

## DIARRHEA

### Description

The passage of an increased number of loose stools is known as diarrhea. The number of stools may vary from one to 30 or 40 a day. Diarrhea is a symptom of an irritation in the bowel and not a disease. The body tries to rid itself of the irritation by increasing peristalsis, which is the wormlike contraction of the intestines. There is more fluid in the intestinal tract because the rapid passage of its contents does not allow for proper absorption.

Increased peristalsis causes the patient to have intestinal cramps. *Tenesmus,* which is painful straining without having a bowel movement, may be present. Nausea, vomiting, a feeling of weakness, and fever are commonly associated with diarrhea. Dehydration occurs in severe cases of diarrhea which results in thirst and dryness of the mouth and skin. An excessive loss of fluid is especially dangerous in infants and small children as it may result in death if allowed to continue.

## Cause

Irritation of the intestinal tract resulting in diarrhea has many causes. Nervousness may produce diarrhea. Many types of laxatives produce an increased number of loose stools. Improper foods, such as spoiled custard, underripe fruit, overripe fruit, and contaminated canned food, irritate the intestines. Infants may develop diarrhea when their formula contains too much sugar. Diarrhea can be a symptom of an intestinal obstruction, infection of the intestines, and colitis which is an inflammation of the colon. Amebic dysentery, typhoid fever, and bacillary dysentery are examples of infections caused by specific microorganisms.

## Treatment and Nursing Care

Rest of both the body and gastrointestinal tract is needed by the patient with diarrhea. If there is a possibility that the diarrhea is a result of infection, the patient is placed in isolation. This includes disinfection of the stools. In severe cases of diarrhea, especially when vomiting is present, the patient is given no food by mouth. As his condition improves, the physician prescribes a nonirritating diet which progresses from liquids, such as tea, weak broth, buttermilk, and boiled milk, to soft foods. Soft-cooked eggs, toast, custard, plain gelatin desserts, and strained cereals are examples of bland foods often ordered by the doctor. The patient is usually left on a bland diet until the diarrhea has been absent for several days. His return to a regular diet should be gradual.

Since dehydration may be a serious complication of diarrhea, it is of vital importance to replace the fluids lost. The practical nurse should encourage the patient to drink fluids allowed by the doctor when nausea and vomiting are not present. If the patient cannot take fluids by mouth, either the physician or, when indicated, the professional nurse gives fluids by injection.

The practical nurse is often asked to collect stool specimens to aid the doctor in determining the cause of the diarrhea. It should be remembered that it is necessary to keep the feces warm in many examinations. The container containing the stool specimen can be placed in a basin of warm water if there is any delay in sending it to the laboratory.

When there is a definite microorganism causing the diarrhea, the doctor prescribes a drug to cure the infection. Perparations of bismuth, kaolin, atropine, and opium are commonly used to relieve the cramps and to check diarrhea.

The nurse should report the approximate amount, color, and consistency of feces, and the frequency of diarrhea. The stool should be examined for mucus, blood, pus, and other abnormalities which might aid the doctor in his diagnosis. Also, the presence of tenesmus and intestinal cramps should be reported.

## CONSTIPATION

### Description

The individual who has fewer stools than is usual for him has constipation. The fecal material is usually hard and dry. Constipation may be a symptom of an organic disease or it may be functional. In an organic disease there is a change in the organ or tissue to explain the patient's symptoms. Functional constipation is more common than organic.

Two types of functional constipation are atonic and spastic. An individual who is habitually constipated usually has decreased muscle tone in his colon. This type of constipation is referred to as atonic. The colon in some nervous individuals may develop an increased muscle tone. Parts of the colon become spastic and prevent the normal passage of feces. This is called spastic constipation.

Functional constipation results from the individual's habits. Repeatedly delaying the desire to have a bowel movement; eating a diet low in roughage, fruit, and vegetables; drinking an insufficient amount of fluids; and lack of exercise cause constipation. Also, a change of daily habits, such as taking a trip or being hospitalized, causes many individuals to become constipated.

### Treatment and Nursing Care

The physician treats the patient with constipation of organic origin for the underlying disease. The treatment and nursing care of a patient with functional constipation are directed toward helping the patient to re-establish normal bowel habits. Often the doctor prescribes an enema or a laxative for temporary relief of constipation.

In severe cases the rectum may become impacted, filled with masses of hard fecal material. This is referred to as a *fecal impaction*. In some cases the doctor orders a small amount of oil placed in the rectum to soften the feces, to be followed by a cleansing enema. Some fecal impactions have to be removed with gloved fingers.

The practical nurse needs to understand that the physician usually does not prescribe laxatives for patients with ulcerative conditions of the intestines, appendicitis, an intestinal obstruction, and inflammatory conditions of the intestines. Also, laxatives are prescribed with caution during the late stages of pregnancy.

There are many simple measures which the practical nurse can use to help the patient in re-establishing normal bowel habits. She can encourage the patient to drink a glass of water before meals, especially breakfast. The patient's request for a bedpan should be fulfilled promptly. Privacy should be provided for the patient at the same time each day. Exercise as allowed by the physician is beneficial. If permitted by the doctor, a diet which includes fresh fruit (especially with the peeling), green leafy vegetables, and coarse cereals aids in relieving constipation. A low-residue diet may be prescribed for the patient with spastic constipation.

## DEHYDRATION

### Description

Dehydration is the loss of water from the body's tissues. Normally water makes up 70 to 75 per cent of the body's weight. Replacement of water is the body's most urgent dietary requirement. Body fluid is lost each day in the form of urine, perspiration, moisture in exhaled air, and feces. Fluid is taken into the body daily by drinking and eating. When a person loses more fluid than he receives, dehydration results. The water balance in his body is disturbed; that is, his intake and output of fluids are not balanced.

The patient who is dehydrated has extreme thirst, dry tongue, parched lips, dry skin, and a scanty amount of urine. His face looks thin and his eyes appear sunken. If the disturbed water balance is not corrected, he will become comatose and die.

# WATER BALANCE

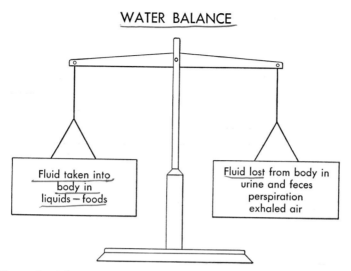

**Figure 1.** The water balance of the body is maintained by an adequate intake and output of fluids.

# DEHYDRATION

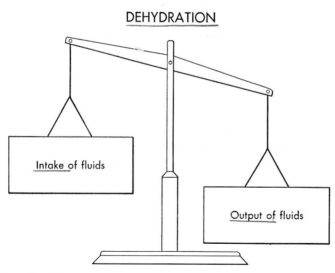

**Figure 2.** The water balance is disturbed when a person does not take in a sufficient amount of fluid or when a person loses too much fluid. This results in dehydration.

33

## Cause

An individual becomes dehydrated when he loses an excessive amount of fluid or when he is unable to drink an adequate amount. Loss of fluid may result from excessive voiding and perspiration, diarrhea, hemorrhage, and persistent vomiting. Inability to drink fluids occurs in unconscious patients and in those with nausea, vomiting, and anorexia. Frequently nausea and vomiting following surgery result in slight dehydration.

## Nursing Care

A dehydrated patient is treated with the administration of fluids which are given by mouth when possible. If the patient is unable to drink or to retain liquid, it may be given subcutaneously (into tissue under the skin) or intravenously (into the vein). The practical nurse is often asked to assist the doctor and sometimes the professional nurse in these procedures.

Frequently the physician requests that the nurse record the patient's intake and output. In this case an accurate record is kept of all fluid taken into the body and all fluid lost from the body. Most hospitals have a special sheet which is kept at the patient's bedside for notations to be made when the patient receives or loses liquids. The total output and the total intake are summarized at the end of 24 hours. The physician uses this important information as a basis for treating the patient.

A record of the fluid intake and output should be kept for patients who are likely to become dehydrated. For example, the practical nurse who is caring for the new postoperative patient should measure and record liquid taken into the body as well as that which is lost. She can also encourage the patient to drink beverages which are permitted by the doctor.

## EDEMA

### Description

Edema is the medical term for dropsy. The patient with edema has a collection of fluid in his tissues which results in swelling. It may be a symptom of heart disease, kidney disease, or a local obstruction of lymphatic or venous circulation.

### Nursing Care

A record of the patient's intake and output should be kept. The practical nurse needs to protect the skin over the edematous area. Decubitus ulcers are likely to occur because of the impaired circulation. Also, the practical nurse may be responsible for weighing the patient daily. The doctor may prescribe a low-salt diet since (salt helps the tissues to hold fluid.) Also, he may prescribe *diuretics*, a group of drugs which increases the flow of urine. Thus, fluid is removed from the tissues. Meralluride (Mercuhydrin) and ammonium chloride are two examples of diuretics.

## CHILL

### Description

When a patient has a chill, he feels cold and shivers and shakes. This increased muscular activity raises the body temperature. It can be compared with the shivering which occurs when a person is cold and is trying to get warm. When the chill is a result of nervousness, the patient generally does not have a fever after the shivering has ended. In general, a chill is a symptom of an infection, such as pneumonia, malaria, and influenza.

### Nursing Care

The practical nurse should make the patient who is having a chill comfortable with warm blankets and a hot beverage. It is important for her to observe and to report the time the chill started and ended and its severity. The patient's temperature should be taken 20 to 30 minutes after the chill has ended.

## FEVER

### Description

The patient with a fever has a body temperature above normal. The average normal temperature varies in different parts of the body.

For example, the average temperature in the mouth is 37° C (98.6° F), the rectum 38° C (100.4° F), and the axilla 36° C (96.8° F). Fever is generally a symptom of an infectious disease. However, an elevated body temperature may result from other factors, such as strenous exercise, heat stroke, and dehydration. Fever is considered to be one of the important defenses of the body against infection. Because of this, measures to reduce fever are not used too frequently except in cases of extremely high temperature.

### Nursing Care

The practical nurse should encourage the patient to drink an increased amount of fluids. A daily cleansing bath and a change of linen, when necessary, add to the feverish patient's comfort. The physician may prescribe an alcohol sponge bath and an icecap to the head when the fever is extremely high. The temperature of the patient with a fever should be checked every two to four hours, depending upon the hospital policy.

## COUGH

### Description

Cough is a violent, involuntary exhalation of air following a deep inspiration. Usually it is a symptom of irritation within the respiratory tract. Occasionally it may be either a nervous habit or a means of attracting attention. Coughing is a symptom of many diseases. A sore throat, tuberculosis, whooping cough, bronchitis, a lung tumor, and congestion in the lungs which is due to heart failure are only a few examples. Also, the inhalation of food particles and of irritating substances such as smoke, dust, ammonia, and chlorine causes coughing.

### Nursing Care

In caring for the patient with a persistent cough the nurse should observe and report the type of cough. A dry cough is one without expectoration. A laryngeal or croup-like cough has a hard, metallic, ringing sound. In a moist or productive cough there is expectoration of sputum. In addition to observing the type of cough, the nurse should note the amount, color, odor, and consistency of the sputum.

The patient should be encouraged to cough into a tissue. A sputum cup can be used for patients with a productive cough. Steam inhalations may be used to soothe the irritated membranes.

## HEMOPTYSIS

### Description

Hemoptysis is the expectoration of blood from the respiratory tract. It may be a symptom of such diseases of the lungs as pneumonia, cancer, and abscess. Hemoptysis may also occur in the patient with heart failure. When his heart fails to pump blood through his lungs properly, the patient has an excess amount of blood in the lungs.

### Nursing Care

The patient with hemoptysis needs reassurance from the nursing team as he is usually frightened. Rest is of extreme importance in helping to check the bleeding. The patient may be turned on the affected side in an effort to prevent blood from entering the healthy lung. For this reason, the practical nurse may be asked to help in keeping the patient turned on one specific side. After determining which side of the lung is bleeding, the doctor generally leaves an order regarding the side the patient should lie on.

When helping to care for the patient with hemoptysis, the practical nurse should observe and report the color and amount of expectoration which may be bright red, brownish, or rusty in color. It may also be foamy in appearance. The amount of expectoration may range from slight streaking of the sputum to a massive hemorrhage. The bloody sputum is measured and recorded. Sputum from the patient with an infectious disease, such as tuberculosis, is disinfected according to hospital procedure before being discarded. The patient with hemoptysis should be observed for symptoms of shock, such as paleness, cold and clammy skin, weak and rapid pulse, rapid and shallow respiration, lowered blood pressure, and cyanosis. The practical nurse reports the presence of any of these symptoms immediately to her team leader or head nurse.

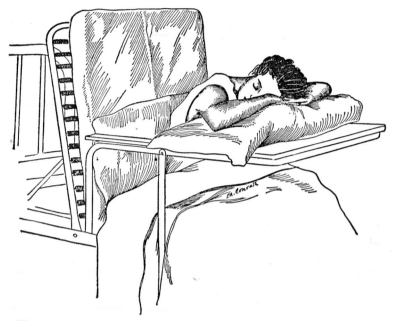

Figure 3.  The patient with orthopnea is often more comfortable in this position. (Jensen, Julius, and Jensen, Deborah: *Nursing in Clinical Medicine,* 4th ed. The Macmillan Company, New York, 1954.)

## DYSPNEA

### Description

The patient with dyspnea has difficulty in breathing or shortness of breath. Dyspnea which causes the patient to sit up to breathe is termed *orthopnea*. Dyspnea may be a symptom of an obstruction in the respiratory tract, lung disease, heart disease, or a blood disease in which the oxygen-carrying capacity of the blood is reduced, such as anemia.

*SOB . shortness of breath*

### Nursing Care

The patient should be placed in a comfortable position. Free circulation of air, but not a draft, is needed. His clothing should be loosened. Since this patient is usually anxious, the nurse should try to relieve this by having a calm, sympathetic, and self-confident attitude. The physician prescribes oxygen if necessary.

## CYANOSIS

The patient with cyanosis has a bluish color of his skin and mucous membranes. It is a symptom of an inadequate amount of oxygen in the hemoglobin of the blood. Cyanosis often occurs when the blood receives an insufficient supply of oxygen from the lungs in patients with either heart or lung disease. It is most noticeable in the patient's nail beds, ear lobes, and lips. Frequently, cyanosis occurs in patients having dyspnea.

## CHEYNE-STOKES RESPIRATION

Cheyne-Stokes respiration is a type of breathing. The patient's respirations show a gradual increase in depth and rate, then a gradual decrease in depth and rate, which is followed by apnea (temporary absence of breathing). Following the apnea, the cycle starts again. A simpler definition of Cheyne-Stokes breathing describes it as periods of deep snoring respirations interrupted by periods of apnea. This type of breathing is a grave sign. It may be a symptom of brain injury, kidney failure, and heart disease.

## EPISTAXIS

### Description

Epistaxis or nosebleed may occur in normal individuals. It may be due to an injury of the nose and to rupture of a blood vessel in patients with high blood pressure. Nose-picking, especially in children, is a common cause of nosebleed. Epistaxis may be a symptom of certain diseases, such as rheumatic fever, measles, influenza, and a disease of the blood in which the clotting time is longer than normal, as well as the excessive use of some drugs such as aspirin.

### Nursing Care

The patient who is bleeding from the nose should be placed at rest in a sitting position. Cold compresses may be placed over the bridge of the nose. Because applications of cold cause blood vessels to constrict, this simple remedy is often effective in relieving a nose-bleed. Gentle pressure may be applied to the soft outer portion of the nose to aid in checking the hemorrhage. The practical nurse should observe and report the time and amount of bleeding. The physician should be called if these simple emergency measures do not relieve the hemorrhage or if the bleeding is profuse.

## BRADYCARDIA

A person with bradycardia has a slow heart action with a pulse rate which is usually below 60. This may be present in normal individuals. Also, it may be a symptom of disease. A patient with kidney failure, an underactive thyroid gland, jaundice, heart disease, and an overdosage of certain drugs, such as morphine and digitalis, may have bradycardia. It is also present in certain brain diseases, such as a brain tumor or head injury, when the pressure within the skull is increased.

## TACHYCARDIA

The patient with tachycardia has a rapid heart action. The prac-tical nurse observes this symptom when she counts the patient's pulse and notices that it is abnormally fast. Tachycardia may be associated with fever, an overactive thyroid gland, emotional excite-ment, hemorrhage, heart failure, and exercise.

A sudden attack of tachycardia which is not associated with the above conditions is known as *paroxysmal tachycardia*. It begins suddenly and ends suddenly. Normally, impulses for the heartbeat begin in the sinus node or pacemaker of the heart. In paroxysmal tachycardia, another area of the heart takes over the starting of impulses and a rapid pulse results.

## PAIN

### Description

Pain is one of the most common symptoms which cause an in-dividual to see his doctor for relief. It results from irritation and stimulation of nerves which carry the feeling of pain to the brain.

Pain is an important protective mechanism of the body. Usually it is a warning that a certain part of the body is either diseased or injured. Pain may occur when neither disease nor injury is present. In other words, the doctor finds no evidence of organic disease. A complaint which has no organic basis is called functional. But it must be remembered that the pain is still real to the patient.

Although pain usually occurs in the region which is diseased, this is not always the case. Pain felt in an area of the body which is not the diseased place is called *referred pain.* For example, pain from a diseased gallbladder may be felt under the right scapula rather than in the gallbladder region. Pain from heart disease may be felt in the left arm.

### Nursing Care

The practical nurse should observe and report the location, the type, and the duration of the patient's pain. Frequently the patient places his hand over the painful area. Words often used in describing the type of pain are dull, sharp, shooting, throbbing, aching, gnawing, and burning. In addition to finding out from the patient the location of his pain and its type, the practical nurse should ask the patient when it began and whether it is constant or intermittent (comes and goes).

It is important for the practical nurse to have a kind and sympathetic attitude toward the patient in pain. After she has reported important factors about the patient's pain to the head nurse or the doctor, she should return to the patient and tell him that it has been reported. Often the registered nurse asks the practical nurse to tell the patient what measures are being taken to relieve his pain. For example, the professional nurse might ask the practical nurse to tell the patient that the doctor is being consulted. In the meantime, the patient's discomfort may be eased by placing him in a comfortable position. Frequently a soothing back rub adds to his comfort.

## CONVULSION                                   10/21/65

### Description

The medical term for a spasm or a fit is *convulsion.* A person having a convulsion has involuntary contractions of the muscles.

Convulsions may be a symptom of such diseases as epilepsy, tetany, brain tumor, brain injury, stroke, and kidney failure causing edema of the brain. Also, some poisons and an overdose of insulin cause convulsions.

### Nursing Care

The patient having a convulsion should be protected from injury. The clothing around his neck should be loosened. Placing something soft between his teeth prevents injury to the tongue. The nurse needs to protect her fingers when placing this in his mouth. A wooden or metal object should not be used *unless* it is well padded. The patient should not be moved while he is having a convulsion. The nurse who is present when the patient is having a convulsion should observe and report important points about the seizure. When did it begin? In what part of the body did the muscular contractions start? What part of the body was involved? Did the muscles relax during the attack? Did the patient stop breathing? Was he cyanotic? Did the patient appear unconscious? Was the patient incontinent? When did it end? The nurse who can observe these factors and give an accurate report of them aids the physician in his diagnosis.

After the convulsion has ended, the patient should be allowed to rest and to sleep if possible. The surroundings should be quiet as sudden noises may cause another attack.

When the nurse is caring for a patient who is likely to have convulsions a mouth gag should be kept available. Also, he should be in a quiet room.

### URINARY RETENTION

### Description

The patient with urinary retention has urine in the bladder but is unable to void. It may be caused by temporary paralysis of the bladder sphincter as a result of anesthesia. Thus, it is commonly seen in patients after surgery and delivery. Other main causes of urinary retention include obstruction of the urethra by a tumor (abnormal growth), enlargement of the prostate gland in men, and emotional tension.

## Nursing Care

The nurse should make every effort to stimulate voiding before catheterizing the patient. Three reasons for avoiding a catheterization if possible are: (1) there is a possibility of carrying an infection into the bladder; (2) there is a danger of injuring the meatus, urethra, and bladder with the catheter; and (3) the patient who has been catheterized once often needs to be catheterized again.

Nursing measures which can be used to stimulate micturition (voiding) are the following: placing the female patient in a comfortable position on a warm bedpan, letting the patient hear water running, putting his or her hands in warm water, giving fluids to drink, and pouring warm water over the female patient's perineum. When it is permitted by the doctor, allowing the male patient to stand by the bed or the female patient to sit on the commode often helps a person to void. When these nursing measures fail, the patient needs to be catheterized as ordered by the doctor.

In some cases, the physician has a catheter left in the bladder to allow for drainage of the urine. This is known as an *indwelling* or a *retention* catheter. If a regular catheter is used, it should be held in place with adhesive tape. Frequently a Foley catheter is used; it has a rubber bag near its tip which is inflated with a sterile solution, such as water, after the catheter has been inserted into the bladder. Because the inflated bag is too large to pass through the meatus, the catheter remains in the bladder. The practical nurse should remember that this type of catheter has a smaller tube within the larger one. The larger channel allows for the drainage of urine and the smaller one leads to the inflatable bag. The large opening is connected to rubber or plastic tubing which leads to the drainage bottle. The tubing should be checked frequently to see that urine is flowing through it. The nurse should measure and record the urine in the drainage bottle at frequent intervals. The bottle should be washed thoroughly before it is returned to the patient's unit.

## SUGGESTIONS FOR STUDY

1. What is meant by the term symptomatic care?
2. What has caused you to have anorexia?
3. What factors should be observed and reported about a patient who is vomiting?
4. What is the cause of diarrhea?
5. In what age group is diarrhea especially dangerous?
6. Discuss ways in which the practical nurse can help the patient with constipation to re-establish normal bowel habits.
7. What is the body's most urgent dietary requirement?
8. Familiarize yourself with the method of recording a patient's intake and output in your hospital.
9. What is the medical term for dropsy? What causes it?
10. How long should the practical nurse wait after a patient's chill has ended before taking his temperature?
11. Discuss the nursing care of a patient with a persistent cough.
12. Review the meaning of hemoptysis, dyspnea, orthopnea, and cyanosis.
13. Review the description of Cheyne-Stokes respiration and try to breathe like a person with this symptom.
14. What nursing measures are used to relieve epistaxis?
15. What is the difference between bradycardia and tachycardia?
16. What should the practical nurse observe and report about a patient having pain?
17. Discuss nursing measures to relieve pain.
18. Convulsions may be a symptom of what diseases?
19. Discuss the nursing care of a patient having a convulsion.
20. What should be observed and reported about a patient having a convulsion?

## REFERENCES FOR CHAPTER 4

Emerson, Charles P., Jr., and Bragdon, Jane S.: *Essentials of Medicine,* 17th ed. J. B. Lippincott Co., Philadelphia, 1955, pp. 51-104.
Faddis, Margene O., and Hayman, Joseph M.: *Care of the Medical Patient.* McGraw-Hill Book Co., New York, 1952, pp. 59-67.
Frohman, I. Phillips: "Constipation," *Am. J. Nursing,* 55:65-67, (Jan.) 1955.

Fuerst, Elinor V., and Wolff, LuVerne: *Fundamentals of Nursing.* J. B. Lippincott Co., Philadelphia, 1956, pp. 298-349.

Gill, Helen Z. (ed.): *Basic Nursing,* 4th ed. The Macmillan Company, New York, 1955, pp. 263-73 and 346-61.

Harmer, Bertha, and Henderson, Virginia: *Textbook of the Principles and Practice of Nursing,* 5th ed. The Macmillan Company, New York, 1955, pp 269-307 and 366-464.

Hobby, A. Worth, "Cough, Its Pathology and Management," *Davis Nursing Survey,* 19:197-200, (July) 1955.

Hull, Edgar, and Perrodin, Cecilia: *Medical Nursing,* 5th ed. F. A. Davis Co., Philadelphia, 1954, pp. 8-13.

Osmun, Paul M.: "Nosebleeds," *Am. J. Nursing,* 56:1411-13, (Nov.) 1956.

*Pain—A Signal.* John Hancock Mutual Life Insurance Co., Boston, 1955.

Phelps, Elbert T.: "Fever—Its Causes and Effects," *Am. J. Nursing,* 56:319-21, (Mar.) 1956.

Chapter 5        *CARING FOR*
*THE SURGICAL PATIENT*

## INTRODUCTION

The practical nurse has many responsibilities in the care of a surgical patient. Although the actual procedures assigned to her may vary in different hospitals, knowledge of the principles underlying the care of a surgical patient serves as a basis for more effective nursing care. In this chapter the nursing care commonly needed by the surgical patient before and after surgery is discussed. *Preoperative care* deals with the nursing care of a patient before surgery, and *postoperative care* deals with the nursing care following surgery.

## PREOPERATIVE CARE

Preoperative care of a patient is aimed toward getting the patient into the best possible condition for surgery. This is the aim of all members of the health team caring for him. The needs of the individual patient help to determine which members are called upon for service. The physician, acting as leader of the team, prescribes for the patient. A thorough physical examination is done by the doctor. Examinations of the patient's urine and blood are done by the laboratory technician. Services of the dietitian are needed for the patient's diet. A social worker may be asked to help the patient with home problems or financial worries. A rabbi, priest, or minister serves as the patient's spiritual adviser. Members of the nursing team give the patient nursing care. A technician in the x-ray department takes x-rays requested by the doctor. The physician, laboratory technician, dietitian, social worker, spiritual adviser, nurse, and x-ray

46

technician are some of the many people working with the preoperative patient. Success of the surgery depends upon the ability of all members of the health team caring for this patient.

## Admission of the Patient

Generally, the patient is admitted to the hospital one or two days before the operation is scheduled so that he can be prepared for surgery. The actual procedure for admitting a surgical patient varies slightly in different institutions. In addition to knowing exactly what is expected of her in a specific hospital when admitting a patient, the practical nurse needs an understanding of feelings often experienced by patients before surgery. She can assume that a patient posted for surgery has emotions regarding his operation. He may have a slight feeling of anxiety or actual fear. Also, members of his family have similar feelings.

Fears often felt by surgical patients are fear of death, disfigurement, disability, feeling the incision made, and waking up before the operation has been completed. The possibility of telling their secrets when reacting from the anesthetic causes apprehension in some patients. Also, fear of the unknown is present in many preoperative patients.

In addition to his concern regarding the operation, the patient is in strange surroundings, away from his family and his home, and meeting new people. Pausing for a moment to consider the probable feelings of the patient, the nurse sees many ways in which she can help him to feel more comfortable. Greeting the new patient in a warm and friendly manner, showing him how a nurse can be signaled, telling him where his clothes are placed, and introducing him to his roommate are only a few examples of seemingly small acts which the thoughtful nurse can do to make the patient feel more at ease.

Procedures assigned to the practical nurse should be done in a manner which gains the patient's confidence. Having confidence in those caring for him is an important factor in the patient's recovery. It also gives the patient needed reassurance.

The surgeon leaves preoperative orders for the patient. Usually his orders include the following factors: area to be prepared for surgery (see Figs. 4-8), laboratory work, a cleansing enema, diet, the time to discontinue giving the patient fluids and food by mouth, the time the patient's operation is scheduled, and preoperative medication. His order for drugs almost always includes a sedative to be given the night before surgery to produce sleep. The medicine to be given immediately before surgery varies. Frequently, atropine and morphine are the drugs prescribed when a general anesthetic is to be given. Because atropine checks the secretion of mucus in the respiratory tract, it reduces the possibility of the patient aspirating excess mucus. Morphine causes relaxation and relieves anxiety. An antibiotic may be prescribed to combat or to prevent an infection.

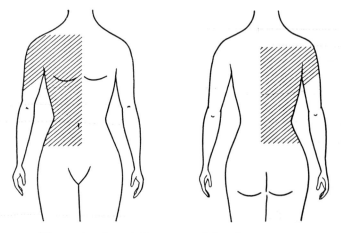

**Figure 4.** Area to be prepared for chest surgery.

After the patient has been admitted, the practical nurse may be asked to assist the physician in taking the patient's history and doing a thorough physical examination. The patient's urine and blood are examined in the laboratory. The practical nurse is often the one assigned to collect the urine specimen. A chest x-ray is customary in many hospitals.

Prior to surgery, permission for the operation must be granted in writing by the patient or his nearest relative. Either the parents or the guardian sign for the patient who is under legal age (a minor). The nearest relative signs for the patient who is unconscious or who is in no mental condition to be responsible for his actions.

## Diet

After determining the nourishment needed by the patient, the physician prescribes the diet. The undernourished patient receives a special diet to improve his condition before surgery. When a patient is unable to take an adequate amount of food and fluid by mouth, he is given them intravenously.

The patient's stomach should be as empty as possible when surgery is done. This is especially important when the patient is put to sleep (loses consciousness from a general anesthetic). The reason for having the stomach empty is to prevent vomiting while the general anesthetic is being given. If the patient vomits while unconscious, he is likely to aspirate some of the food and fluid into his lungs. Vomitus in the lungs can cause serious complications, such as pneumonia or lung abscess.

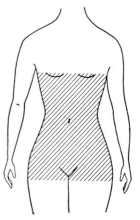

**Figure 5.** Area to be prepared for abdominal surgery.

Usually the last meal eaten by the patient before the operation consists of easily digested food. In some types of surgery this kind of food is given for several days before the operation. When surgery is planned for the next morning, the patient should eat no food after the evening meal. Most surgeons allow their patients to drink fluids until either bedtime or midnight on the night before the operation. The practical nurse needs to find out from the head nurse when she should stop giving the patient fluids.

## Elimination

The lower intestine should be as empty as possible before surgery in order to prevent fecal incontinence during the operation, and postoperative discomfort from gas in the intestines. Also, a full colon interferes with an abdominal operation. The physician prescribes

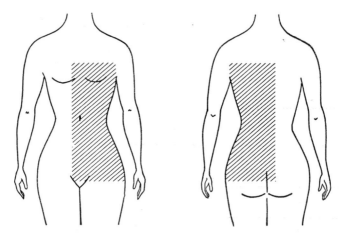

Figure 6.   Area to be prepared for kidney surgery.

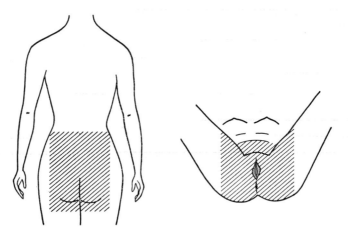

Figure 7.   Area to be prepared for perineal surgery.

enemas to empty the colon. According to the doctor's preference, the enemas are given either the night before surgery or in the early morning before the operation. It is important for the nurse giving the enema to be certain that all of the solution has been expelled.

### General Hygiene

An important part of preoperative care is a thorough cleansing bath and good oral hygiene. Cleanliness helps to prevent postoperative infections. When permitted by the physician, the practical nurse can assist the patient in taking a tub bath. If not, a bed bath should be given. The patient's nails should be clean and free of polish. The patient's mouth should be cleansed thoroughly.

### Local Preparation

The purpose of skin care of the operative field is to make it as clean and free of bacteria as possible without harming the skin. A large area around the future wound should be cleaned thoroughly and shaved. Generally, this procedure is done the night before surgery. It is important that all hair over the area be removed because of the bacteria present on it. Soap

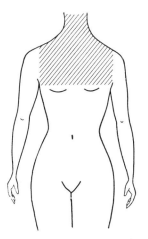

**Figure 8.** Area to be prepared for neck surgery.

and warm water are the agents most often used in cleaning the operative area. The procedure of local preparation for surgery in some hospitals calls for the application of an antiseptic agent after the area has been cleaned and shaved. Either benzene or ether may be used in removing oily dirt and adhesive if the patient does not object to the odor. The practical nurse needs to familiarize herself with the procedure used in the institution in which she is nursing.

### Immediate Care before Surgery

The care of the patient immediately before surgery should be arranged so that he is not upset by hurrying and by poorly planned work. Following the bath and good mouth care the nurse should put a cotton hospital gown on the patient. The hair should be combed and hairpins removed. A woman's long hair can be plaited into two braids. The patient's hair is covered with a cotton head covering in some hospitals.

The temperature, pulse, and respiration are taken and recorded. It is important for the practical nurse to report any abnormality in the temperature, the pulse, or the respiration to her team leader or to the head nurse. An increased temperature may indicate an infection of the respiratory tract. An increased pulse and respiratory rate may be symptoms of excess anxiety or fear. A marked change in the patient's temperature, pulse, and respiration may cause the surgeon to postpone the operation.

The practical nurse should observe and report other symptoms of undue apprehension. Also, the patient should be observed for signs of an upper respiratory infection, such as sneezing, coughing, hoarseness, and sniffling. The surgeon may decide to delay surgery if the patient has an upper respiratory infection or is too apprehensive.

The doctor's orderbook will specify whether false teeth are to remain in the patient's mouth or to be removed before going to surgery. However, the anesthetist may request that the dentures be left in the patient's mouth. This may help the anesthetist to apply the mask more securely when giving the anesthetic. If false teeth are removed, they should be placed in a container, clearly labeled, which is then put in a safe place, such as the drawer of the bedside table. Jewelry and other valuables should be handled according to hospital procedure for safekeeping. A ring may be secured with either adhesive tape or bandage.

After the patient has received his preoperative medication, he should remain in bed. His surroundings should be quiet.

The patient's bladder should be emptied before he is transferred to surgery to prevent incontinence during anesthesia. After the patient has voided, the practical nurse measures and records the amount of urine and the time. Inability to void should be reported as the surgeon may want the patient catheterized.

The patient is transferred to the operating room on a stretcher or in his bed. Adequate covering is needed to prevent chilling. The practical nurse may be asked to accompany the patient to surgery.

Having a familiar person with him reassures the patient. The patient should not be left unattended while on a stretcher. A strap is placed across the patient's thighs and secured to the stretcher as a safety measure in some hospitals.

## POSTOPERATIVE CARE

After the patient has been transferred to the operating room, the unit should be prepared for his return. The recovery bed is made according to the hospital's procedure. Rearrangement of the furniture may be necessary so that the stretcher can be rolled directly to the bedside. Windows and screens are adjusted to avoid drafts.

### The Anesthetized Patient

The anesthetized patient has lost the ability to feel because of a drug which is given. This loss of feeling, which may be general or local, is produced by a drug which is called an *anesthetic*. When a patient has a general anesthetic, his entire body is affected, and he loses consciousness. Ether, nitrous oxide, and cyclopropane are examples of drugs which produce general anesthesia by inhalation. Thiopental sodium (Pentothal sodium) is given intravenously to produce general anesthesia. A local anesthetic causes a loss of sensation in a part of the body, and the patient does not lose consciousness. Local anesthesia is produced by the injection of a drug, such as procaine (Novocain). In a spinal anesthetic, the drug is introduced into the spinal canal. This causes paralysis of the nerves as they leave the spinal cord.

Usually, the patient who has had a local anesthetic has no symptoms resulting from the drug except in the case of a spinal anesthetic. The nurse caring for the patient who has had a spinal anesthetic should check his blood pressure, pulse, and respiration frequently. The patient should be kept quiet and flat in bed for six to eight hours, or for as long as this is ordered. The nurse should observe the return of movement and feeling in the patient's legs and feet. The patient is considered to be recovered from the spinal anesthetic when there is a complete return of movement and feeling in his toes.

The patient who has had a general anesthetic may be transferred to a recovery room or to his unit. This varies with the physical plan of the hospital. The patient should be lifted gently from the stretcher to the bed. After the patient is covered adequately, the top bedding is tucked under the mattress. Usually the patient is placed on his back with his head turned to the side, or on his side, to aid the drainage of vomitus and mucus from his mouth. It is of extreme importance for this patient to be attended at all times by the nurse until he has reacted fully from the anesthetic.

Since the practical nurse is asked frequently to assist the professional nurse in caring for the anesthetized patient, she needs to know the important factors to observe. The pulse, the respiration, and the blood pressure are usually taken and recorded every 15 minutes, or as ordered. The dressing is checked frequently for bleeding and drainage. Observation of the patient's color is another important point. It is essential that the practical nurse report any unusual symptoms promptly to her team leader or the head nurse.

Drainage tubes should be attached to the proper equipment. For example, an indwelling catheter is to be attached to rubber tubing leading to the drainage bottle.

Respiratory difficulty is a dangerous complication which occurs frequently while the patient is reacting from general anesthesia. Depression of the respiratory center in the brain, the falling back of the tongue into the throat, and the collecting of mucus or vomitus in the throat are examples of common causes of respiratory difficulty. The rate of breathing is decreased when the respiratory center is depressed. The physician prescribes a respiratory stimulant when marked depression is present. Keeping the patient's head in good position often keeps the tongue from falling back in the throat. Also, leaving the airway in the mouth and throat until the patient reacts sufficiently to push it out prevents the tongue from falling back. When the tongue slips back into the throat, the nurse can pull it into normal position after she has protected her hand with gauze or a piece of clean cloth. Turning the patient's head to the side and gently swabbing the patient's mouth helps to rid the patient of excess mucus.

A patient often becomes restless and talks incoherently as he begins to react from the anesthetic. As the patient is not aware of what he is saying or doing, it is the nurse's responsibility to protect him from injury. The actions or sayings of the patient during this stage should not be discussed with him after his recovery from anesthesia. Although the patient may not be able to answer the nurse, he can often be quieted if she tells him repeatedly that the operation is over and he is back in his bed. It is amazing how this simple measure reassures the patient.

## The Reacted Patient

The nurse should not leave the patient alone until he has regained full consciousness. Before leaving the reacted patient, the nurse should make him as comfortable as possible. Gently washing his face and hands, helping with mouth care, giving a soothing backrub, and changing his position are nursing measures which increase his comfort. Using pillows for support after the position has been changed is helpful. Extra bedclothing placed on the bed for its use during recovery should be removed. The patient's gown and linen should be changed, if necessary. The safe practice of using side rails on the bed of a patient who has recently reacted is used regularly in many hospitals. If side rails are used, they should be placed in position before the nurse leaves the patient.

Although the patient has reacted from a general anesthetic, the nurse is still responsible for checking his condition. His temperature, pulse, respiration, blood pressure, and bandage should be checked frequently during the first 24 hours or for as long as ordered. The nurse also measures and records the amount of urine voided by the patient during the first 24 hours or for a longer period, if necessary. If the patient is unable to void in the first 8 to 12 hours, the physician prescribes a catheterization.

The patient is given water and food as allowed by the doctor. Intravenous fluids are given until the patient is able to take adequate liquids by mouth. The practical nurse should check with the head nurse before giving the patient water to drink. Frequently patients ask for crushed ice following their surgery. Some surgeons prefer their patients to have tap water or cracked ice during the first few days instead of ice water. It is thought that ice water increases postoperative discomfort from gas.

The patient should be encouraged to move around in bed and to take deep breaths. These measures are helpful in preventing postoperative complications which are discussed next in this chapter.

Usually the patient is helped to sit on the side of his bed to dangle his feet before getting out of bed. Since patients are allowed out of bed soon after surgery, the patient needs the nurse's assistance until he is capable of getting out by himself.

## POSTOPERATIVE DISCOMFORTS AND COMPLICATIONS

### Pain

Pain is often the first discomfort experienced by the postoperative patient. In addition to the nursing measures used to relieve pain, drugs, such as morphine, meperidine (Demerol), and pantopon, are given by injection. The observation and care of a patient having pain are discussed on pages 40 to 41.

### Hemorrhage

The hemorrhaging patient is losing blood from his blood vessels. Bright red blood which spurts with each heartbeat indicates that the blood is coming from an artery. Dark red blood which flows in a continuous stream indicates that the blood is coming from a vein. Blood coming from capillaries flows slowly and steadily. The practical nurse should summon help immediately when a patient is hemorrhaging. It may be necessary to apply pressure over the bleeding area until help arrives. When the patient is bleeding internally, the first symptoms to be noted are those of shock. Also, symptoms of shock occur in cases of external hemorrhage.

### Shock

#### Description

A patient in shock has an insufficient amount of blood circulating in his body, especially in the vessels of the outer part of his body. It may be due to an actual loss of blood during a hemorrhage or it may be due to a marked dilation of the blood vessels. Blood is pooled within the body when the surface vessels are dilated. The exact cause of this is not clearly understood. Extreme pain, burns, marked fear, injury, hemorrhage, and surgery are some of the common causes of shock.

## Symptoms

It is of vital importance for the practical nurse to develop the ability to observe early symptoms of shock. If this condition of collapse is profound and is not observed and treated, the patient is likely to die. The patient in shock is pale, apprehensive, and restless. In some cases the patient is listless. His skin feels cold and clammy, the pulse is weak and rapid, and his respiration is rapid and shallow. The patient may become cyanotic. The blood pressure is lowered. In profound shock the blood pressure cannot be determined. Frequently the patient complains of thirst. His eyes may be expressionless or staring.

## Treatment and Nursing Care

Help must be summoned at once. The immediate care of a patient in shock includes the application of warm blankets. If hot-water bottles are prescribed, the nurse should use extreme caution in placing them next to the patient as he can be burned easily while in shock. The foot of the bed may be elevated in an effort to force blood from the extremities to the vital centers of the brain. The patient is given additional fluid, usually intravenously, to fill the blood vessels. When shock results from hemorrhage, the lost blood may be replaced by blood transfusion. The physician also treats the hemorrhaging area.

## Abdominal Distention

## Description

Abdominal distention is a common discomfort following surgery, especially an abdominal operation. After the patient has reacted from the anesthetic, peristalsis may be slow in returning. Fluids and gases collect in the gastrointestinal tract, causing an enlargement of the stomach and intestines, which is called distention.

### Symptoms

The patient with abdominal distention has a swollen abdomen, a feeling of fullness, and cramping pains in his abdomen. Nausea and vomiting may occur. In extreme cases pressure on the diaphragm causes difficult breathing.

### Treatment and Nursing Care

The patient's position should be changed frequently. Many surgeons request that their patients be given tap water, warm fluids, and crushed ice instead of ice water and other cold fluids. The basis for this request is the idea that warm fluids stimulate the return of peristalsis better than cold liquids and that crushed ice when it reaches the stomach is the temperature of the body. The practical nurse should encourage the patient to eat the diet prescribed for him. When the flatus (gas) is in the lower colon the insertion of a rectal tube helps the patient expel the flatus. The outer end of the rectal tube can be placed in either a small basin, a urinal, or a urine specimen bottle. This is done to prevent the patient's bed from becoming soiled by fecal material which is likely to be expelled with the flatus. Frequently, an enema is prescribed to stimulate the return of peristalsis. The application of heat to the abdomen is ordered sometimes in the form of turpentine stupes, heating pad, or hot-water bottle. When the above methods do not relieve abdominal distention, gastrointestinal suction may be used. In this case, the physician inserts a tube into the upper gastrointestinal tract and attaches it to an apparatus which produces suction. Thus, gas and fluid are removed from the gastrointestinal tract. Gastrointestinal suction is discussed in detail on pages 222 to 223.

### Respiratory Complications

### Prevention

Respiratory complications are both frequent and serious in the surgical patient. An important function of the nurses caring for this patient is prevention of these complications. This prevention starts with the preoperative care and is continued through the convalescence.

As stated on page 52 of this chapter, the patient should be observed for symptoms of a respiratory infection while he is being prepared for surgery. Generally, the surgeon does not perform surgery on a patient with a respiratory infection except in an emergency. The patient with an infection, such as a cold, is likely to develop more serious complications after surgery.

Another preoperative nursing measure to prevent pulmonary complications postoperatively is good oral hygiene to prevent the aspiration of food particles and infected material during anesthesia. The patient's stomach should be empty to avoid aspiration of vomitus.

It is the nurse's responsibility to keep the patient comfortably warm.

After the patient has reacted from the anesthetic, the nurse should change his position frequently. When he is capable of moving by himself, the nurse should remind and encourage him to move around. Early ambulation, or getting the patient out of bed within the first few days following surgery, is considered an important factor in reducing respiratory complications. The nurse needs to assist the patient in getting out of bed until he has regained adequate strength to do so by himself. In some cases the patient is lifted from the bed to a chair by the nurse and other assistants.

Another important measure in the prevention of respiratory complications is to encourage deep breathing. This is particularly important when the patient is taking shallow breaths because it hurts his incision when he breathes deeply. The physician frequently prescribes deep breathing exercises every hour. In this case, the nurse has the patient take at least 10 deep breaths every hour. Some surgeons have their patients blow up a paper bag or balloon a certain number of times each hour. A great percentage of the respiratory complications discussed in the following paragraphs can be prevented by these measures.

### Bronchitis

The patient with bronchitis has an inflammation of the mucous membrane lining the bronchial tubes. His chief symptom is a cough.

The act of coughing is painful for the postoperative patient, especially if he has had chest or abdominal surgery. For this reason he tries to avoid coughing. If the cough is productive, he should be encouraged to cough and to expectorate the mucus. Having the patient hold his hands over his bandaged incision when coughing often relieves some of the discomfort. The nursing care of a patient with a persistent cough is discussed on pages 36 to 37.

### Pneumonia

Pneumonia, which is inflammation of the lungs, is a frequent postoperative complication. It occurs often in the older individual and in the one whose preoperative condition was poor. An increasing amount of surgery is being performed on elderly people. The older person is more likely to have a chronic disease of his lungs such as bronchitis. Also, he may have a heart condition which causes the blood to flow more slowly through his lungs. Because of this, he is more likely to develop pneumonia when he stays in one position too long. This kind of pneumonia is known as *hypostatic pneumonia*. Knowing these facts, the practical nurse can realize the importance of turning the older patient more frequently. He also needs to be encouraged to take deep breaths and to cough. Early ambulation is especially important in the care of this patient.

Fortunately, this disease can be prevented in many instances by the nursing measures used to prevent respiratory complications which were discussed in the above paragraph and on pages 58 to 59 in this chapter. The physician now has many antibiotics from which he can select the proper one to combat a particular type of pneumonia.

### Pulmonary Embolism

An embolus is a foreign body in the blood stream. It is usually a blood clot or part of a blood clot which is carried by the blood stream to another part of the body. When the embolus reaches a blood vessel which is too small for it to pass through, it lodges there and causes an obstruction in that vessel. If the embolus lodges in an artery in the lungs, it is called *pulmonary embolism*. As a result, the lung tissue supplied by the affected artery has an insufficient blood supply.

Pulmonary embolism is a grave postoperative complication. It occurs most often when the patient is convalescing. The patient is attacked suddenly with sharp chest pain, cyanosis, and dyspnea. If a large pulmonary artery is closed by the embolus, death results within a short period of time. When a small branch of the pulmonary artery is obstructed, the patient may recover.

Since the practical nurse is the one who is frequently assigned to care for the patient during his convalescence, she should observe her patients for symptoms of pulmonary embolism. This is especially important when she is helping the patient out of bed for the first few times. Help should be secured immediately when a patient develops these symptoms. Drugs, such as morphine or meperidine (Demerol), are given to relieve the patient's pain and anxiety. Oxygen therapy is used also.

### Phlebitis and Thrombophlebitis

Phlebitis is an inflammation of a vein. In thrombophlebitis the vein is inflamed and a blood clot forms. The femoral vein, which is a large vein in the leg, is affected frequently.

Measures to prevent this complication include an adequate intake of fluids to prevent a concentration of the blood, changing the patient's position often, encouraging the patient to move his feet and legs while in bed, and early ambulation. Pressure on the legs by tight straps and leg holders during surgery should be avoided. The symptoms, treatment, and nursing care are discussed on pages 149 to 150.

### Nausea and Vomiting

Nausea and vomiting are discomforts which occur frequently in the postoperative patient. For this reason, it is customary for the nurse to place an emesis basin in a convenient place when preparing the recovery bed. When vomiting occurs, the nurse turns the patient's head to the side to aid in preventing aspiration of vomitus. The nursing care of a patient with nausea and vomiting is discussed on pages 28 to 29.

### Urinary Retention

Urinary retention occurs frequently in postoperative patients. The care of a patient with this symptom is discussed on pages 42 to 43.

The amount of urine voided by the postoperative patient should be measured and recorded for at least the first 24 to 48 hours after surgery. When the practical nurse notices that a patient is voiding frequently and in small amounts, she reports this fact. Usually the passage of 30 to 60 ml* (1 to 2 oz) of urine every 20 to 30 minutes is a symptom of an overdistended bladder which is not being emptied when the patient voids. This condition is referred to as "retention with overflow." The doctor frequently requests the nurse to have the patient void and then do a catheterization when this condition is suspected. The amount of urine removed by catheter varies, but it may be as much as 600 to 900 ml (20 to 30 oz).

## Wound Infection

Occasionally, a patient's wound (incision) becomes infected. His symptoms vary with the amount of infection. When an area around one of the skin sutures (stitches) is infected, it is called a *stitch abscess*. The physician may open the involved area to allow it to drain.

*Dehiscence - separation of wound edges, without protrusion of organs*

*Pinkish on dressing - call head nurse or doctor.*

## SUGGESTIONS FOR STUDY

1. Discuss ways that the practical nurse can make the newly admitted surgical patient feel more at ease.
2. What fears are common in patients before surgery?
3. Why should the patient's stomach be empty before surgery? Why should the patient's bladder be empty before surgery?
4. Why is an area larger than the future wound cleaned and shaved before surgery?
5. What symptoms should be reported in caring for a preoperative patient?
6. Discuss the responsibilities of the nurse caring for a patient recovering from a general anesthetic and a spinal anesthetic.
7. When should an airway be removed from the postoperative patient's mouth?

---

* Because in the fifteenth revision of the *United States Pharmacopeia* and the tenth edition of the *National Formulary* (both officially published in 1955) cubic centimeter (cc) was replaced by milliliter (ml) for liquid measurement, this change has been made throughout the text.

*Evisceration - separation of wound edges plus organ protrusion occur within 6-8 day*

8. What are the symptoms of shock? How is shock treated?
9. What can be done to prevent abdominal distention? What measures are used for its relief?
10. Discuss ways of preventing respiratory complications following surgery.
11. What is pulmonary embolism?
12. Discuss nursing measures to prevent thrombophlebitis.
13. Why should a catheterization to relieve retention be avoided if possible?
14. What symptoms does the patient have when he has "retention with overflow"?

## REFERENCES FOR CHAPTER 5

Bird, Brian: "Psychological Aspects of Preoperative and Postoperative Care," *Am. J. Nursing,* **55:**685-87, (June) 1955.
Eliason, Eldridge; Ferguson, L. Kraeer; and Sholtis, Lillian A.: *Surgical Nursing,* 10th ed. J. B. Lippincott Co., Philadelphia, 1955, pp. 52-158.
Harmer, Bertha, and Henderson, Virginia: *Textbook of the Principles and Practice of Nursing,* 5th ed. The Macmillan Company, New York, 1955, pp. 989-1047.
Lam, Conrad R.: "What Is Shock?" *Am. J. Nursing,* **51:**116-17, (Feb.) 1951.
Maddock, Walter G.: "Gastrointestinal Distention," *Am. J. Nursing,* **56:**893-95, (July) 1956.
Proudfit, Fairfax T., and Robinson, Corinne H.: *Nutrition and Diet Therapy,* 11th ed. The Macmillan Company, New York, 1955, pp. 358-68.
Stafford, Edward S., and Diller, Doris: *Surgery and Surgical Nursing,* 3rd ed. W. B. Saunders Co., Philadelphia, 1958, pp. 54-93.
West, John P.; Keller, Manelva W.; and Harmon, Elizabeth H.: *Nursing Care of the Surgical Patient,* 6th ed. The Macmillan Company, New York, 1957, pp. 81-161.
Young, Helen, and Lee, Eleanor: *Lippincott's Quick Reference Book for Nurses,* 7th ed. J. B. Lippincott Co., Philadelphia, 1955, pp. 27-29, 37-38, and 176-86.

*Place sterile dressing & sterile Normal Saline over organs to prevent drying of organs. Get nurse or doctor.*

*Responsibilities*
*of the Practical Nurse*
*in Caring for*
*the Patient with*
a *General Disease*
*Condition*


PART II

# Chapter 6

# THE PATIENT WITH AN INFLAMMATION

## INTRODUCTION

Inflammation is a defensive reaction of the body to any injury. Injury is produced by a blow, a foreign body, a chemical; also by electricity, heat, cold, or a pathogenic microorganism (pathogen). A microorganism is a tiny living body which is visible only through a microscope. When this minute cell causes disease, it is spoken of as a *pathogen.* The inflammatory process produced by a pathogen is called an *infection*.

The suffix "-itis" means "inflammation of." The hundreds of medical terms ending with "-itis" indicate the frequency with which a practical nurse is called upon to nurse a patient with an inflammation. Appendicitis, tonsillitis, poliomyelitis, colitis, and sinusitis are only a few examples. The first part of the above words indicates the part of the body whch is inflamed. Since inflammations occur so often, the practical nurse must have a basic understanding of the changes which occur in the patient's body.

Many inflammations result from disease-producing microorganisms such as those which cause tuberculosis, typhoid fever, and pneumonia. Also, the inflammatory reaction of the body to other injuries is often complicated by pathogens as in an infected burn or cut. Since inflammation is so frequently associated with pathogenic organisms, this chapter deals primarily with inflammation resulting from infection or associated with an infection.

## HOW MICROORGANISMS CAUSE DISEASE

All microorganisms do not produce disease. These which do not cause disease are referred to as nonpathogenic microorganisms. Many are beneficial to man, such as the yeast which causes bread to rise or the mold from which penicillin is derived. These minute particles of life may be compared with the families in your community. Members of certain groups have similar characteristics just like the family who lives next door to you. They have group or family names. Members of the animal kingdom called protozoa cause malaria and amebic dysentery. The virus family has such small members that they are visible only with the high-powered electron microscope. A virus can reproduce only when it is within another living cell. Smallpox, measles, and mumps are caused by different members of the virus group.

Yeast and molds belong to the vegetable kingdom. A member of the mold family produces athlete's foot and an offspring of the yeast group causes thrush. Members of another family in the plant kingdom are called bacteria. Typhoid fever and tuberculosis are produced by bacteria. Since bacteria produce most of the infectious diseases which the practical nurse encounters, it is necessary for her to learn more about them.

A common classification of bacteria is based upon their shapes. (1) Those which are rod-shaped are called "bacilli." Tuberculosis is an infection resulting from the tubercle bacillus. (2) Bacteria in the form of a corkscrew are referred to as "spirilla" or "spirochetes." Syphilis is caused by a spirochete. (3) Bacteria having round forms are referred to as "cocci." This group is further classified according to the way cocci grow in groups. (a) The oval-shaped bacteria which grow alone or in pairs are diplococci. A disease resulting from diplococci is pneumococcal pneumonia. (b) Streptococci grow in chain formation. Scarlet fever is one of the many infections caused by streptococci. (c) Other members of the cocci group grow in clusters and are called staphylococci. An infection produced frequently by members of this group is a skin abscess or boil. Some bacteria produce toxins, which are poisonous substances. Toxins secreted by the living microorganisms are referred to as exotoxins. Poisons stored within the organism and given off after the bacterium's (singular, for bacteria) death is an _endotoxin_. Production of toxins by bacteria within the patient's body accounts for much of his general malaise.

A bacterium may go into a period of rest. During this time the protoplasm is concentrated into a small round body and is covered with a tough membrane. Such a microorganism is spoken of as a spore. Spore-forming bacteria are difficult to kill during this resting stage. Thus, longer exposure to heat or to a disinfectant is required to kill them. The bacillus causing (tetanus or lockjaw) is spore-forming.

The practical nurse will hear bacteria referred to as being gram-negative or gram-positive. This method of grouping bacteria is based upon their reaction to Gram's stain. This specially prepared blue stain is used in the laboratory to aid the pathologist in identifying the microorganism. The gram-positive bacterium retains the blue color of the stain, and the gram-negative bacterium does not retain the blue color. The (tubercle bacillus is gram-negative)

Microorganisms enter the body in the food we eat, the water we drink, and the air we inhale. Also, they may enter through a break in either the mucous membrane or the skin. However, a few pathogens can pass through the unbroken skin. Amebic dysentery is caused by the ameba which enters the mouth and continues down the gastrointestinal tract which is lined with mucous membrane. The virus of the (common cold and the tubercle bacillus) may produce an infection after entering the body through inhaled air. The Anopheles mosquito punctures the person's skin and deposits the microorganism responsible for malaria. Staphlococci sometimes pass through the (hair follicles of the unbroken skin and cause a boil) After the pathogenic microorganism enters the body through the skin or mucous membrane it may be carried to another part of the body by circulating body fluids or it may remain at the point of entry.

## THE BODY'S DEFENSES

The human body has an amazing and quite effective protective mechanism against these invaders from the microbe world. The skin and the mucous membrane make up the body's first line of defense. Usually, pathogens are unable to penetrate the unbroken skin. The mucous membrane increases its secretion of mucus when

attacked by invading microorganisms. Cilia also help to protect
the body. These are hairlike projections of mucous membrane in
various parts of the body. For example, (the cilia lining the nose,
trachea, and bronchi remove excess mucus and foreign bodies from
the upper respiratory tract by their waving motion) Hair lining the
**margins of the nostrils helps to** remove foreign material from the air
we breathe. Following an injury, whether it is caused by a foreign
body, cut, blow, or a pathogenic microorganism, the defensive army
of the body is called into action. Important members of the body's
protective team are antitoxins, antibodies, white blood cells, and
the lymph-vascular system. First, let us examine a simple inflammatory process which is not caused by a pathogen as in the case of
the incision made by the surgeon's sterile knife.

(Tissues surrounding the incision respond immediately to the
injury by starting a mild inflammatory process) The first reaction is
an increased blood supply to the area. Blood vessels dilate, and the
flow of blood within this area is slower. The walls of the blood vessels adapt themselves to allow white blood cells and serum to leave
the blood stream and go directly to the injured part. The increased
blood supply is spoken of as _congestion_. Since no pathogens are present, the inflammation begins to subside. The white blood cells or
leukocytes take up the dead cells and return to the blood stream. The
excess fluid is reabsorbed into the blood. The wound edges grow to
gether, and the area soon heals.

When inflammation is caused by, or complicated by, pathogenic
microorganisms, the body's defensive reaction starts in the same
manner as described in the simple inflammatory process. After leaving the blood stream, the leukocytes try to kill the invading organisms. (Antitoxins and antibodies) are two important immune substances which are carried to the area by blood serum. (They act
against the invader and counteract the toxins excreted by the pathogens.) The battle between the defensive army and the invader has
begun. If the immune substances and leukocytes are strong enough
to kill the invader, inflammation begins to disappear.

When the body's resistance is too weak or the pathogens too
strong, many tissue cells and leukocytes are killed. A collection of
dead tissue cells, bacteria, and dead white blood cells is called _pus_.
This process of pus formation is called _suppuration_. Infected particles

# AN ABSCESS

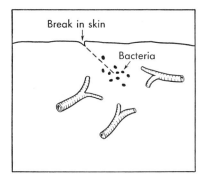 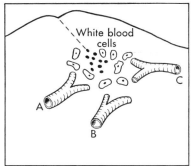

**Figure 9.** (*Left*) A break in the skin allowing bacteria to enter.

**Figure 10.** (*Right*) Blood vessels, A, B, and C dilate following an injury. White blood cells and serum containing antitoxins and antibodies go to the injured part. The increased blood supply causes the area to swell.

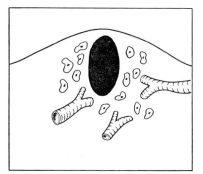 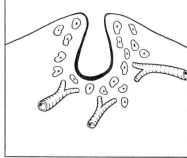

**Figure 11.** (*Left*) Pus forms when tissue cells, white blood cells, and bacteria are killed. White blood cells form a wall around the collection of pus which is called an abscess. It spreads into the tissue which offers the least resistance.

**Figure 12.** (*Right*) The abscess ruptures when it reaches the surface. The defenses of the body overcome the infection, and the wound heals.

which escape the area of battle are picked up by the lymph-vascular system. When these invaders reach the lymph nodes, specialized cells within the nodes try to render the bacteria harmless. At the same time the body attempts to build a wall of white blood cells and tissue around the collection of pus. This collection of pus surrounded by a wall is known as an *abscess* or a *boil.* The abscess tends to enlarge as more pus is added and likewise tends to spread into the tissue which offers least resistance. If the abscess spreads toward a surface, it eventually ruptures. The physician may have to incise the area to let it drain. Another possible way in which the infection may terminate is for the abscess to be absorbed gradually into the lymph stream. The defenses of the body have successfully overcome the invader.

## SYMPTOMS

### Local Symptoms

The local symptoms which the patient with an inflammation experiences are redness, swelling, heat, pain, and loss of function. The extent to which these symptoms are noticed depends upon the virulence of the microorganism, the body's resistance, and the part of the body affected. Redness, swelling, and heat can be noticed by the observer when the battle site is on the body surface. The area is red, swollen, and warm because of increased blood to the injured part. This increased amount of fluid presses on the sensitive nerve endings and produces pain. The inflamed part loses its ability to function efficiently because the increased fluid makes it difficult to move and the movement increases the pain.

### General Symptoms

The patient with an infected foot is not separated from the part of his body which is inflamed. His entire body is influenced by the battle being waged in his foot. If one state in our country were attacked by an invading army, the entire country would exert its efforts toward aiding the state in distress. Also, the other states would feel the effects of the war. So it is with the patient's body. His whole body feels the results of infection. Severity of the general symptoms of inflammation depends upon the ability of his body to combat the pathogens and the amount of toxins which are absorbed into his blood stream.

The patient usually has a <u>fever, an increased pulse and respiratory rate, headache, dry skin, flushed cheeks,</u> an increased white blood cell count, and malaise. *Malaise* is a general and indefinite feeling of discomfort or illness. The <u>elevated temperature is another defense</u> mechanism of the body to aid in combating infection. As the temperature rises, the pulse and respiratory rate are also increased. The patient's headache can be associated with the fever or with the toxins in his blood stream. <u>The dry skin and red cheeks</u> are also <u>associated with temperature elevation.</u> General malaise results from the fever as well as the toxins. The body produces more leukocytes since they are the fighting cells of the blood.

*leukocytosis*

## NURSING CARE

The practical nurse assumes an important role in caring for a patient with an infection. As a member of the nursing team she is guided by the professional nurse who receives specific instruction from the physician. The practical nurse needs an understanding of the basic principles involved in nursing a patient <u>with an infection</u> if she is to fulfill her obligation as a team member.

### Local Care

The <u>aim</u> of local nursing measures ordered by the physician is to <u>relieve the pain and aid nature in healing the inflamed area.</u> The <u>part is elevated, put to rest, and hot or cold applications are applied.</u>

### *Elevation*

The person who has had an infected finger remembers the relief obtained when the finger was elevated. The throbbing pain was eased almost immediately. <u>Elevating the inflamed part, also, relieves swelling. Drainage from the dilated blood vessels is increased by the force of gravity.</u> As the stagnant blood is carried away, fresh blood with an increased amount of immune substances and leukocytes is brought to the site. The <u>extremities,</u> head, and neck are parts of the body which are <u>most easily elevated</u>. In raising an extremity, the entire part should be raised. For example, in elevating the foot, the entire leg should be raised with the foot higher than the knee, and the knee higher than the hip. Plastic-covered pillows should

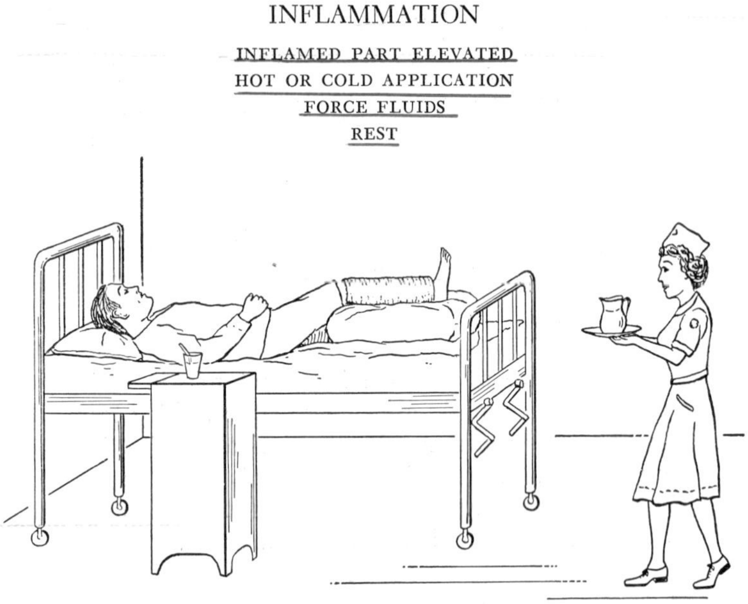

## INFLAMMATION

<u>INFLAMED PART ELEVATED</u>
HOT OR COLD APPLICATION
<u>FORCE FLUIDS</u>
<u>REST</u>

Figure 13.   Nursing the patient with an inflammation.

be arranged under the extremity for support. An ambulatory patient can have his infected arm elevated in a sling. In this case, the patient's hand should be approximately 10 to 12.5 cm (4 to 5 in.) higher than the level of the elbow.

### Rest

<u>Nature causes the patient to rest the infected area because of the pain involved when moving it</u>. Additional rest aids in the healing process. It allows more of the body's defenses to be directed into the battle zone. Delayed healing of a cracked lip illustrates how movement of an inflamed part slows down the process of recuperation.

## Heat

Local applications of heat are prescribed by the physician to increase the amount of blood to the inflamed area, to relax the muscles, or to relieve pain. The practical nurse should remember that some patients are more sensitive to heat than others. Extreme caution is necessary when applying heat to infants, aged persons, patients with diabetes and arteriosclerosis, and unconscious patients. Dry or moist heat may be ordered by the doctor.

## Dry Heat

HOT-WATER BOTTLE. The hot-water bottle, electric heating pad, and heat cradle are three common methods of applying dry heat. The nurse often hears the patient complain that his hot-water bottle is not warm enough when it is applied. However, the water must not be too hot as it may burn the patient. In order to prevent burning him, the practical nurse should check the temperature of the water to be used in the hot-water bottle with a thermometer. In general, the temperature of the water should not be higher than 48.9° C (120° F) for an adult. The temperature should be 43.3° to 46.1° C (110° to 115° F) for a child. The hot-water bottle should be warmed first by filling it with hot water and then emptying it. This simple measure helps to prevent cooling the water when it is poured into the hot-water bottle which is then suitably covered. The practical nurse should remember that some body areas, such as the inner aspect of the arms and thighs, are more sensitive to heat. She should observe the area beneath the hot-water bottle frequently for symptoms of burning, such as increased redness and warmth. These should be reported promptly to the team leader or head nurse.

The hot-water bottle should be filled one-third to one-half full, depending upon the site of application. When the weight of a half-filled bag is too much for the inflamed area, the bag should be one-third full. Removal of excess air, also, decreases the weight.

ELECTRIC HEATING PAD. An electric heating pad is prescribed when the physician wants the heat applied over a larger area for a longer period of time. Using moisture with an electric heating pad is a dangerous practice as fluid may cause a short circuit. It is necessary for the pad to be covered with waterproof material. Putting a pin through the pad is another hazardous practice. If a safety pin is used to secure a flannel cover over the pad, care should be used to avoid puncturing the heating pad. It is important to observe the patient frequently to avoid a burn from an overheated pad.

HEAT CRADLE. A heat cradle is another method of applying heat to an inflamed area. The warmth is often produced by electric bulbs in the ceiling of the cradle. This treatment is frequently used for patients with chronic inflammatory conditions of the muscles and the bones, such as arthritis. The actual technique of using a heat cradle varies with the type of equipment available as there are innumerable sizes and shapes. The practical nurse should seek specific instructions regarding the number of bulbs, the wattage to be used, and the distance of the heat cradle from the inflamed area. A thermometer is suspended inside the cradle as a guide for regulating the temperature. The nursing team should maintain the temperature of air within the cradle as prescribed by the doctor. As with other methods of applying heat, the danger of burning the patient is present. The patient should be observed frequently for increased redness and warmth of the part being treated.

## Moist Heat

Moist heat produces effects similar to those of dry heat. Although the results are similar, moisture increases the effect of heat. Why does a humid hot day cause you to feel the effects of heat more than a dry hot day? Moisture is a conductor of warmth. Also, the increased amount of water in the air slows down the evaporation of perspiration from a person's body. Therefore, it is essential to remember that moist heat burns more quickly than dry heat. A warm solution applied to a bandage burns more quickly than if it were placed on the skin, because the rate of evaporation is slower and the moisture increases the effect of heat.

HOT WET DRESSINGS OR HOT COMPRESSES. Hot wet dressings or hot compresses may be applied by putting warm solution on the part which is already bandaged or by applying compresses saturated with a heated solution and then wrung out. Moisture is retained in these dressings by wrapping the area with a thin piece of rubber or plastic

material, heavy waxed paper, or oilcloth. Warmth is maintained
by applying a hot-water bottle or covering the part with a heat
cradle. It is necessary to use sterile technique when the inflamed part
has an open lesion.

When a continuous hot wet dressing is prescribed, the bandage
needs to be changed when it starts to dry. If a hot-water bottle is the
method used to supply warmth, it should be changed as it begins to
cool. The inflamed part of a patient receiving continuous moist heat
should be examined frequently for early symptoms of injury by heat.

SITZ BATH. Having the patient sit in a bath of warm water from
5 to 60 minutes is known as a sitz bath. A temperature of 40.6°
to 43.3° C (105° to 110° F) is recommended. This type of moist heat
provides much relief to patients following rectal and perineal surgery.
It is also used in the treatment of patients with an acute inflammatory disease of the pelvis.

It is important to observe the patient for signs of exhaustion during
this treatment. If the practical nurse remembers that a hot bath for a
well person may cause temporary weakness, she should have little
difficulty in realizing the effect which a sick person may experience
from a sitz bath. The bath should be discontinued if the patient
shows signs of weakness. For example, the patient may have an increased pulse rate, perspire excessively, or complain of feeling weak.

LOCAL SOAKS. Immersion of an infected extremity is often indicated. The type of solution, temperature, and length of time are
ordered by the doctor. Sterile solution and a sterile basin are used
when there is an open lesion on the infected part.

## Cold

Local application of cold constricts blood vessels. Because of its
constricting action on blood vessels, it reduces the amount of blood
in the inflamed area. Cold relieves pain caused by the pressure of
increased fluid on the delicate nerve endings. Since the blood vessels
become smaller, hemorrhage and the inflammatory process are checked.
The effects of moist cold are greater than those of dry cold.

Prolonged application of cold can endanger the life of the area,
just as a person's life is endangered during a long period of time in
an extremely cold temperature. The site of application should be

examined frequently by the nurse for danger signals of tissue damage. The area becoming endangered by cold is bluish purple, has a mottled appearance, and feels numb and stiff. These symptoms should be reported immediately.

The ice bag or icecap is used to apply dry cold to an area. Moist cold is frequently applied by use of moist gauze. The gauze is dipped into a cold solution, wrung out, and applied to the inflamed area. It is necessary to replace the compress with another cold moist one every few minutes. This procedure is often used in applying moist cold to the eyes.

### General Care

Elevation, rest, and the application of heat or cold are the three main local treatments of an inflamed area. The patient with an acute localized infection or one with a generalized inflammation needs more than these three treatments to aid nature in the healing process

### *Rest*

The patient needs mental and physical rest. Keeping the patient in bed reduces the work of the heart and lungs. This enables the body's energies to be directed toward combating the infection. The practical nurse is an important figure in helping the patient to obtain rest. She can increase his comfort by simple but effective nursing measures, such as a bath, back rub, and change of position.

### *Fluids and Nutrition*

The diet indicated is one which is easily digested and assimilated. Liquid and soft foods are usually given to the patient with a high fever. The physician may order a diet higher in calories and protein, since the metabolic needs of the body are increased. This need may be compared with that of a furnace. As the furnace gives off more heat, it needs more fuel. When the body uses more energy and gives off more heat, it needs more food. The fluid intake of the patient should be increased to 3000 ml (3 qt) or more during a 24-hour period. Forcing fluids increases production and excretion of urine. Since the kidneys are responsible for ridding the body of many bacterial toxins, an increased fluid intake aids in eliminating the toxins. A greater intake of fluid also aids in counteracting the dehydrating effects of fever.

### Drugs Commonly Used

Drugs frequently used to aid nature in combating infection are the sulfonamides and antibiotics. The idea that penicillin cures most infections is not true. The practical nurse needs an understanding of why the physician selects streptomycin instead of penicillin or oxytetracycline (Terramycin) instead of chlortetracycline (Aureomycin). After determining the cause of the infection, he then selects the antibiotic or the sulfa drug which is known to be most effective against the invading microorganism. Certain pathogens are killed by a specific drug whereas other microorganisms are not affected by that drug. For example, penicillin is more effective against the bacteria causing a "strep throat" than it is against the virus which produces the common cold. The physician has a long list of drugs from which to select the appropriate one for a specific pathogen or group of pathogens.

Analgesic medicines are often prescribed to relieve the patient's pain. Members of the salicylate family, such as aspirin, are widely used as pain relievers. Opiate derivatives and meperidine (Demerol) are used for more severe pain. Morphine, pantopon, codeine, and dihydromorphinone (Dilaudid) are members of the opiate family.

### SUGGESTIONS FOR STUDY

1. How many words can you list from memory which end with "-itis"?
2. What causes inflammation? What inflammations have you had which were caused by these different factors?
3. The microorganism causing malaria belongs to what group? Thrush? Tuberculosis?
4. What is a spore-forming bacterium? Why is it difficult to kill?
5. What important defenses does the body have against invading pathogens?

6. What is pus?

7. Review the local and general symptoms of inflammation.

8. What local measures are used in caring for an inflamed area?

9. Does dry heat burn more quickly than moist heat? What is the reason for your answer?

10. When is it necessary for the practical nurse to use sterile technique in applying hot compresses?

11. What effect does the application of cold have on an inflamed area?

12. Why is bed rest important for the patient with an acute infection?


## REFERENCES FOR CHAPTER 6

Eliason, Eldridge; Ferguson, L. Kraeer; and Sholtis, Lillian A.: *Surgical Nursing*, 10th ed. J. B. Lippincott Co., Philadelphia, 1955, pp. 12-31.

Emerson, Charles P., Jr., and Bragdon, Jane S.: *Essentials of Medicine*, 17th ed. J. B. Lippincott Co., Philadelphia, 1955, pp. 729-55.

Faddis, Margene O., and Hayman, Joseph M.: *Care of the Medical Patient*. McGraw-Hill Book Co., New York, 1952, pp. 33-47.

Goodale, Raymond: *Nursing Pathology*, 2nd ed. W. B. Saunders Co., Philadelphia, 1956, pp. 15-39.

Harmer, Bertha, and Henderson, Virginia: *Textbook of the Principles and Practice of Nursing*, 5th ed. The Macmillan Company, New York, 1955, pp. 940-65.

Jensen, Julius, and Jensen, Deborah: *Nursing in Clinical Medicine*, 4th ed. The Macmillan Company, New York, 1954, pp. 55-74.

Krause, Marie: *Nutrition and Diet Therapy*, 2nd ed. W. B. Saunders Co., Philadelphia, 1957, pp. 180-87.

Muller, Gulli L., and Dawes, Dorothy E.: *Introduction to Medical Science*, 4th ed. W. B. Saunders Co., Philadelphia, 1958, pp. 81-131.

Proudfit, Fairfax T., and Robinson, Corinne H.: *Nutrition and Diet Therapy*, 11th ed. The Macmillan Company, New York, 1955, pp. 369-78.

Stafford, Edward S., and Diller, Doris: *Surgery and Surgical Nursing*, 3rd ed. W. B. Saunders Co., Philadelphia, 1958, pp. 26-39.

*Granulation*

Chapter 7

# THE PATIENT
# WITH CANCER

*Chapter*
*Outline*

TUMOR
PREVALENCE
SOCIETY'S METHOD OF COM-
    BATING THE PROBLEM
PREVENTION

DANGER SIGNALS
DIAGNOSIS
TREATMENT
NURSING CARE

## TUMOR

### Definition

Normally cells of the body grow in an orderly manner and have certain duties to perform. Each day millions of cells in the human body disintegrate and are replaced by new ones which have the same shape and functions. When these new cells assume a new type of growth which makes them incapable of fulfilling their role in the body, they are referred to as a *tumor*. This tumor or abnormal growth of cells which is known as either a neoplasm or a tumor contributes nothing in return for the nourishment it receives from the body. The patient with a tumor has a *neoplastic disease*. The tumor may be either benign or malignant.

### Types

A benign or nonmalignant tumor grows slowly, does not spread, and is usually surrounded by a covering or capsule. Looking at an orange with its peeling or outer covering helps one to visualize the covering of a benign tumor. When a nonmalignant tumor is removed, it is not likely to grow back again. Moles and warts with these characteristics are good examples of benign tumors; however, some moles and warts may later become malignant.

A malignant tumor is referred to as *cancer* or a *malignancy*. It grows rapidly, is not surrounded by a covering, and spreads to other parts of the body. These abnormal cells invade nearby tissue. They

81

are also carried to other parts of the body by the lymph and blood. This transfer of malignant cells to another part of the body is called *metastasis*. The new growth which is started from the transported cells is referred to as a *metastatic growth*. This rapid and uncontrolled growth of body cells eventually threatens the individual's life.

## TUMORS

DIAGRAMS ILLUSTRATING THE DIFFERENCE BETWEEN
A BENIGN AND A MALIGNANT TUMOR

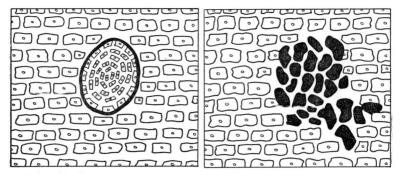

**Figure 14.** (*Left*) Benign tumor: grows slowly; does not spread; usually surrounded by covering or capsule.

**Figure 15.** (*Right*) Malignant tumor: grows rapidly; does spread, not surrounded by covering or capsule.

A malignant tumor is classified according to the type of tissue from which it grows. The two main groups of cancer are carcinoma and sarcoma. A malignancy of epithelial cells, which are located in the skin, mucous membrane, and serous membrane, is called *carcinoma*. *Sarcoma* is the term used in referring to cancer of connective tissue such as bone, cartilage, fat, and tendons. These two main classifications are further subdivided according to the particular kind of tissue involved. Two examples of sarcoma are given for illustration. Osteosarcoma indicates a malignancy of the bone, and liposarcoma indicates a malignancy of fatty tissue.

### Cause

The exact cause of cancer is not known. Research reports show that a malignancy is not inherited. It is believed that an individual may inherit a tendency toward cancer. In other words, the child of parents with cancer is more likely to develop it than the child of parents without cancer. However, this does not mean that the child of parents with cancer necessarily will develop a malignancy. Studies also show that prolonged irritation may lead to cancer. For example, irritation of the lip from prolonged pipe smoking may result in cancer. Another example is cancer of the skin resulting from long exposure to the sun.

## PREVALENCE

Cancer is the second leading cause of death in the United States. Approximately 220,000 persons die each year from a malignancy. It affects persons of all age groups but is more common during and after middle age. The number of cases of cancer is increasing. Two main factors contributing to this fact are that people are living longer and are more likely to develop cancer and better methods of diagnosis have increased the number of cases discovered.

Research has shown that individuals in certain age groups are likely to develop cancer of specific organs, and malignancy of certain organs is more common in one sex than in the other. For example, cancer of the lung occurs more often in men than in women. Also, men between the ages of 40 and 50 are more likely to develop lung cancer than men between the ages of 30 and 40. The most common sites of malignancy in women are the breast, uterus, and skin; whereas the most common sites in men are the skin, stomach, lung, and prostate gland. Children are more likely to have cancer of the bone, blood, kidney, and eye. Cancer leads other diseases as the cause of death in children between 4 and 15 years of age.

It is estimated that cancer will affect one out of four Americans. Although this one statement might be depressing, the picture is not so gloomy as one might think. Another estimate brightens this dark picture; one-half of these individuals who develop a malignancy could be cured if the diagnosis were made early and proper treatment started promptly. Approximately one-third of the patients now dying of cancer could have been cured if correct treatment had been started early.

## SOCIETY'S METHOD OF COMBATING THE PROBLEM

*Early* is the keyword for improving the prognosis, which is the possible outcome of the patient with cancer. Early recognition of the symptoms, an early diagnosis by the doctor, and early treatment are of vital importance in curing the patient.

Programs are being developed in numerous health departments for early diagnosis and prompt treatment of patients with cancer. Agencies have been established throughout the United States to aid in combating the problem. The American Cancer Society is one example of these agencies. Realizing that early recognition is the first step which must be taken by the patient, this organization has as one of its aims education of the public regarding the early symptoms as well as the importance of a prompt visit to the doctor. It also helps by emphasizing to members of the medical profession the importance of looking for early signs of cancer, by establishing facilities for early diagnosis and proper treatment, and by doing research in an effort to discover the cause of cancer.

As a member of the health team, the practical nurse also has an important part to play in the problem of combating cancer. She is in an important position to aid in detecting cancer symptoms in her patients as she spends most of her time with them. She should report an early sign of malignancy to the person to whom she is directly responsible, such as the team leader, head nurse, or physician. For example, a practical nurse heard her middle-aged male patient complain of mild indigestion. She asked how long he had been bothered with it. He told her that he had been bothered with it for several weeks before being admitted to the hospital for a broken leg. Knowing that persistent indigestion especially in middle-aged men might be an early symptom of cancer, she promptly reported this to the head nurse. The doctor in turn was notified, and a curable cancer was found.

The practical nurse's friends and relatives often discuss their ailments with her. If they have a symptom which might indicate cancer, she should advise them to consult their doctor. She also needs to know the facilities available in the community for both diagnosis and treatment.

## PREVENTION

Because the specific cause or causes of a malignancy are not known, it is difficult to prevent an individual from developing cancer. The few factors which predispose to the development of cancer can be avoided. The two main examples are constant irritation of any one body area and prolonged exposure to the sun. Although little can be done at present to prevent the development of cancer, much can be done if it is detected early.

Members of the health team, as well as the general public, should know the danger signals of a malignancy. To be aware of these symptoms is not enough. The person may know that he has a symptom of cancer but may be afraid to consult his doctor because of the idea that there is no hope for anyone with this condition. The information that many malignancies can be cured when an early diagnosis is followed by prompt treatment should help to combat this fear.

Reducing the large number of deaths resulting from cancer is based upon the keyword *early*, as mentioned previously. Early recognition of symptoms, early diagnosis, and early treatment are the three vital steps. Since the symptoms are often vague at first, an annual, thorough physical examination is recommended. Men over 45 years of age should have a chest x-ray every six months. Women over 35 years of age should have a pelvic examination every six months.

## DANGER SIGNALS

It is important for the practical nurse to know the early danger signals commonly associated with cancer. Although these symptoms do not necessarily indicate cancer, the presence of one or more of them should cause an individual to consult his physician. The early symptoms are: (1) any sore which does not heal, especially around the mouth; (2) any lump or thickening, particularly in the breast; (3) irregular bleeding or discharge from a natural body opening; (4) any progressive change in a wart or a mole, especially in regards to the color or size; (5) indigestion or difficulty in swallowing which persists; (6) persistent hoarseness and cough; and (7) unusual change in bowel habits.

Since cancer may affect any part of the body, the symptoms vary with the area affected. Generally, after the patient has noticed one of the above-mentioned warning signals, he experiences weakness, anorexia, and loss of weight. This is true especially with a malignancy of the digestive system. Anemia, a decrease of the red blood cells or the hemoglobin, is another common symptom. Fever occurs in advanced cases as a result of complicating infections. Pain is usually a late sign.

## DIAGNOSIS

The physician makes a tentative diagnosis of cancer by taking a history of the patient's complaints and doing a thorough physical examination. Various laboratory procedures, as well as x-ray studies, may be a part of the doctor's examination. For example, if a patient complains of persistent indigestion, the doctor may have a gastric analysis (laboratory procedure) done. A lack of hydrochloric acid in the patient's stomach secretions may indicate cancer. An x-ray examination of the upper gastrointestinal tract may show a growth which resembles cancer. A positive diagnosis is made only when the cells from this growth are identified as malignant ones under the microscope.

Microscopic examination of cells contained in the body's secretions to determine the presence of malignant cells is called the cytologic test for cancer. This type of test is also known as the Papanicolaou smear. Secretions from the uterus, bladder, kidney, bronchi, lungs, and stomach can be examined for malignancy. The cytologic test for cancer is especially beneficial in detecting unsuspected cases of cancer of the uterus. During a pelvic examination, the doctor removes a small portion of the cervical discharge and places it on a glass slide. This small amount of uterine secretion is then examined under the microscope by the pathologist. When abnormal cells are found, it indicates that cancer may be present somewhere in the reproductive system. The doctor would then do a biopsy, which is the removal of a small portion of tissue for microscopic examination. Thus, a sample of the tumor must be obtained and examined under the microscope by the pathologist before a positive diagnosis of malignancy can be made. The physician may remove the tissue to be examined by surgical excision or by aspiration. In an aspiration, he removes a small amount of tissue by means of a large needle and syringe with suction.

## TREATMENT

The patient with cancer may be treated with either surgery or radiation therapy. The use of energy which is given off in the form of rays is known as *radiation therapy* or *radiotherapy*. Since these rays have the ability to penetrate and to destroy tissue, they can be used to destroy malignant growth. X-ray, radium, and other radioactive substances are used in radiotherapy. Surgery and radiotherapy may be used together or singly in treating the patient with a malignancy. These are the only approved methods of curing cancer. This disease cannot be cured by injection, oral medicine, or ointment as falsely advertised. Male and female hormones and chemical substances, such as nitrogen mustard, are used mainly to make the patient more comfortable. These measures also aid in slowing down the progress of a malignancy in some cases. The treatment is selected by the physician on the basis of such factors as the type of malignancy, its location, and its extent.

### Surgery

When a malignancy is diagnosed early, has not metastasized, and is in an operable region, the chances of cure by surgery are good. The surgeon removes the tumor as well as much of the surrounding tissue, especially the lymph glands. This is necessary because cancer cells may have invaded the neighboring tissue. If a malignancy has already metastasized, surgery is sometimes done in an effort to make the patient more comfortable.

### Radiotherapy

X-ray and radium are the two main ways of treating a malignancy by radiotherapy. The x-ray machine produces rays referred to as x-rays. *Radium* is a metallic element which gives off rays; thus, it is radioactive. The rays of radium and x-ray kill cells, especially malignant ones. A cancer may be completely destroyed or its growth slowed down without much damage to surrounding tissue. Radiotherapy is often used in inoperable cancer as well as in connection with a surgical procedure.

Since x-rays penetrate deeper into body tissues than radium, it is often used for deep therapy when internal organs are affected. X-ray can be used in treating larger areas than radium. Thus, a widespread malignancy of the skin would more than likely be treated with x-ray.

Either radium or radon is often used in treating surface and easily accessible cancer of such sites as the cervix, larynx, esophagus, and lips. *Radon* is the gas given off by radium which is collected and sealed in tiny glass or gold tubes. These tubes, which are called *seeds* or *implants*, are often buried in the tissue. Since radium rays injure normal tissue, it should never be handled with the bare hands. Long forceps and special lead containers are provided for the handling and care of radium.

Other substances are now being used in radiotherapy. For example, radioactive cobalt and radioactive iodine may be used. These substances have the ability to absorb and to give off radioactive rays after having been placed in an atomic furnace. Rays from radioactive cobalt can penetrate deeply into the tissue. For this reason, it may be used when deep radiation therapy is needed. Radioactive iodine is helpful in treating some types of malignant tumors of the thyroid gland. Remembering that iodine is concentrated in the thyroid gland, the practical nurse can readily understand that radioactive iodine will be concentrated there also.

## NURSING CARE

As stated previously, the physician selects the method of treatment which offers the best chances of recovery for the patient. Nursing care is planned within this framework.

### Surgical Patient

The practical nurse plays an important part in the preoperative and postoperative care of the patient with cancer. She is often the one who has the longest period of contact with the patient. Fear of the pending operation may be noticed while she is doing such nursing procedures for him as bathing him or making the bed. Of course, fear of surgery should be reported to the team leader or the head nurse as excessive anxiety may hinder the success of surgery since a very apprehensive patient is more difficult to anesthetize than a reasonably relaxed person.

As surgery for the treatment of cancer is usually extensive, patients are frequently admitted to the hospital several days in advance for mental and physical preparation. This period helps the patient to start becoming adjusted to the loss of a part of his body. For example, if the patient is to have a colostomy, formation of an artificial anus in the abdominal wall, this extra time gives him an opportunity to become oriented to a marked change in his body. Also, it gives the patient an opportunity to develop confidence in members of the nursing team. In addition to the general principles of nursing the surgical patient which were discussed in Chapter 5, the practical nurse should realize that the patient with a malignancy often needs to have his general state of health improved before the operation. A special diet to supply deficiencies such as protein and vitamins is often prescribed; vitamins may also be given either by mouth or by injection.

## Patient Receiving Radiotherapy *inserted in seeds*

Patients often have a fear of x-ray therapy and radium therapy. Knowing that the rays cause no pain and that the patient feels no heat from them, the practical nurse can answer his questions more intelligently and help to allay his fear.

The patient may have a reaction to radiotherapy called *radiation sickness.* Symptoms such as nausea, vomiting, anorexia, malaise, diarrhea, chills, and fever are often associated with radiation sickness. Nursing care is aimed toward relieving these discomforts. The dosage of radiation may be reduced if these symptoms are marked.

In x-ray therapy, the skin over the treated area is often marked with indelible ink as a guide for the therapist. These are referred to as *portal of entry marks* and should not be removed when bathing the patient. While the patient is receiving x-ray treatment, the skin covering the treated area should be kept dry and free from further irritation, such as the rubbing of bedclothes. X-ray therapy may cause the skin to turn pinkish and to have the appearance of a sunburned area. Powders and oinments which contain metals should not be

*Prevent irritation    No ointment with metal*

*Keep dry    Not remove portals of entry marks*

used on the site as these increase the dose of x-ray to the skin. For example, zinc oxide is a metallic substance frequently used in many powders and oinments. However, the practical nurse may be asked to dust the area with powder containing metallic substances, such as zinc oxide, *after* the radiotherapy has been completed. Since the skin covering the area being treated with x-ray should be kept as dry as possible, it is not to be cleaned with soap and water.

The practical nurse caring for a patient who has radium inserted needs to remember that it is an expensive element. The cost of radium ranges from $20,000 to $23,000 a gram. Knowing the expense of radium will help her to remember that dressings should be inspected for this element before being discarded. The physician calculates the length of time the radium should remain in contact with the area being treated. He accepts the responsibility for removing it.

### Mental Aspects

The nurse's personal attitude toward cancer is reflected in the type of nursing care she gives to these patients. If she has a fatalistic viewpoint, she is less able to give understanding care to the patient and his family when it is needed. The nurse who realizes the possibilities of cure or relief is better equipped to care for the patient who has a cancer.

As the practical nurse is often the one spending long periods of time with the patient, she is the one he often turns to for kindness. The ability to put oneself in the patient's place and to imagine how he feels is an important basis for kindliness and understanding in the care of any patient.

Disfigurement may result from the treatment of a malignancy as well as from the tumor itself. The patient may react to this in a number of ways. For example, he may be depressed, irritable, or resentful. The nurse who understands that these reactions are the patient's response to his disfigurement is more capable of being tolerant, especially of the patient who shows resentment toward doctors and nurses. The nurse should do all within her power to make the disfigurement less unsightly. For example, a malignancy of the face can be covered with a dressing when permitted by the doctor. Arranging the lighting in the room so that a shadow falls on the area is also helpful. A small tumor near the hairline can often-times be covered with a change of hair styling. Many advances have been made in plastic surgery for the permanent removal and correction of disfigurements.

Some physicians tell selected patients of their true diagnosis. This is an individual matter between the doctor and his patient. The nurse should assume that the patient does not know his diagnosis unless the doctor makes it known that he has told the patient. A fear of dying may be present in patients who know their diagnosis as well as those who do not. The nurse should be capable of listening to the patient when she sees that he wants to discuss his worries.

### Diet and Fluids

As stated previously, the general nutritive state of the patient with cancer is often affected. The doctor prescribes a diet to meet the needs of each particular patient's body. For example, one patient may need a high-protein diet and another one may need a diet high in vitamins. The patient with a malignancy of the gastrointestinal tract often cannot digest solid food and may be given small liquid feedings. The patient's choice should always be considered as far as possible.

An adequate intake of fluids is essential. When the patient is unable to take a sufficient amount of liquid by mouth, the practical nurse is called upon frequently to assist in giving fluids intravenously (in the veins) or subcutaneously (under the skin).

### Comfort Measures

The patient with cancer needs expert skin care as his tissues do not repair themselves so quickly as they did when he was well. Measures to avoid decubitus ulcers prevent much discomfort. He needs a daily cleansing bath with special attention paid to the affected area. This site may need to be cleaned in a prescribed manner. Dressings may also need to be changed frequently.

In addition to the nursing measures to relieve pain and discomfort which were discussed on page 41, the doctor prescribes analgesic drugs necessary for the patient. Meperidine (Demerol), morphine, and dihydromorphinone (Dilaudid) are examples of drugs used to relieve pain.

## The Patient with Terminal Cancer

As the present-day treatment of cancer does not always result in a cure, the practical nurse frequently is responsible for nursing the patient in his terminal illness. In addition to the nursing care already discussed in this chapter, the patient with terminal cancer needs additional care depending upon the stage of his illness. He is kept ambulatory, not confined to bed, as long as possible with suitable diversions. The patient's comfort is the primary objective of all persons caring for him during his last days. Often the measures to relieve his discomfort seem to prolong his life for a short while. For example, the administration of fluids intravenously to prevent or to relieve discomfort from dehydration may appear to lengthen life.

The bedridden patient should be in a clean, pleasant, bright, and cheerful room which is free of unpleasant odors. Slough or death of the tissues causes an undesirable odor. The nurse should make every effort possible to remove the odor. Keeping the patient and his room clean, maintaining good ventilation, changing dressings frequently, and removing used dressings immediately from the room help to reduce the odor. Deodorants are used in some hospitals. Commercial products which absorb odors are available for use in electric dispensers and in bottles containing wicks.

As life ebbs, the inner resources of the nurse are tapped for comfort, understanding, and support needed by the patient and his family. If the nurse imagines how she would like to have the person dearest to her cared for if he were in the condition of the patient, she can develop an excellent guide for the nursing care needed.

*TEST FRIDAY*

## SUGGESTIONS FOR STUDY

1. What is a tumor?
2. In what three ways does a benign tumor differ from a malignant one?
3. Why is the number of cases of cancer increasing?

4. Does your community have a local cancer society? If so, what are its functions?

5. Discuss the responsibilities of the practical nurse in combating cancer.

6. What are the danger signals of cancer?

7. How does the doctor make a definite diagnosis of cancer?

8. What are the approved methods of treating a malignancy?

9. Review the nursing care of a patient receiving radiotherapy.

10. Discuss the mental aspects of nursing the patient with a malignancy.

## REFERENCES FOR CHAPTER 7

American Cancer Society, Inc.: *X-Ray, Radium, Surgery: The Three Approved Methods of Cancer Treatment.* The Society, New York, 1952.

————: *A Cancer Source Book for Nurses.* The Society, New York, 1956.

Eliason, Eldridge; Ferguson, L. Kraeer; and Sholtis, Lillian A.: *Surgical Nursing,* 10th ed. J. B. Lippincott Co., Philadelphia, 1955, pp. 195-204.

Esau, Margaret; Fallon, Barbara R.; Frentzos, Kathryn G.; Phillips, Elisabeth C.; and Tourtillott, Eleanor A.: *Practical Nursing Today, Attitudes–Knowledge–Skills.* G. P. Putnam's Sons, New York, 1957, pp. 315-35.

*Facing the Facts about Cancer.* Public Affairs Committee, Inc., Pamphlet No. 38, New York, 1953.

Goodale, Raymond: *Nursing Pathology,* 2nd ed. W. B. Saunders Co., Philadelphia, 1956, pp. 81-101.

Kelly, Dorothy N.: "Practical Nurse Students and the Cancer Patient," *Am. J. Nursing,* **55**:454-56, (Apr.) 1955.

Knapp, Margaret F.: *Cancer Nursing: A Manual for Public Health Nurses.* National Cancer Institute, Public Health Service, Department of Health, Education, and Welfare, Washington, D. C., and the New York State Department of Health, Albany, 1955.

————: "Cancer—A Review," *Am. J. Nursing,* **56**:440-43, (Apr.) 1956.

Richmond, Clara E.: "The Practical Nurse and the Cancer Patient," *Practical Nurses Digest,* **2**:20-22, (Sept.) 1955.

West, John P.; Keller, Manelva W.; and Harmon, Elizabeth H.: *Nursing Care of the Surgical Patient,* 6th ed. The Macmillan Company, New York, 1957, pp. 45-56.

*What Are the Facts about Cancer? What Are We Doing about Cancer?* National Health Education Committee, Inc., New York, 1956.

*11/16/65*

## Chapter 8      *THE PATIENT WITH AN ALLERGY*

## DESCRIPTION

The patient with an allergy is hypersensitive or overly sensitive to a substance which usually does not affect most individuals. The substance to which this person is overly sensitive is known as an *allergen*. The body generally responds to this irritant by a dilation of the small blood vessels in the involved area. This results in redness, which can be observed when the area involved is on the surface. Fluid seeps through the capillaries causing edema (swelling). In some cases hemorrhage may occur.

## CAUSE

An allergic reaction may be caused by digestion, by inhalation, or by injection of the irritating substance, or by contact with it. For example, foods frequently causing an allergy include milk, wheat, eggs, fish, strawberries, tomatoes, and chocolate. Aspirin is an example of a drug taken by mouth which may cause an allergic reaction. Inhalation of ragweed pollen, dust, and other substances can result in a reaction. The injection of morphine, penicillin, tetanus antitoxin, and other medications can cause an allergic reaction in some individuals. It can be caused by contact with an irritating substance, such as poison ivy. An individual may also develop an allergy from a chronic infection such as bronchitis and sinusitis. It is believed that proteins are the main offenders.

94

Allergic reactions may occur during specific seasons of the year in which case it is *seasonal*. However, there may be no relationship between the allergy and the season. Although an individual does not inherit an allergy, he may inherit a tendency toward developing it. A person who has no past history of allergy in his family may develop this condition. In this case the disease is said to be *acquired.* An allergic person may have a reaction only when he is emotionally upset or is extremely tired.

## TYPES

The patient with an allergy may have one or more conditions as a result of his allergy. He may develop bronchial asthma, hay fever, urticaria, dermatitis, angioneurotic edema, and anaphylactic shock. He may also have gastrointestinal symptoms, such as indigestion, nausea, vomiting, and diarrhea, as a result of an allergy.

Various parts of an allergic patient's body usually have different degrees of hypersensitiveness. This can result in the patient's having a variety of symptoms. For example, the allergic individual may have digestive disturbances, hay fever, and a skin rash after eating a food to which he is allergic. Individuals may also respond differently to the same substance; one person may respond to strawberries by having hay fever, and another one by having asthma.

## TREATMENT AND NURSING CARE

Members of the nursing team are responsible for helping the physician in his diagnosis. Because of this, the practical nurse needs an understanding of methods commonly used. The physician bases his diagnosis on a careful history of the patient, a thorough physical examination, and special tests for allergy. The patient's health history and that of his family are of extreme importance to the doctor. Remembering that an allergy is more likely to develop in the person with a family history of it helps the practical nurse in understanding why the doctor takes such a detailed history. Also, the history may give the physician a clue regarding the allergen. In addition to doing a complete physical examination, the doctor pays particular attention to the areas involved.

Tests to determine specific allergens which may be performed are *skin tests*, an *ophthalmic test*, and an *elimination diet test*. Although specific procedures vary in different clinics and hospitals, the practical nurse needs a basic understanding of them.

*Skin tests* are used frequently to determine specific causes of allergy. The physician makes scratches on either the patient's back or arm and drops a solution containing a specific allergen into each of them. This is known as the *scratch test*. Solutions containing known allergens may be injected intradermally (between the skin layers) also. This is known as the *intradermal test*. The person has a positive reaction when the area around a particular scratch or site of injection becomes swollen. Knowing the allergens which were used and the site of application, the physician can determine the patient's reaction to the various substances. Unfortunately skin tests are not always successful in helping the doctor determine which substances cause the patient to have a reaction. The patient may have a negative reaction to certain substances when tested and give a history which definitely indicates that he is sensitive to them. Or he may have a positive reaction to an allergen when tested and develop no symptoms when he actually comes in contact with it.

In the *ophthalmic test*, an allergen is dropped into the conjunctival sac, which is the mucous membrane lining the eyelids and covering the front part of the eyeball. The membrane becomes reddened and swollen when the patient is allergic to that particular substance.

In an *elimination diet test* the patient is given foods which usually do not cause an allergy. This is used frequently when a food allergy is suspected. The physician indicates the specific foods which are to be added gradually to the patient's diet. The practical nurse should remember that the patient is to be served only the foods allowed by the doctor. The patient is observed for symptoms of an allergic reaction, such as itching, swollen areas, sneezing, and difficult breathing, after a new food has been added to his diet. If he has an allergic reaction after eating a new food, he may be allergic to that one. Sometimes a particular food may cause the patient to have a reaction one day and may cause no reaction on another day.

When the practical nurse is responsible for assisting in the care of a patient undergoing diagnostic tests, she should learn the procedures of that particular institution or clinic. She should observe and report symptoms of an allergic reaction as mentioned previously. For example, she may notice that the patient began sneezing after the maid had cleaned the room. Although this symptom may or may not have any relation to the cleaning of his room, it should be reported. Similar observations made by the nurse help the doctor in establishing the diagnosis.

After determining the substances which cause the patient to have an allergic reaction, the physician attempts to eliminate them from the patient's environment. Members of the nursing team are asked to assist in achieving this goal. For example, if feathers are the offender, pillows and other sources of feathers are removed from the room. The patient who is allergic to flowers cannot have these in his room. Air conditioning may be helpful to the person who is sensitive to pollen and dust. In some cases, the doctor may advise the patient to move to another climate in order to avoid contact with certain allergens. Foods to which the patient is allergic are eliminated from his diet. The practical nurse may be asked to use a special soap when bathing the patient. This is necessary when the soap contains substances to which he is allergic.

Another method of treatment which the doctor may use is *desensitization,* or *hyposensitization.* He tries to reduce the patient's sensitivity by giving him injections of extracts made from the allergens. This is done to help the patient build up a tolerance to that substance. The length of time required by the patient to build up a tolerance to an allergen varies. It may take one person weeks to develop a tolerance and another person months or years. Some patients never build up a tolerance.

Hormones and antihistamines are drugs which may be prescribed for symptomatic relief. Two hormones, ACTH (adrenocorticotropic hormone) and cortisone, may be used in severe allergic reactions to relieve the symptoms. Three examples of antihistamines are diphenhydramine (Benadryl), tripelennamine (Pyribenzamine), and antazoline (Antistine). The patient with an allergy frequently has an increased amount of histamine in the tissues which are reacting to the irritant. This results in localized swelling. For example, swelling of the mucous membrane of the nose is known as hay fever and of the skin as hives. Antihistamines are prescribed to counteract the effect of histamine in the tissues. In many cases the symptoms of patients with hives, dermatitis, and hay fever have been relieved with antihistamines. These have not been so effective in relieving asthmatic sufferers.

Drugs which act as vasoconstrictors may be ordered for the patient having an acute allergic reaction. The action of these drugs is to constrict the blood vessels which are dilated. This offers symptomatic relief from the swelling and redness. Epinephrine (Adrenalin) and ephedrine are two examples of these drugs, which offer relief to the asthmatic patient because they dilate the bronchi in addition to their action as vasoconstrictors.

The patient having an acute allergic reaction needs to be in quiet surroundings. Undue excitement may aggravate the condition. Frequently visitors are either restricted or limited during this period.

## ASTHMA

### Description

An individual with asthma has attacks of dyspnea, which is difficult breathing. Two main types of asthma are cardiac and bronchial. Cardiac asthma occurs when failure of the left ventricle results in congestion of the lungs (p. 110). Bronchial asthma, which is a severe form of allergy, is herein discussed.

The mucous membrane lining the bronchioles of a patient with asthma is hypersensitive. This membrane within the bronchioles becomes swollen when an allergen reaches it. The muscles around the bronchioles become spasmodic. The swollen mucous membrane and the muscle spasms cause the tiny air passages to become even smaller. Thus the patient has wheezing and difficult breathing.

### Symptoms

As stated above, the patient having an attack of asthma has difficult breathing. In addition to this, he has a feeling of tightness in his chest. He seems to have more trouble in expiration (breathing out) than in inspiration (breathing in). The wheezing sounds associated with his breathing can be heard across the room. Wheezing is caused by air going through thick fluid which is collecting in the constricted bronchioles. His sputum is clear and gluey. After the attack has ended, the patient feels well until the next attack.

## Treatment

The patient having an attack of asthma should be placed in a quiet room. Drugs such as epinephrine (Adrenalin), ephedrine, and aminophylline may be prescribed. Cortisone and ACTH (adrenocorticotropic hormone) are used in some severe cases. Oxygen therapy may be used also.

The physician directs his treatment toward preventing or reducing the frequency of further attacks. Measures used to determine the allergen and to treat the patient with an allergy, discussed earlier in this chapter, apply to this patient.

Unfortunately the irritant cannot always be determined. In this case the aim of treatment is to reduce the frequency of attacks and to alleviate them when they occur. A room with filtered air is beneficial to many of these patients. The doctor may recommend that the mattress and pillows be made of sponge rubber or be covered with plastic cases. Factors in the patient's environment which cause anxiety should be either alleviated or removed. Psychotherapy is used in some cases.

## HAY FEVER

The patient with hay fever has an allergic reaction of the mucous membrane lining his nose, sinuses, and eyelids. The membrane becomes swollen. The patient complains of itching, sneezing, and a watery discharge from his nose and eyes. Frequently hay fever is associated with the season of the year.

## URTICARIA

The patient with urticaria has *hives* or *nettle rash.* At first he usually complains that his skin itches. This is followed by the appearance of *wheals,* which are swollen areas. The wheals may tingle, burn, or itch. These vary in size and may come and go quickly.

## DERMATITIS

A person with dermatitis has an inflammation of his skin. Although there are many causes of dermatitis, this discussion deals with the condition resulting from an allergic reaction. The allergen may have come in direct contact with the skin or it may have entered the body by either the respiratory or the digestive tract. The patient's skin becomes red and frequently itches.

## ANGIONEUROTIC EDEMA

An individual with angioneurotic edema has localized, swollen areas of either his skin or his mucous membrane. Although these swollen areas may resemble those of urticaria, they are larger and deeper. Angioneurotic edema may sometimes be caused by a food **allergy.** The swelling frequently occurs about the face, hands, and feet. The tongue and larynx (voice box) may be affected also. The area itches or burns and soon begins to swell. Most frequently the edema (swelling) lasts for a day or two and then disappears.

## ANAPHYLACTIC SHOCK

A person may go into anaphylactic shock following the injection of a substance to which he is sensitive. For example, the administration of certain drugs such as tetanus antitoxin, local anesthetics, and penicillin to an individual who is allergic to them may result in this condition. Certain drugs are known to produce a high degree of sensitivity in man. It is for this reason that a patient may be given a small amount of a drug which is known as a *test dose* before the full dosage is administered. If the practical nurse is told by a patient that he is allergic to a certain drug, she should report it to her team leader or head nurse.

The patient in anaphylactic shock needs immediate help. Sudden death may occur. In addition to having symptoms of shock, the patient may lose consciousness and have difficult breathing. Injections of epinephrine and antihistamines are used frequently in this emergency.

## SUGGESTIONS FOR STUDY

1. Describe the body's reaction to an allergen.
2. What are some of the foods which frequently cause an allergic reaction?

3. How may the doctor determine substances to which a patient is hypersensitive?

4. What conditions have you seen which were caused by an allergy?

5. Describe the breathing of a patient having an attack of asthma.

6. What happens to the bronchioles of an individual having an attack of asthma?

7. Which allergic reaction is most likely to result in sudden death?

8. Why is it important for the practical nurse to report information about a drug to which a patient is allergic?

9. Discuss the nursing care of a patient having an allergic reaction.

REFERENCES FOR CHAPTER 8

Berger, Arthur J.: "Sensitivity Reactions," *Am. J. Nursing,* **55**:948-49 (Aug.) 1955.

Emerson, Charles P., Jr., and Bragdon, Jane S.: *Essentials of Medicine,* 17th ed. J. B. Lippincott Co., Philadelphia, 1955, pp. 507-20.

Faddis, Margene O., and Hayman, Joseph M.: *Care of the Medical Patient.* McGraw-Hill Book Co., New York, 1952, pp. 514-25.

Hull, Edgar, and Perrodin, Cecilia: *Medical Nursing,* 5th ed. F. A. Davis Co., Philadelphia, 1954, pp. 597-611.

Jensen, Julius, and Jensen, Deborah: *Nursing in Clinical Medicine,* 4th ed. The Macmillan Company, New York, 1954, pp. 179-96.

Krause, Marie: *Nutrition and Diet Therapy,* 2nd ed. W. B. Saunders Co. Philadelphia, 1957, pp. 239-46.

Peshkin, M. Murray: "Some Facts about Allergies," *Practical Nurses Digest,* **3**:14, (Jan.) 1956.

Proudfit, Fairfax T., and Robinson, Corinne H.: *Nutrition and Diet Therapy,* 11th ed. The Macmillan Company, New York, 1955, pp. 506-15.

Unger, Albert H., and Unger, Leon: "Modern Treatment of Bronchial Asthma," *Am. J. Nursing,* **54**:1367-72, (Nov.) 1954.

Test  2-22  -  <u>82</u>

3- 7        76

4. 7        56

5. 9        94

5. 25

Average on May 27

<u>83</u>

# Nursing the Patient
# with a Disease of
# the Circulatory System

## PART III

Med. Surg. II

1-25-66 - 6-8-66

✓Thursday 2-10-66 conference on patient
Cardiac if possible
CUA

Care Study - PAR

75 hours

$$\begin{array}{r} 25\overset{4}{\phantom{2}}1 \\ 105 \\ \hline 146 \end{array}$$

Chapter 9

# THE PATIENT
# WITH A DISEASE OF
# THE HEART

## STRUCTURE AND FUNCTION

A basic understanding of the structure and function of the circulatory system is necessary for the practical nurse if she is to give
intelligent nursing care to the cardiac patient. The heart and circulation of the blood are discussed in this chapter as a review for the
student before she begins her study of heart disease.

In order to live, all tissues of the body must receive oxygen and
food materials. They must also have waste products removed. These
essential functions are carried out by the circulatory system. The
pumping action of the heart causes the blood to circulate continuously
through a closed set of tubes known as blood vessels. This continuous flow of blood picks up oxygen from the lungs, food material
from the digestive system, and important secretions produced in
certain parts of the body. These substances are then carried to other
tissues of the body by the flow of blood. Waste products are removed
from the cells and carried to the lungs, kidneys, intestine, and skin
to be excreted. The flow of blood has additional functions to perform, such as helping protect the body from harmful microorganisms
and to regulate the body's heat.

*105*

### Heart

The heart is the organ which has the vital function of pumping the blood by its rhythmical contractions. This organ is located within the thoracic cavity between the two lungs. The heart is approximately the size of one's closed fist. Knowing that the heart accomplishes its function by contracting rhythmically, the practical nurse can readily understand why it is composed mainly of muscle tissue. This muscle tissue is known as *myocardium*. A membrane called *endocardium* lines the inside of the heart. The membranous sac surrounding the heart is the *pericardium*. Blood vessels supplying the heart with oxygen and food are called *coronary arteries*.

The heart is a hollow organ which is divided into a right and left side. These two sides normally have no direct passageway to each other following birth. Each side is further divided into two cavities. The upper chambers are called atria (auricles), and the lower chambers, ventricles. The atria receive blood, and the ventricles force blood from the heart. Openings between the atria and ventricles, and between the ventricles and arteries, are protected by valves. These valves open to permit passage of blood from the atria to the ventricles and from the ventricles to the arteries. They close to prevent the blood from returning.

The *tricuspid valve* is located between the right atrium and right ventricle. The *bicuspid*, or *mitral*, *valve* is situated between the left atrium and left ventricle. The opening between the right ventricle and the pulmonary artery, which carries blood away from that chamber of the heart, is protected by the *pulmonary valve*. The opening between the left ventricle and the *aorta*, the large artery leading from that chamber of the heart, is guarded by the *aortic valve*.

Blood is returned to the heart by blood vessels known as *veins*. The *superior* and *inferior venae cavae* are large veins which empty into the right atrium. The left atrium receives blood from four veins known as *pulmonary veins*. The two ventricles force blood outward through blood vessels called *arteries*. The pulmonary artery leads from the right ventricle to the lungs, and the aorta leads from the left ventricle. Thus, blood is carried away from the heart by the arteries and returned by the veins. Many veins have valves to keep the blood flowing toward the heart.

Both the left and the right atria contract at approximately the same time forcing blood into the ventricles. Then both ventricles contract pumping blood into the arteries. The right ventricle forces blood to

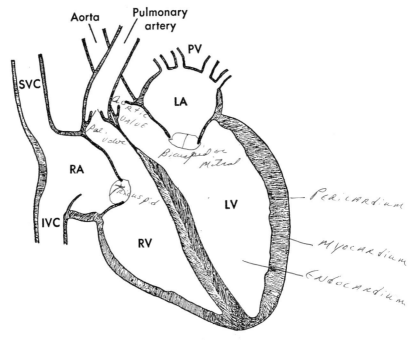

**Figure 16.** A diagram to show the four chambers of the heart, seen from the front. Blood containing a fresh supply of oxygen is brought from the lungs by the pulmonary veins (PV) to the left atrium (LA). Blood is forced through the bicuspid valve into the left ventricle (LV). Contraction of the left ventricle forces blood through the aortic valve into the aorta. From there, it flows into smaller blood vessels. Blood is returned by way of the superior vena cava (SVC) and the inferior vena cava (IVC) to the right atrium (RA) of the heart. After being forced through the tricuspid valve into the right ventricle (RV), blood is then pumped through the pulmonary artery to the lungs. (Kimber, Diana C.; Gray, Carolyn E.; Stackpole, Caroline E.; and Leavell, Lutie C.: *Textbook of Anatomy and Physiology*, 13th ed. The Macmillan Company, New York, 1955.)

the lungs and the left ventricle pumps blood through the aorta into arteries leading to all parts of the body. The practical nurse feels the wave of blood as it is forced through the artery when she takes the pulse of a patient. The *pulse* is a change in the shape of an artery caused by contraction of the left ventricle which forces blood through the aorta into smaller arteries. The practical nurse may be surprised to know that before she feels the pulse again, the heart will have dilated, rested, and then contracted. These three phases make up the *cardiac cycle.* In other words, the term cardiac cycle is used to refer to a complete heartbeat. The period during which the heart contracts is called *systole* and the period during which it dilates is known as *diastole.* The third phase of the cardiac cycle is known simply as the *rest period.*

## Circulation

Blood which contains a fresh supply of oxygen is brought from the lungs by the pulmonary veins to the left atrium. After passing through the bicuspid valve, blood is pumped from the left ventricle over the aortic valve into the aorta and then into smaller arteries. These divide into smaller blood vessels called *arterioles* which connect with even smaller vessels known as *capillaries.* Through the thin walls of tiny capillaries, oxygen and food are exchanged for carbon dioxide and other waste products. The blood which has picked up waste products and given up some of its oxygen flows from the capillaries into small blood vessels called *venules.* These lead to veins. Blood is returned to the right atrium by large veins known as the *superior* and *inferior venae cavae.* It flows over the tricuspid valve into the right ventricle. Contraction of the right ventricle forces blood through the pulmonary valve into the pulmonary artery and then into the lungs. Here the blood gives up carbon dioxide and receives oxygen. It is then returned to the left atrium through the pulmonary veins.

Since the practical nurse may hear other members of the health team refer to pulmonary circulation, she needs to know its meaning. *Pulmonary circulation* refers to the flow of blood from the right side of the heart, through the lungs, to the left side of the heart. *Systemic circulation* refers to the flow of blood from the left ventricle, through arteries, arterioles, venules, veins, and back to the heart again. When

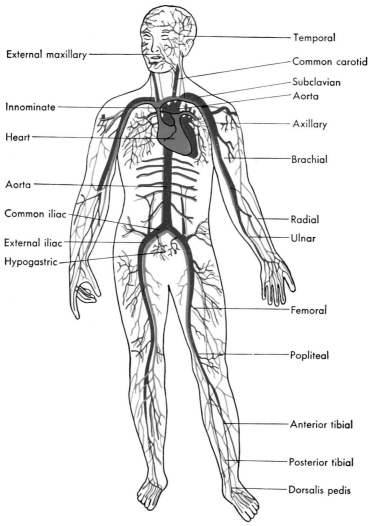

External maxillary

Innominate

Heart

Aorta

Common iliac

External iliac

Hypogastric

Temporal

Common carotid

Subclavian

Aorta

Axillary

Brachial

Radial

Ulnar

Femoral

Popliteal

Anterior tibial

Posterior tibial

Dorsalis pedis

**Figure 17.** A general diagram of the circulation. Many arteries are named. (Kimber, Diana C.; Gray, Carolyn E.; Stackpole, Caroline E.; and Leavell, Lutie C.: *Textbook of Anatomy and Physiology*, 13th ed. The Macmillan Company, New York, 1955.)

blood flows through the various systems of the body, it also goes to the kidneys. These organs act as filters and remove waste products. Blood picks up food substances as it flows through the digestive organs.

## WHAT IT MEANS TO THE PERSON TO HAVE "HEART TROUBLE"

The practical nurse needs to be keenly aware of the emotional impact which the diagnosis "heart trouble" has on the patient and his family. These words have a frightening effect. Fear and anxiety are among the first emotions felt by the patient and his relatives when the doctor informs them of the diagnosis.

As heart disease is a leading cause of death, fear of death can be expected. The diagnosis of heart disease does not mean necessarily that the outcome will be fatal. Advances made in the care and treatment of cardiac patients have made it possible for a great number of these patients to be returned to a comparatively healthy state.

When the patient recovers from the acute phase of his illness, worries and problems associated with chronic disease are often present. The patient may be concerned over paying his bills, supporting his family, and being able to return to his job. In addition, he will want to know how much activity he will be able to assume, what he can do for diversion during his convalescence, and what he will be allowed to eat. Because of the chronicity and frequency of heart disease, the practical nurse has an important place on the health team which cares for these patients.

## PREVALENCE

Diseases of the heart and blood vessels (cardiovascular diseases) are the leading cause of death in the United States. The death rate from this group of diseases continues to increase. One factor contributing to this increase is that the number of deaths from other diseases, such as pneumonia, tuberculosis, and acute communicable diseases, has been markedly decreased. Thus, people are living longer and are more likely to develop a disease of the circulatory system.

Heart disease affects all age groups. Infants who are born with an abnormal heart have congenital heart disease. Great strides have been made recently in the surgical treatment of some of these cardiac abnormalities. Children and young adults are subject to rheumatic heart disease.

*Head elevated*
*skin care*
*extremities elevated*
*diuretics - edema*

## CONGESTIVE HEART FAILURE

### Definition

Heart failure occurs when the heart is unable to perform its pumping function efficiently. This results in a collection of fluid in the tissues which is referred to as *edema*. Since most of the symptoms of heart failure are caused by congestion, the condition is called *congestive heart failure*. It is also referred to as *cardiac failure* or *cardiac decompensation*.

The practical nurse must realize that the term "heart failure" does not mean necessarily that the patient is doomed to die. Present-day treatment and nursing care are effective in aiding the return of many of these patients to a compensated condition. The compensated heart has made up for the disease which produced the failure. For example, the heart may enlarge in an effort to meet the extra demands made upon it by disease.

### Symptoms

It is important for the practical nurse to have a basic understanding of symptoms associated with cardiac failure. A majority of her patients with heart disease develop congestive heart failure.

### Failure of the Left Side · *pulmonary*
*right.*

When the left side of the heart is not functioning properly, the blood being returned to the left atrium through the pulmonary veins becomes congested in the lungs. This may result in *cardiac asthma* (p. 98) in which the patient has spells of dyspnea especially at night. An increased amount of blood in the lungs causes dyspnea. If the patient's condition continues, he is likely to have *pulmonary edema* which is a collection of fluid in the air sacs and lung tissue. The patient may become cyanotic, expectorate frothy, blood-tinged sputum, and have rales. *Rales* are abnormal sounds in the air passages.

The patient with pulmonary edema is likely to have rales which have a bubbling sound. This is caused by air passing through fluid in the air passages. These sounds may sometimes be heard by the nurse.

### Failure of the Right Side

When the right side of the heart is functioning improperly, the blood being returned to the right atrium backs up into the inferior vena cava. Edema develops in the parts of the body drained of its venous flow by this large vein. Thus, the organs below the heart are subject to a collection of fluid in their tissues. This edema develops in the lower areas of the body first. Edema progresses from the ankles, to the legs and thighs, and then into the abdomen. A collection of fluid in the peritoneal cavity is called *ascites*.

Edema of the abdominal organs, such as the stomach and intestines, causes loss of appetite, indigestion, and flatus (gas in the gastrointestinal tract). *Oliguria,* a decreased amount of urine, occurs because a decreased amount of blood is pumped through the kidneys. In addition, edema of the kidneys may be present, decreasing their ability to function.

The patient with congestive heart failure usually has a combination of right- and left-sided failure with one side weaker than the other. More than likely he has most of the symptoms described above. The severity of his symptoms depends upon the degree of cardiac inefficiency. In the early stage of heart failure, or mild cardiac failure, the patient experiences fatigue, dyspnea following slight exertion, and edema of his feet and ankles. The edema usually disappears after a night's rest. A slight cough, with a small amount of expectoration, may be present. Also, the patient may awaken at night with dyspnea, which is relieved by sitting up.

The patient in an advanced stage of heart failure has the above-mentioned symptoms to a greater degree. His dyspnea is acute even while at rest. He may have orthopnea, a condition in which there is need to sit up to breathe more easily (see Fig. 3). He coughs and expectorates frothy, blood-tinged sputum. Cyanosis is present. There is marked edema of the feet, legs, back, and abdomen. The urinary output is decreased. Mental processes are affected when the blood supply to the brain is inadequate. The patient may have lapses of memory, drowsiness, or restlessness because of this.

## Treatment

As nursing care is planned within the framework of treatment prescribed by the physician, the practical nurse needs an understanding of commonly used treatments. Important principles of treating specific cardiac diseases are discussed within the area dealing with that particular disease. The over-all nursing care of acutely ill and mildly ill cardiac patients is discussed later in this chapter.

The patient with advanced congestive heart failure is placed at absolute or complete bed rest in a comfortable position. A low-salt, easily digested diet and digitalis (drug causing the heart to beat stronger and slower) are usually prescribed. Oxygen therapy is administered when needed. Diuretics (drugs which increase urinary output) are used when edema is present.

Similar treatment is prescribed when the heart is in an early stage of failure. The patient is allowed as much activity as his heart can handle. Ability of the heart is balanced with the amount of exertion the patient is permitted. This is true also when a person with advanced heart failure begins to improve.

## CORONARY HEART DISEASE

The patient with coronary heart disease usually has arteriosclerosis of the coronary arteries, called *arteriosclerotic heart disease*. Over a period of time, particles of lime salts are deposited in the inner layer of the arterial wall. Formation of lime salts is called *calcification*. The affected artery becomes hard and thick, and loses its elasticity. The passageway within the artery is narrowed, and the heart muscle receives less blood. When the blood supply is temporarily inadequate to the part of the heart being fed by the affected artery, the patient has an attack of *angina pectoris*. Arteriosclerosis may lead to the formation of a blood clot, which is known as a *thrombus*. If the artery channel is completely closed by the blood clot, the patient has a heart attack which may be called either a *coronary occlusion, coronary thrombosis, myocardial infarction*, or "*a coronary*."

Fortunately the network of coronary arteries has an amazing

method of compensating for the narrowing of some of its members. While some of the arteries become smaller and less efficient, others feeding the same area get larger so they can carry more blood to the muscle needing it. Small new branches of these healthier arteries are formed. This method of compensation is called collateral circulation. Following a heart attack caused by closure of a coronary artery,

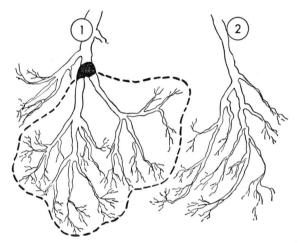

**Figure 18.**   Diagram showing a section of the outside of the heart. Coronary artery (1) supplying this portion has been closed by a blood clot. The myocardium within the dotted line will suffer from lack of nourishment and oxygen. Coronary artery (2) is sending small new branches to supply the stricken area with blood. This is known as collateral circulation.

collateral circulation plays an important part in the recovery of the patient.

**Angina Pectoris** - M E N   over 40

### Cause

The patient with angina pectoris has attacks of chest pain caused by an insufficient blood supply to the heart muscle. The myocardium needs more blood than it is receiving by means of the coronary arteries. When the blood supply to any muscle is inadequate, it begins to ache. For example, if a tourniquet is left on a patient's arm

*Vaso . constuctor & dialates vessels*

too long, he complains of pain. This discomfort is relieved when the tourniquet is removed and fresh blood flows into the arm.

Attacks of angina pectoris may result from spasm or arteriosclerosis of the coronary arteries. The most common cause is arteriosclerosis. The exact cause of arteriosclerosis is not known. The heart's blood supply may be adequate when it is not working hard, but when the work load is increased by exercise or by emotion the supply is not sufficient.

### Symptoms

Symptoms of this condition occur more often in men over 45 years of age. An attack is usually preceded by physical activity or an emotional upset such as anger or anxiety. The outstanding symptom is a squeezing pain which starts under the sternum (breastbone). It frequently spreads to the left shoulder and down the inner side of the left arm. Severity of the pain ranges from a discomfort to an immobilizing pain. The patient usually feels all right after the acute pain has subsided. However, the outcome may be fatal if a large area of the heart has an inadequate blood supply for too long a period of time.

### Treatment

As the pain is caused by an insufficient blood supply to the heart muscle, the aim of the physician's treatment is to increase the blood to the aching muscle. Rest and vasodilators, drugs which cause the blood vessels to dilate, are the two main measures used to accomplish this aim. The amount of work required of the heart is reduced when a person is at complete rest.

Nitroglycerin and amyl nitrite are two examples of drugs commonly used to relieve the pain of an attack of angina pectoris. These drugs cause the coronary arteries to dilate, enabling them to carry more blood to the affected area, and, thus, the pain is relieved.

The physician advises the patient regarding regulation of his daily activities in an effort to prevent further attacks. Efforts are made to balance the demands made on the heart by exercise and emotional strain with the activity allowed by his cardiac blood supply. Overeating, overactivity, rushing, and worry must be avoided. The patient should learn to live within the restrictions placed on him by the condition of his coronary arteries.

## Coronary Occlusion

### Description

The patient with a coronary occlusion has an obstruction in a coronary artery. The area of his heart fed by the diseased artery suffers from an insufficient blood supply. As previously stated, this disease, which may also be referred to as myocardial infarction, coronary thrombosis, or "a coronary," occurs when an artery is closed. Closure of the artery results in death to tissue supplied by that artery. This type of heart attack is the most common cause of sudden death from cardiac disease. Although myocardial infarction affects both men and women, it seems to be more common in men especially 50 years of age and over.

If a small blood vessel is obstructed and the collateral circulation is good, the patient may experience few symptoms, and chances of recovery are excellent. When the obstructed artery is a large one, and the collateral circulation is poor, the patient may die immediately.

### Symptoms

The beginning of a myocardial infarction is often sudden, and, unlike an anginal attack, the patient is usually at rest. The patient experiences a severe vise-like pain under the lower part of his sternum and shortness of breath. Nausea and vomiting are frequently present. His pulse is rapid and weak, and may be irregular. Symptoms of shock often present are paleness, cyanosis, cold and clammy skin, and a drop in blood pressure. A day or two after the attack the patient has a low-grade fever and an increase in his white blood cell count.

The doctor makes his diagnosis of coronary occlusion by careful examination of the patient. Electrocardiographic tracings are important aids in helping him to confirm his diagnosis. This tracing is a graphic record of the electrical activity of the heart which shows the condition of the heart muscle.

### Treatment

Absolute bed rest is essential. Medication, such as morphine, is prescribed for the relief of pain. Oxygen therapy is often used to decrease the work of the heart and to relieve cyanosis. *Anticoagulants,* drugs which prolong the clotting time of blood and help to prevent further clot formation, may be ordered. Bishydroxycoumarin (Dicumarol) and heparin are two such drugs. The patient is kept at rest until the affected area of his heart has healed and sufficient scar tissue has formed. His return to activity must be gradual.

## RHEUMATIC HEART DISEASE

### Description

Rheumatic heart disease is a form of rheumatic fever. This is an infection occurring most often in childhood and early adulthood. The patient frequently has an infected throat caused by the hemolytic streptococcus (member of streptococcal family of bacteria) before developing rheumatic fever. The specific cause of this disease is unknown.

### Symptoms and Complications

The patient has a migrating inflammation of one joint after another; in other words, the inflammation moves from one joint to another. For example, the knee joints may be inflamed first and in a short while an elbow joint becomes inflamed. The inflammation of the first joints to be affected disappears. Symptoms of inflammation, which are discussed in Chapter 6, such as fever, malaise, and local pain and swelling of the joints are present. Rheumatic infection may affect the endocardium, myocardium, or pericardium. Symptoms vary with the part of the heart which is inflamed.

The endocardium is most often involved. Since this membrane lines the valves, the patient may develop a heart murmur. The valves, which are normally smooth, become hard and scarred. Blood flowing over a diseased valve makes an abnormal sound called a *murmur*. A diseased valve may be unable to fulfill its function of keeping blood from returning to the cavity which is pumping it on. This valve, which does not close properly, allows blood to flow in the wrong direction, and is referred to as a *leaking valve*. When a valve does not open properly, it is stenosed (narrowed).

The mitral valve between the left atrium and left ventricle is most often involved. Stenosis of this valve is called mitral stenosis. Mitral insufficiency occurs when the mitral valve flaps are so scarred and shrunken that they cannot close the opening. Congestive heart failure may develop during the acute phase, or after many years have passed.

### Treatment

Treatment is aimed toward relieving the symptoms, preventing permanent heart damage, and preventing another attack. The most important factor during the acute stage is rest. Salicylates, such as aspirin and sodium salicylate, are used to relieve joint pain. Penicillin and cortisone are helpful in some cases.

The patient with marked mitral stenosis can often be aided by a new surgical procedure, called *commissurotomy*. This operation is performed after the inflammation has subsided.

## ENDOCARDITIS

### Description

Inflammation of the endocardium may be caused by a rheumatic infection or by bacteria; when caused by bacteria, this condition is called *bacterial endocarditis*. When it is caused by bacterial infection, local areas of inflammation result in the formation of tiny masses, called *vegetations*. When these vegetations form on valve flaps, abnormal functioning of the valve occurs. Scar tissue forms in the areas of vegetation after the inflammatory process has subsided. When scar tissue affects the functioning of a valve, the patient has *valvular heart disease*.

### Symptoms

Symptoms usually associated with an inflammation are present: fever, chills, fast pulse rate, increased white blood cell count, and malaise. A murmur is often heard by the physician.

### Treatment

In addition to bed rest, drugs are used to combat the infection. The physician selects the drug which is most effective against the bacteria causing the infection. Although the infection can usually be cured by drugs, valvular damage is not improved.

## MYOCARDITIS

Myocarditis, inflammation of the myocardium, may develop as a complication of such diseases as diphtheria, scarlet fever, and typhoid fever. It may also be associated with a rheumatic infection of the heart.

Since the major function of the heart is dependent upon muscular activity, an acute inflammation of this muscle is serious. Often the first signs noted are symptoms of rapidly developing heart failure. Measures for the care of a patient with congestive heart failure are employed (p. 112).

## PERICARDITIS

The patient with pericarditis has an inflammation of the pericardium. It can be caused by a rheumatic infection of the heart or an infection of the lungs, such as tuberculosis and pneumonia, which may spread to the pericardium. This inflammation may also be caused by pathogenic microorganisms brought in by the blood stream.

Functioning of the heart is affected when fluid collects in the pericardial sac and presses on the heart. A procedure performed by the doctor to remove the fluid is called a *pericardial tap*. He places a needle into the fluid and aspirates it.

## NURSING CARE

### The Acutely Ill Patient

The practical nurse is called upon frequently to assist in caring for the acutely ill cardiac patient. This patient has congestive heart failure, or he may be on the verge of developing it.

### Rest

Rest is of vital importance for the acutely ill cardiac patient. The heart, which has added strain placed upon it by disease, needs maximum relief from normal demands of body functions. It is the nursing team's responsibility to help the patient obtain the maximum amount of mental and physical rest. Anxiety and restlessness increase the strain placed on the heart. Problems which worry the patient should be reported to the team leader or head nurse.

The patient should be in a quiet, well-ventilated room. Complete

or absolute bed rest is usually prescribed. In this instance the patient
is not allowed to exert himself. He is bathed, turned, lifted, and fed.
Sedatives, drugs having a quieting or soothing effect, are often ordered
as an aid in producing rest. Bromide, phenobarbital, and chloral
hydrate are three examples. Morphine and other opium derivatives
are used because they produce an exaggerated sense of well-being
(euphoria) and relieve pain.

Straining when having a bowel movement increases the heart's work
load. This should be avoided. It is for this reason that either an
enema or a mild laxative is ordered. Of course, the enema must be
given with gentleness and skill.

### Diet

The physician frequently orders a low-salt diet, because salt helps
to retain fluid in body tissues. The doctor wants to aid nature in
eliminating excess fluid as well as to prevent the collection of more
fluid in the edematous patient. Also, the feedings are usually small
and served frequently as it may tire the patient to eat.

Foods which are more difficult to digest, as well as those which are
gas-producing, such as cabbage, beans, and peas, should be avoided.
Flatus (gas) in the stomach causes pressure on the diaphragm which
increases the patient's dyspnea.

Overeating and gaining weight put added strain on the heart.
Overweight patients are often placed on a diet low in calories.

The practical nurse is frequently responsible for some aspect of the
diet therapy. It may be the preparation of the food in the home, or
serving and feeding the patient in the hospital. Foods cooked without
salt are unappetizing to the average person who is accustomed to
seasoning. Patients who understand the importance of a restricted
diet are more likely to be cooperative.

Meals must be made as appetizing as possible within the limitations outlined by the physician. For example, a poached egg cooked
without salt and not served immediately would not tempt the patient's appetite. Of course, the patient on a low-salt diet is not allowed
to have salt on a poached egg, but it certainly could be served warm.

### Fluids

A record of the fluid intake and output is frequently requested by the
doctor. An accurate account of the amount of liquids taken into

the body, and those excreted from the body, is an important guide for the physician in planning his treatment. For example, if the patient's intake for a 24-hour period was 2000 ml (2 qt) and his output for the same period was 250 ml (8.3 oz), the doctor might order a diuretic; whereas, if the output was 1000 ml (1 qt), he probably would not prescribe this drug. The intake and output record aids the physician in determining the patient's condition.

The fluid intake of the patient is often restricted to a certain number of milliliters or ounces within a 24-hour period. Although the amount of liquids is usually decreased, some doctors increase the intake for patients on a low-salt diet. It is the nursing team's responsibility to keep the amount of fluids within the range prescribed.

Frequent weighing of the patient indicates an increase or decrease of edema. For example, a loss of several pounds in a 24-hour period shows an improvement. For accuracy, the patient should be weighed on the same scales, at the same time each day, and he should have on the same amount of clothing.

### Attitude of the Practical Nurse

The nurse who has a genuine feeling of compassion and kindliness for her patient and his family renders an invaluable service. Of course, this is true in the case of all patients, but is even more so when the patient is desperately ill. This patient needs reassurance, which is best demonstrated by the nurse's calmness, skillfulness, self-confidence, and ability to anticipate the patient's needs. These personal characteristics help the patient to feel more secure.

Simple explanations of treatments before they are started aids in obtaining cooperation as well as relieving apprehension. The patient's condition should not be discussed within his range of hearing.

As the patient improves, he may need to be encouraged to increase gradually his activity as prescribed by the doctor. The protective attitude shown during the more acute stage of illness needs to be reduced.

### Position

The practical nurse should assist in placing the patient in the position most comfortable for him. He is usually more comfortable with his head elevated if dyspnea is present. Supporting the head, arms, and back with pillows increases his comfort. Weight from the bedclothing on his feet can be prevented by using a bed cradle or a footboard.

When the practical nurse is helping to care for a critically ill cardiac patient, she should seek specific instructions before changing the patient's position. In some cases the doctor does not want the patient to be turned for a certain length of time. In the absence of this request from the physician, the patient's position needs to be changed frequently.

### Personal Hygiene

Oral hygiene is especially important for the mouth-breathing dyspneic patient. Restricted fluids also increase dryness of his mouth. The nurse is responsible for cleaning the patient's mouth when he is on absolute bed rest.

Particular attention must be paid to the patient's skin when edema is present. Edematous tissue is more likely to develop decubitus ulcers.

### The Mildly Ill Patient

Basically, the nursing care of the cardiac patient when mildly ill is similar to that given him during an acute phase. He continues to need rest, a daily bath, special skin care, and an easily digested diet. The chief difference in nursing the acutely ill patient and the mildly ill patient is that the latter is allowed to do more things for himself as he improves. For example, instead of being turned by the nurse he turns himself.

As the symptoms of the acute cardiac condition disappear, the patient feels more comfortable. Often the patient is overly anxious to resume previous activities. His return to normal activity must be gradual. The bed patient is usually allowed to progress from self-help in bed to dangling his feet, sitting in a chair, and then walking. His pulse should be taken and reported before and after each of these exertions.

Observing the patient for symptoms of congestive heart failure is a part of the nurse's responsibility. A record of intake and output and daily weight may be continued into the convalescent period. He must be protected against colds and other infection as an inflammatory process increases the work load of the heart.

## Diversions

Helping the patient to amuse or entertain himself during a period of relative inactivity is indeed a challenge to the nursing team. The practical nurse with imagination, ingenuity, interest, and enthusiasm can contribute much toward his diversional activities.

Factors to consider in selecting diversions for the patient include the amount of activity permitted by the physician, personal preferences of the patient, and available facilities. During the more acute phase of his illness the patient's entertainment may consist mainly of nonexciting radio and television programs, and reading aloud by the nurse. Preparing attractive trays with a miniature vase of flowers, or with tray favors, gives the patient something to anticipate. Arranging his get-well cards so he can see them gives many hours of pleasure. Watching activities of goldfish and observing the growth of flowers are additional sources of passive entertainment.

As the patient improves and is allowed more freedom of activity, he may enjoy playing cards, working puzzles, collecting articles of interest such as stamps and rocks, observing activities of birds, writing, painting, and knitting. These are only a few examples of diversions which the nurse can help the patient to enjoy.

Many large hospitals have departments of occupational therapy. The occupational therapist helps to plan diversional activities as well as suitable occupations for patients. This member of the health team is of great importance to the person who is a partial invalid because of a heart condition.

## The Patient Receiving Oxygen Therapy

Oxygen is frequently prescribed for the cardiac patient. However, oxygen therapy is used for persons affected by other diseases also. A discussion of the general principles of oxygen therapy is included in this chapter, since it contains one of the first discussions of a major disease condition frequently treated with oxygen therapy. The general principles of oxygen therapy rather than the actual procedures are included. The role that oxygen plays in the body, the characteristics of oxygen, the cause of oxygen deficiency, and the symptoms of oxygen deficiency are discussed first in order to help the practical nurse to understand her responsibilities in caring for the patient receiving oxygen therapy.

## Introduction

Oxygen is a gas necessary for life; in fact, it can truly be called the breath of life. Under normal conditions, the body's tissues receive an adequate amount of oxygen. This vital gas is taken into the lungs by inhalation (breathing in). Oxygen passes from the lungs into the blood, which carries it to all of the body cells. Carbon dioxide, which is a waste product of the cells, is taken by the blood and carried to the lungs. There it is removed by expiration (breathing out). The body needs a continuous supply of oxygen since it does not store this essential gas.

Different tissues of the body vary in their reaction to an insufficient amount of oxygen. For example, there is permanent damage of the brain when it is deprived of oxygen for five to seven minutes. When the heart receives no oxygen for a period of 30 to 40 minutes, it too has permanent changes. Skeletal muscles can be deprived of this gas for several hours and then regain their function when the supply is re-established.

Oxygen is prescribed by the physician when the cells of the patient's body do not receive an adequate supply. The responsibility for safe and effective oxygen therapy is shared by members of the nursing team, and in some hospitals, by a technician specially trained for this. As the practical nurse is an important member of the nursing team, she shares this responsibility. She also spends a great proportion of her time at the individual patient's bedside. Thus, the practical nurse needs a thorough understanding of the principles and techniques involved. Continued study is necessary in order to learn of advances in oxygen therapy. The practical nurse should use additional literature, such as equipment manuals, hospital procedure sheets, recent magazine articles, and other texts, to increase her knowledge of specific types of oxygen therapy.

The practical nurse needs a basic understanding of oxygen in order to assist with oxygen therapy. It was stated earlier in this discussion that oxygen is a gas. It makes up approximately 20 per cent of the air around us. Although oxygen does not burn, it is necessary for combustion (burning) to take place. A fire is not possible without oxygen. The simple experiment of placing a lighted candle under a glass illustrates this fact. The candle stops burning when there is no more oxygen in the glass.

A fire burns more rapidly when the amount of oxygen is increased. For instance, a lighted cigarette smoldering in an ash tray will burst into flames when oxygen in the air around it is increased. Thus, the danger of fire in oxygen therapy is an ever-present one.

Another characteristic of oxygen which the practical nurse needs to know is that it has a drying effect. She will see equipment used to add humidity (moisture) to the oxygen in some methods of administration. When oxygen is administered by a nasal catheter, additional moisture is needed. This is necessary because the flow of oxygen is so direct. Humidity is increased by having the oxygen flow through water. With mask therapy, the moisture in the exhaled air collects on the inside of the face piece. This moistens the inflow of oxygen into the mask. However, additional humidity may be needed for mask therapy, especially when a high concentration of oxygen is given over a long period of time. When a tent is used, the exhaled air from the patient usually contains adequate moisture which is picked up by the oxygen flow and recirculated.

### Oxygen Deficiency

#### Cause

The individual with an oxygen deficiency has *hypoxia*. This condition occurs when the cells are unable to use this vital gas or when the cells receive an inadequate amount of it. An example of hypoxia caused by an inability of the cells to use oxygen is seen in the patient suffering from cyanide poisoning. Certain conditions of the lungs, heart, blood, and central nervous system cause the cells to receive an inadequate amount of oxygen. Diseases of the lungs, such as pneumonia and asthma, can prevent oxygen from passing through the lungs to the blood. An example of heart disease causing hypoxia is seen in the patient with cardiac failure, which prevents the heart from pumping blood rich with oxygen to the tissues. An individual has an insufficient amount of blood cells to transport oxygen when he has severe anemia or a massive hemorrhage. An example of hypoxia caused by a central nervous system condition may be seen in the patient with a stroke. Also, depression of the functions of the brain by an overdose of sedatives or opiates can cause a person to have this deficiency. His respirations become so slow that his blood receives an insufficient amount of oxygen to supply the cells.

*Symptoms*

The patient with hypoxia may have a variety of symptoms. The degree of oxygen deficiency influences his symptoms. His pulse and respiratory rate usually increase as his need for oxygen becomes greater. However, in severe cases, the pulse and respiratory rate decrease and may become irregular. Restlessness is another common symptom of hypoxia. The patient may have a combination of additional symptoms, such as sighing, yawning, headache, nausea, vomiting, anxiety, dyspnea, cyanosis, and impaired vision. Mentally, he may become confused and lose consciousness. The patient may have muscle twitching or even convulsions.

*Methods of Administration*

Oxygen is supplied in a cylinder (tank) or in an oxygen-piping system in some hospitals. A device which is called a *regulator* or a *reducing valve* must be attached to the cylinder before oxygen can be administered to the patient. The regulator is necessary because the oxygen is stored in the tank under such high pressure. This device also makes it possible for the operator to control the amount of oxygen flowing from the cylinder. Two gauges are attached to the regulator. One shows the amount of oxygen in the cylinder and the other one, which is called a *flow meter*, shows the flow of oxygen in liters per minute. In an oxygen-piping system, the oxygen is already at an acceptable pressure; therefore, only a flow meter is needed.

Oxygen can be administered by a variety of methods; but the most common are tent, nasal catheter, and face mask. The doctor determines the method of administration and the concentration of oxygen necessary. He takes into consideration the patient's condition, the amount of oxygen needed by the patient, and the equipment available.

## Oxygen Tent

An oxygen tent is a chamber in which the patient's head and upper part of his body are enclosed. Oxygen is forced into the tent. The practical nurse may find it helpful to think of an oxygen tent as an

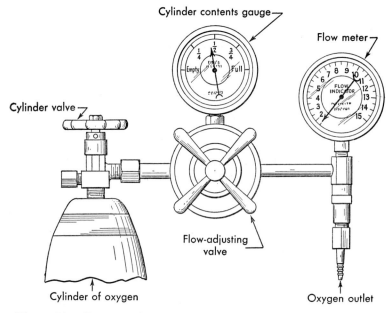

Cylinder contents gauge

Flow meter

Cylinder valve

Flow-adjusting valve

Cylinder of oxygen

Oxygen outlet

**Figure 19.** Diagram of an oxygen regulator. (Courtesy of Linde Co., Division of Union Carbide Corp., New York City.)

air-conditioned unit with an increased amount of oxygen flowing through it. The older models are cooled by ice and the newer ones by refrigerated coils. Most tents in use today are electrically operated and have dials to regulate the temperature according to the individual patient's needs. A tent is used to administer a concentration of approximately 50 per cent oxygen. This method of oxygen therapy requires more oxygen than either a mask or a nasal catheter since the air in the canopy must be enriched with oxygen before the patient receives benefit from it. Oxygen is also lost when the nurse opens the canopy to care for the patient.

### Nasal Catheter

The patient receiving oxygen by nasal catheter has a small tube inserted into his nose. This tube may be inserted deeply so that its

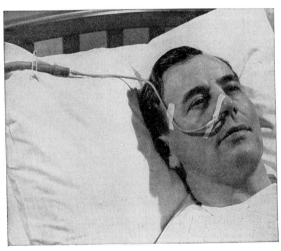

**Figure 20.** The patient receiving oxygen by nasal catheter. Notice that the tubing is secured to the patient's face by tape. The tubing is anchored to the bed clothes by a safety pin. The safety pin should be placed so that the tubing is sufficiently slack to allow the patient free movement of his head. (Courtesy of Linde Co., Division of Union Carbide Corp., New York City.)

tip rests in the back of the throat, or less deeply so that the tip rests in the patient's nostril. Oxygen is forced through a *humidifier*, which is a jar containing water, into the catheter. The purpose of the water is to humidify the oxygen and thus prevent the mucous membrane of the nose and throat from becoming dry.

The location of the tip of the catheter influences the oxygen concentration which the patient actually receives. The patient with a catheter inserted into the back of his throat can receive a concentration of 30 per cent oxygen with a flow of 4 to 5 liters per minute; 40 per cent, when the flow is 6 to 7 liters; and 50 per cent, when the flow is 8 to 9 liters. The patient with the tip of the catheter in his nostril receives a lower concentration of oxygen.

### Face Mask

Two main types of masks are available for the administration of oxygen. One type covers the nose only and the other type covers the nose and mouth. However, there are many different varieties of these two types of masks. For example, some have a meter to mix air with oxygen; some have a rebreathing bag in which the patient inhales part of the air which he exhaled; and others exert pressure during inhalation, exhalation, or both. A greater concentration of oxygen can be obtained by the use of a mask than with either a tent or a nasal catheter. A concentration of oxygen ranging from 30 per cent to nearly 100 per cent is possible with a mask.

### Nursing Care

#### Preparation for Oxygen Therapy

The patient needs an adequate explanation of oxygen therapy before he receives it. Some individuals still believe that oxygen is given as a last resort and become upset over it. The practical nurse must realize that this is not true if she is to help him adjust to oxygen therapy. Frequently a simple explanation regarding the benefit he will receive from the oxygen or the fact that it will hasten his recovery reassures the patient. For instance, the patient with difficult breathing will feel relieved to know that this can be eased.

It may help the practical nurse to have a better understanding of the patient's feeling, if she pauses for a few moments and imagines that her oxygen supply suddenly becomes inadequate. Instead of being able to obtain a sufficient amount of oxygen by her own power, she must depend on a mechanical device controlled by another person. Having used her imagination to help her understand the possible reaction of a patient with hypoxia, the practical nurse can appreciate more fully the importance of an adequate explanation to the patient.

In addition to this, the patient also needs to feel confidence in the person handling the equipment and caring for him. The equipment can be brought to the patient's bedside after he has been told that he is to receive oxygen therapy. In certain emergencies, of course, this time would be shortened. The nurse responsible for assisting in the administration of oxygen should remain with the patient until he seems to be making an adjustment to it.

### Safety Measures

Both the patient and his family should be told that no smoking and no open flame, such as a candle, are allowed. Other patients in the same room should also receive these instructions. Cigarettes, matches, or other smoking materials should be removed from the patient's unit. NO SMOKING signs should be posted in plain view in the patient's unit and on the door.

The practical nurse needs to remember that oil and grease should not be used on oxygen equipment. Either of these substances coming in contact with oxygen stored under high pressure can burn rapidly. The nurse who has either oil or grease on her hands should wash them thoroughly before handling oxygen equipment.

Electrical equipment can cause a fire when the patient is receiving oxygen. For this reason, signal lights and electric heating pads should not be used. It is necessary to make special arrangements for the patient to call the nurse, such as by the use of a tap bell. Some hospitals are equipped with safety attachments to be added to the electric call system. This is especially convenient for the patient in an oxygen tent.

It is important for the tank of oxygen to be kept in an upright position. If it falls, the cylinder could cause injury to people in that vicinity, or it could be damaged. An oxygen cylinder should be placed in a location where it cannot be knocked over accidentally. Strapping it to the bedpost or placing it in a protected spot, such as a corner, helps to reduce this danger. Some hospitals are equipped with cylinder stands which are used to hold the cylinder in a safe, upright position. Also, some oxygen tents have a special space with a protecting door into which the cylinder can be placed.

## Oxygen Tent

Manufacturers supply information about the use of their oxygen tents. Members of the nursing team should consult the operating instructions of a particular tent before using it. Many newer models have directions printed on them. In general, the motor should be started and the flow of oxygen set at 15 liters per minute before the canopy is placed over the patient. The temperature within the tent can be adjusted by the temperature control dial so that the patient is comfortable. However, the temperature in the tent should not be more than 10° to 15° F below that of the room during hot weather.

After the nurse has placed the patient under the canopy, she should tuck it securely under the mattress. If the front of the canopy is not long enough to tuck under the foot of the bed, it can be tucked with a sheet or a bath blanket. In either case, the canopy should be made as leakproof as possible.

After placing the patient in a tent which has a flush valve, the practical nurse should depress it for a few minutes. The patient should be warned that this makes a rushing noise. When she is using a tent which does not have a flush valve, the nurse should allow the oxygen flow to remain at 15 liters per minute for 20 to 30 minutes. The purpose of either of these activities is to increase the concentration of oxygen within the tent in a short period of time. After the practical nurse has flooded the tent with oxygen, she should regulate the liter flow as prescribed by the doctor. In general, the flow of oxygen for an adult in a tent should be approximately 10 to 12 liters per minute.

Instead of prescribing a specific flow of liters per minute, the doctor may request that the nursing team keep the concentration of oxygen at a certain level. Generally, the desired concentration ranges around 50 per cent. The concentration of oxygen in a tent is determined by the use of an oxygen analyzer. An analysis should be made at regular intervals and after the canopy has been opened for patient care. The practical nurse may be requested by her team leader or head nurse either to increase or decrease the liter flow after the amount of oxygen within the canopy has been determined.

The patient in an oxygen tent should not be removed without

the doctor's permission. The canopy has openings on the sides which allow the nurse to reach into the tent to care for the patient. However, opening the canopy allows oxygen in the tent to be diluted with room air. Knowing this helps the practical nurse to remember the importance of planning nursing care so that the canopy is not opened unnecessarily. When reaching her arm through the opening to care for the patient, the practical nurse should close it around her arm as much as possible to prevent excess loss of oxygen. The practical nurse can slide the canopy up around the patient's neck and tuck it under his pillow when she is doing a procedure such as a bath. Increasing the flow of oxygen for a few minutes after the tent is closed helps to re-establish the proper concentration more quickly.

Members of the nursing team responsible for the care of this patient should visit him frequently. Both the patient and the equipment should be observed. These visits help the patient to realize that the nurses are interested in him. Symptoms which indicate a change in his condition, such as his pulse and respiratory rate, a change in restlessness, difficult breathing, and his color, should be noticed and reported. The equipment should be checked for the amount of oxygen remaining in the tank, the number of liters flowing per minute as shown on the gauge, and the tucking in of the canopy. The patient's unit should be observed for possible fire hazards, such as a visitor smoking in the room, electric call bell within the canopy, or an insecure cylinder. A small light should be left on in this patient's room at night so that the nurse can continue her observations.

The patient's position should be changed frequently unless otherwise ordered. The nurse should not rub the back of the patient in a tent with either alcohol or oil because of the danger of fire. If it is permitted by the doctor, the oxygen can be discontinued while the nurse is using these substances. In some cases a facial apparatus for oxygen administration is substituted while the nurse rubs the patient's back with either alcohol or oil. The nurse should wash her hands to remove either substance before handling the oxygen equipment.

The patient in a tent needs good oral hygiene as his mouth and lips usually become dry. His temperature should be taken rectally instead of orally because a patient in an oxygen tent is frequently a mouth breather. He may also be having dyspnea.

The patient is usually removed from the tent gradually as his condition improves. The practical nurse should observe him for symptoms of oxygen deficiency, which were discussed on page 125. The presence of any of these symptoms should be reported to the team leader or head nurse.

After the oxygen tent has been discontinued, it should be adequately cleaned. The canopy can be cleaned by washing it thoroughly with soap and water. Particular attention should be paid to the inside of the canopy. It should be examined for tears which would permit oxygen leakage during the next usage. After the canopy is thoroughly dry, it should be stored.

### Nasal Catheter

In caring for the patient receiving oxygen by nasal catheter, the practical nurse should check the patient and the equipment frequently. Just as in the care of a patient receiving oxygen by tent, it is important to observe and to report symptoms which indicate a change in the patient's condition. In addition to checking the equipment for the proper liter flow, the amount of oxygen in the cylinder, and safety hazards, the practical nurse should observe the amount of water in the humidifier. It should be filled to the water-level mark. Tap water in some localities contains substances which clog the humidifier. For this reason the practical nurse may be asked to use distilled water instead of tap water. The presence of leaks in tube connections or in the humidifier should be reported. Kinked tubing should be straightened.

The amount of oxygen should be kept at the prescribed liter flow. This generally ranges from approximately 4 to 6 liters of oxygen per minute.

The catheter should be changed every 12 hours or as ordered by the doctor. It is then replaced in the other nostril by a freshly lubricated catheter. Since oily or greasy substances are not to be used on oxygen equipment, the catheter should be lubricated with a water-soluble lubricant. Water is sometimes used for this purpose.

The humidifier, the catheter, and the connector should be washed thoroughly after being used. The catheter must be sterilized before it is used for another person.

*Face Mask*

Since there are different varieties of face masks, the practical nurse should receive specific directions regarding the use of a particular one. However, she needs to know certain important factors which apply to most patients receiving oxygen by face mask.

As in the care of a patient receiving oxygen by other methods of administration, members of the nursing team should check the patient and the equipment at frequent intervals. In addition to checking the equipment for the proper liter flow, the amount of oxygen in the cylinder, safety hazards, and the amount of water in the humidifier when one is used, the practical nurse should observe the connections for leaks. Kinked tubing should be straightened. The mask must be in a leakproof and comfortable position for effective therapy. The strap which is placed around the patient's head to hold the mask in place should be adjusted so that it does not press on the ear. If the practical nurse notices that oxygen is blowing into the patient's eyes, she should adjust the mask to a more leakproof position. Sponge rubber disks present on the sides of some masks may become moist and reduce the efficiency of the treatment. The practical nurse should report this so that the disks can be replaced by dry ones. Another important observation for the practical nurse to make pertains to the bag when one is attached to the mask. In general, if the bag does not move as the patient breathes or if it collapses completely, this should be reported to the team leader or the head nurse.

A mask which covers the patient's nose and mouth must be removed when the patient eats or drinks. If the mask covers the patient's nose only, he may need to be reminded not to breathe through his mouth as this would reduce the amount of oxygen received.

The mask should be removed, washed, and dried thoroughly approximately every two hours. This should be done more often if secretions collect in the mask. Washing the patient's face and giving mouth care when the mask is removed make him more comfortable. Powder may be applied to his face at this time.

The practical nurse should have the patient exhale as she puts the mask on his face. Placing a thin piece of gauze or cotton under the edge of the mask may be necessary to prevent irritation of the bridge of the patient's nose.

When the use of a face mask is discontinued, it should be cleaned and made ready for use by another patient. This can be accomplished by taking the mask apart, washing it thoroughly with soap and water, rinsing it well, and boiling the parts for five minutes. The parts should be dried, reassembled, and stored in a clean place.

## SUGGESTIONS FOR STUDY

1. What other terms may the physician use when referring to congestive heart failure?

2. The practical nurse can expect a patient with failure of the left side of his heart to have congestion in what part of his body? Where does congestion occur in a patient with failure of the right side of his heart?

3. Observe the symptoms of a patient with mild cardiac failure. How do they compare with those discussed in this chapter?

4. What is arteriosclerotic heart disease?

5. What part of the heart is affected by angina pectoris?

6. What causes a patient with angina pectoris to have attacks of pain? What drugs are commonly used to relieve the pain?

7. Review the symptoms of a patient with a myocardial infarction. What treatment can the practical nurse expect the doctor to prescribe?

8. Why is the patient with rheumatic heart disease likely to develop a heart murmur?

9. Discuss the responsibilities of the nursing team for an acutely ill cardiac patient in regard to rest, diet, fluids, and position.

10. How can a nurse reassure the cardiac patient?

11. Review the factors to consider in selecting diversions for a cardiac patient.

12. Compare the approximate percentage of oxygen in the air you breathe with the concentration of oxygen generally received by the use of a tent, a nasal catheter, and a face mask.

13. What is hypoxia?

14. Discuss some of the common causes of hypoxia.

15. What symptoms may occur as a result of hypoxia?

16. How long can the brain be deprived of oxygen before it is permanently damaged? The heart?

17. With what type of equipment for oxygen therapy is a humidifier usually used?

18. Why is a regulator necessary when administering oxygen from a cylinder?

19. Discuss the factors which are important for the practical nurse to remember when she is helping to start oxygen therapy.

20. Review the responsibilities of the nursing team for a patient receiving oxygen by tent, nasal catheter, or mask.

21. Why would the clothing of a patient in an oxygen tent burn rapidly? What precautions should be taken to prevent fire?

REFERENCES FOR CHAPTER 9

Barnes, B. de S.: "Some Facts about Oxygen Therapy," *Practical Nurses Digest*, **4**:3-6, (Jan.) 1957.

Brown, Amy F.: *Medical Nursing*, 3rd ed. W. B. Saunders Co., Philadelphia, 1957, pp. 109-38, 169-71, and 201-79.

Cooley, Denton A.: "Open Heart Surgery in Children," *Am. J. Nursing*, **58**:200-202, (Feb.) 1958.

Davidson, Sidney: "Diet and Cardiovascular Disease," *Am. J. Nursing*, **57**:194-96, (Feb.) 1957.

Eliason, Eldridge L.; Ferguson, L. Kraeer; and Sholtis, Lillian A.: *Surgical Nursing*, 10th ed. J. B. Lippincott Co., Philadelphia, 1955, pp. 257-60.

Emerson, Charles P., Jr., and Bragdon, Jane S.: *Essentials of Medicine*, 17th ed. J. B. Lippincott Co., Philadelphia, 1955, pp. 245-53 and 273-308.

Faddis, Margene O., and Hayman, Joseph M.: *Care of the Medical Patient*. McGraw-Hill Book Co., New York, 1952, pp. 153-98.

Ferree, John W., "The Practical Nurse and the Heart Patient," *Practical Nurses Digest*, **2**:12-13, (Apr.) 1955.

Fleming, Mildred: "Rheumatic Fever and Cortisone Therapy," *Am. J. Nursing*, **56**:728-31, (June) 1956.

Groom, Dale: "Drugs for Cardiac Patients," *Am. J. Nursing*, **56**:1125-27, (Sept.) 1956.

Hull, Edgar, and Perrodin, Cecilia: *Medical Nursing*, 5th ed. F. A. Davis Co., Philadelphia, 1954, pp. 169-219.

"If You Ask Me—About Helping Patients Accept Low Sodium Diets," *Am. J. Nursing*, **56**:68, (Jan.) 1956.

Jensen, Julius, and Jensen, Deborah: *Nursing in Clinical Medicine*, 4th ed. The Macmillan Company, New York, 1954, pp. 221-302.

Klocek, Joseph J.: "The Oxygen Therapy Supervisor," *Am. J. Nursing*, **57**:68-70, (Jan.) 1957.

Krause, Marie: *Nutrition and Diet Therapy*, 2nd ed. W. B. Saunders Co., Philadelphia, 1957, pp. 296-304.

Livingstone, Huberta M.: "Nursing Care in Oxygen Therapy," *Am. J. Nursing,* **57**:65-68, (Jan.) 1957.

Marple, Charles D.: "Cyanosis," *Am. J. Nursing,* **58**:222-25, (Feb.) 1958.

Modell, Walter, and Schwartz, Doris R.: *Handbook of Cardiology for Nurses,* 3rd ed. Springer Publishing Co., New York, 1958.

*Oxygen Therapy Handbook,* 4th ed. Linde Co., Division of Union Carbide Corp., New York, 1957.

Peyton, Alice B.: *Practical Nutrition.* J. B. Lippincott Co., Philadelphia, 1957, pp. 202-9.

Proudfit, Fairfax T., and Robinson, Corinne H.: *Nutrition and Diet Therapy,* 11th ed. The Macmillan Company, New York, 1955, pp. 458-77.

Sachs, Bernard A.: "Arteriosclerotic Heart Disease," *Am. J. Nursing,* **55**:838-41, (July) 1955.

Sadler, Sabra S.: *Rheumatic Fever—Nursing Care in Pictures.* J. B. Lippincott Co., Philadelphia, 1949.

Silber, Earl N.: "Medical Management of Angina Pectoris," *Am. J. Nursing,* **55**:168-69, (Feb.) 1955.

Terry, Florence J.; Benz, Gladys S.; Mereness, Dorothy; and Kleffner, Frank R.: *Principles and Technics of Rehabilitation Nursing.* C. V. Mosby Co., St. Louis, 1957, pp. 137-47.

Wortham, Elizabeth D., and Ritchie, Geraldine: "Nursing Care of Children after Open Heart Surgery," *Am. J. Nursing,* **58**:203-4, (Feb.) 1958.

*Chapter 10*

# THE PATIENT
# WITH A DISEASE OF
# THE BLOOD VESSELS

## ARTERIOSCLEROSIS

### Description

Arteriorsclerosis is commonly known as hardening of the arteries. Normally, these vessels which carry blood containing food and oxygen to the cells are elastic, soft, and rather thin. The patient with arteriosclerosis has a thickening of the walls of his arteries because soft fatty substances have been deposited on the inside of the blood vessels. Over a period of time calcium is deposited in these fatty areas making the artery rigid, hard, brittle, and less elastic. These changes can be compared with those seen in rubber hose. The new hose is elastic and soft; whereas the old one is rigid, hard, and brittle. The term for fatty deposits in the innermost wall of the artery is *atherosclerosis*.

### Cause

The exact cause of arteriosclerosis is not known. It is often associated with diabetes mellitus, chronic nephritis (inflammation of the kidney), and high blood pressure. Many physicians believe that a moderate amount of arteriosclerosis is associated with growing older. Although older people are most often affected, it may also be found in young individuals. There appears to be a tendency for members of certain families to develop arteriosclerosis at an earlier age.

Since arteriosclerosis is know as a degenerative disease, the practi-

137

cal nurse needs to know that this type of disease occurs most often in older people. The patient with a degenerative disease has a change in the normal structure of his cells. The cells deteriorate, fibers grow in the affected part, and calcium is often deposited.

## Symptoms

The patient with arteriosclerosis may have symptoms of inadequate blood supply to the area of his body supplied with food and oxygen by the diseased arteries. As the artery's wall becomes thicker because of deposits, the inside of the vessel gets smaller; therefore, less blood is forced through it. Parts of the body often affected by arteriosclerosis are the heart, brain, kidneys, and lower extremities.

The patient who has arteriosclerosis of the coronary arteries may develop arteriosclerotic heart disease. Symptoms resulting from disease of arteries nourishing the brain vary. The patient may have a poor memory. Often he forgets recent events, but remembers his childhood. This change is frequently seen in older people. He may become irritable, unable to concentrate, and moody. When the kidney arteries are affected, the kidneys lose their ability to function properly. The patient with arteriosclerosis in his feet and legs may experience coldness, numbness, and pain. These symptoms are usually increased by walking because the muscles need more blood during exercise.

A thrombus, blood clot, is likely to form in the arteriosclerotic artery (see Fig. 21). Two main factors which aid in thrombosis (blood clot formation) are (1) the blood is being carried more slowly through the artery and (2) surfaces of the deposits in the artery's wall are rough. When thrombosis occurs, the area being supplied by that artery has symptoms of inadequate blood supply. If either a large or a vital artery is closed by a thrombus, the result may be quite serious. When the patient has a thrombus in an artery of his brain, it is called cerebral thrombosis (stroke). The patient with a clot in a coronary artery has coronary thrombosis.

## Treatment and Nursing Care

Treatment is aimed toward improving the circulation to the organs or parts of the body affected and relieving the symptoms. For example, the patient with arteriosclerosis of the feet and legs may have special kinds of exercises, warm baths, and massage prescribed in an effort to improve the flow of blood to his extremities. Since the amount of blood needed by an organ is increased with the amount of usage, the patient's mental and physical activity is adjusted to his vascular limitations.

The nursing care of the patient with arteriosclerosis is also determined by his symptoms. In general, sufficient rest and relaxation, good hygiene, moderate living, and freedom from worry are important.

The physician may recommend gradually increasing amounts of exercise for the patient with sclerosis of the arteries in his lower limbs. For example, the patient may be advised to walk at a leisurely pace for an increasing length of time each day. He should stop and rest for a few minutes if he has pain in his legs. Realizing that the active use of a muscle increases its blood supply, the practical nurse can more easily understand how walking can increase the circulation in the feet and legs. When the practical nurse is helping this patient to walk, she should make arrangements for him to rest if he develops pain and numbness. The practical nurse should remember that this **patient is prone to develop gangrene** (death to the part) because of poor circulation. His feet and legs should be cared for in the manner similar to that of the diabetic patient's which is discussed on pages 296 to 297.

The patient with cerebral arteriosclerosis needs to have his physical and mental activities limited. His efforts should be adjusted to his ability. The diet should be served in frequent small quantities in order to avoid the strain of digesting large quantities of food.

## HYPERTENSION

### Description

The patient with hypertension has high blood pressure. The circulatory system was described in Chapter 9 as a closed set of tubes through which blood was pumped by the heart. An artery carrying blood away from the heart may be compared with a garden hose. When the nozzle at the end of a hose is turned to decrease the size of the outlet, water pressure is greater. Arteries possess the ability to constrict. As they become smaller, the patient's blood pressure increases. The patient with a persistent systolic pressure above 140 mm of mercury or a diastolic pressure of more than 90 mm of mercury has hypertension.

The seriousness of high blood pressure depends mainly upon the changes resulting in the heart and arteries. Hypertension lasting over a period of time results in enlargement of the heart, especially of the left ventricle. This enlargement is a result of the increased work load placed on the heart as it tries to force the same amount of blood through smaller arteries. When heart disease results from hypertension, it is referred to as *hypertensive heart disease.*

Hypertension also affects the arteries. Their walls become thicker, and the size of the passageway becomes smaller. Thus, less blood reaches the body's cells. The kidneys usually suffer the most as a result of the diseased arteries. Because of this, many patients with hypertension have symptoms of impaired kidney function. Also, arteries may rupture because of the increased pressure. A ruptured blood vessel in the brain is called a *cerebral hemorrhage* (stroke).

### Cause

Hypertension is often a symptom of kidney disease, arteriosclerosis, hyperthyroidism, toxemia of pregnancy, and tumor of the adrenal gland. A great percentage of patients with high blood pressure do not have these diseases. When none of these diseases is present in a patient with high blood pressure, his condition is called *primary* or *essential hypertension.*

Although the exact cause of essential hypertension is not known, it seems to run in families. It occurs more often in overweight individuals. Essential hypertension occurs in both men and women. Emotional stresses are important factors in some cases. Severe cases of essential hypertension are known as *malignant essential hypertension.* The life expectancy of a patient with malignant essential hypertension is usually several years, whereas the patient with essential hypertension may live 10, 20, or more years.

### Symptoms

The patient with essential hypertension usually has few early symptoms. Headache, nervousness, dizziness, and visual disturbances are some of the more common ones. As hypertension progresses, the patient develops symptoms of disease in the organ which is affected most as a result of the diseased arteries. He may develop symptoms of heart disease, kidney disease, or cerebral hemorrhage.

When hypertension occurs as a symptom of another disease, the patient can be expected to have symptoms associated with that condition. For example, the patient with kidney disease has symptoms of this illness. His high blood pressure is only one of the symptoms.

### Treatment and Nursing Care

The patient whose hypertension is a symptom of another disease is treated for that condition rather than just for the elevated blood pressure. Since a specific cure for the individual with essential hypertension is not known, the treatment is mainly symptomatic. The physician usually advises the patient with essential hypertension to lead a fairly quiet life with frequent rest periods as a part of his daily living. Since emotional stress is considered an important factor, a valuable part of the treatment is the relief and avoidance of worrisome situations. Psychotherapy has proven of value to some of these patients.

A reducing diet is usually prescribed for the overweight patient. Another type of diet frequently ordered is one which is low in salt. Some physicians have had success with the Kempner rice diet which consists of rice, certain fruits, and sugar. The practical nurse can make the patient's special diet more palatable by the use of substitute seasoning agents, such as lemon, paprika, herbs, and vinegar, when these are allowed by the doctor.

A surgical procedure called *sympathectomy* is done occasionally to relieve severe cases of essential hypertension. In this operation a part of the sympathetic nervous system is excised in an effort to produce dilatation of the constricted arteries. This experimental treatment has been successful in some patients, but it appears to be slipping rapidly into the background now with the discovery of hypotensive drugs.

Hypotensive drugs produce a drop in the patient's blood pressure. Because of this change the practical nurse may be called upon to make periodic checks on the patient's blood pressure. Hexamethonium, hydralazine (Apresoline), pentolinium tartrate (Ansolysen), reserpine (Serpasil), and alkavervir (Veriloid) are examples of drugs used for their hypotensive effect.

Sedatives, such as phenobarbital, and bromide, may be prescribed by the physician. These drugs have a soothing effect which aids in preventing further increase of pressure. A relaxed patient is more likely to have a decrease in blood pressure.

## CEREBRAL VASCULAR ACCIDENT

### Definition

The patient with a cerebral vascular accident has a disease of the arteries in his brain. This results in an inadequate blood supply to

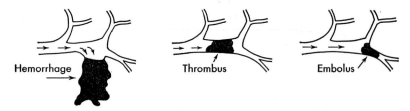

Figure 21.   The three causes of a cerebral vascular accident are hemorrhage, a thrombus, or an embolus. The portion of the brain nourished by the affected blood vessel has an inadequate supply of blood.

the part of the brain nourished by the affected blood vessel. Apoplexy, stroke, and cerebral vascular accident are names commonly used in referring to this disease.

### Cause

The three causes of a cerebral vascular accident are hemorrhage, a thrombus, or an embolus. When the stroke results from a hemorrhage, it is referred to as a cerebral hemorrhage. The patient with apoplexy caused by a thrombus has cerebral thrombosis, and the one caused by an embolus has cerebral embolism.

Rupture of a cerebral artery, or cerebral hemorrhage, results from a disease of the artery. Hypertension and arteriosclerosis are the most common causes of this disease. A congenital weakness in the wall of the blood vessel may also result in cerebral hemorrhage. Cerebral thrombosis is usually a result of arteriosclerosis or syphilis. In this case a clot forms in the diseased vessel. Cerebral embolism occurs when a particle of foreign matter, such as a blood clot and cardiac vegetations being carried through the blood stream, lodges in an artery too small for its passage.

## Symptoms

The onset of a cerebral accident is usually sudden. In general, it is more sudden in a patient with a cerebral hemorrhage than in the one with cerebral thrombosis. Some patients experience headache, a feeling of fullness in the head, and dizziness before other symptoms are evident. If the patient is awake he may collapse into a coma, or he may lose the use of a part of his body without loss of consciousness. The sleeping individual may lapse into unconsciousness without awakening, or he may fall when getting out of bed. The patient may regain consciousness in a few minutes, hours, or days or he may die without regaining consciousness.

The comatose or unconscious patient usually has a flushed face. His breathing is slow, deep, and noisy, and his cheeks flap each time he exhales. The presence of Cheyne-Stokes breathing is considered an ominous sign. His pulse is full and bounding. The patient with hypertension usually has no significant change in blood pressure. Incontinence is often present. Convulsions may occur. The patient may also develop a fever. When the temperature is high and remains so, the patient's prognosis is grave.

The patient most likely to survive this attack regains consciousness within 12 to 48 hours. It is upon the patient's return to consciousness that the presence of *paralysis,* which means loss of function,
 is most often evident. The amount of paralysis is determined by the location of the diseased cerebral artery and the size of the area involved. For example, the patient with a large thrombus in the left side of his brain is paralyzed on the right side of his body. When the thrombus is small, the patient may have a small amount of paralysis or none at all. When paralysis occurs it is present on the side opposite the cerebral accident because the fibers of the

brain cross over to serve the opposite side of the body. _Hemiplegia,_ which is paralysis of _one entire side_ of the body, is a frequent result of cerebral vascular accident. When the lesion is near the speech center in the brain, the patient has _aphasia,_ which is either the loss of speech or an impairment of speech. ʸRⁱGₕₜ

As the patient's condition improves, there may be a partial or complete return of function of the paralyzed part. However, the patient is usually left with some damage, such as difficulty in walking, impaired function of the hand, or a speech defect. Unfortunately the patient is likely to have another stroke because the condition, such as hypertension and arteriosclerosis, which caused the accident still exists.

## Treatment

The care of this patient is discussed in two phases: (1) the acute stage and (2) the convalescent stage. During the acute stage the treatment is directed toward saving the patient's life. Following this, treatment is prescribed which should enable him to regain the greatest amount of use possible of the affected part. Other members of the health team, such as the physical therapist, speech therapist, and occupational therapist, are often called upon to assist with the patient's rehabilitation.

## Nursing Care

The welfare of a patient with a cerebral vascular accident is largely dependent upon the nursing care which he receives. Because of the frequency of strokes and the patient's chronic condition following the accident, the practical nurse is an important person in his care. The practical nurse needs a deep understanding and appreciation of the mental and emotional problems of this patient and his family as well as the ability to give physical care.

### Acute Stage

The patient who has just been stricken with a cerebral vascular accident should be put to bed in a quiet room. His clothing should first be loosened, especially around the neck, and then removed.

✗ as edema of brain subsides use or partial use is regained.

A vital responsibility of the nurse is to keep the air passage clear. The patient's head should be turned slightly to one side to prevent the relaxed tongue from falling back. The nurse should remove dentures and any other loose object in the mouth which could cause suffocation. The use of an airway may be necessary. Excess mucus can be removed by suction. The head of the bed may be elevated slightly unless otherwise ordered.

It is the nurse's responsibility to protect the patient from injury. Side rails are used to prevent the patient from rolling out of bed. The convulsing patient needs additional care which is discussed on page 42.

The practical nurse should not assume that the patient cannot hear what is said because of unconsciousness. A simple explanation of what she is going to do for the patient before doing it often seems to comfort and to quiet him. Answering the family's questions about the patient should be done outside of the patient's range of hearing.

The patient's position should be changed frequently to prevent further complication, such as hypostatic pneumonia. It is important to keep his body in good alignment. The prevention of deformities should be started during the acute stage. A small pillow placed in the axilla of the paralyzed side aids in preventing the shoulder from turning toward the patient's chest. A sandbag placed on the outside of the leg keeps it from turning outward. The fingers should be extended to prevent deformity. A footboard is helpful in preventing foot drop, or the patient's feet and legs can be protected from the weight of the bedclothing with a bed cradle.

The patient who is unable to swallow is given fluid and nourishment in other ways. A common method of administering liquid nourishment is by gavage. Either the physician or the professional nurse usually inserts a tube through the nose into the stomach. After the prescribed formula has been warmed to body temperature, it is poured through the tube at periodic intervals. A small amount of water should be poured through the tube following the feeding to rinse the tube. This also gives the patient additional fluid. Intravenous injection of fluids may also be ordered.

When the patient is able to swallow, fluids and food are given by mouth. When the practical nurse is feeding a paralyzed patient, she should turn the patient's head slightly toward the unaffected side. The food should be placed in the side of the mouth which is not paralyzed.

The practical nurse needs to check the comatose patient for voiding and defecation. He may have retention of urine, which is the inability to void; or he may have incontinence, which is involuntary voiding and defecation. The physican requests that the patient with retention be catheterized. The incontinent patient should be kept clean, dry, and free from odor. The skin needs special attention to prevent decubitus ulcers. Oil or lotion may be applied to dry areas after they have been cleaned with warm water and mild soap. Changing the patient's position frequently helps to prevent excess pressure on any one area of the body. Absorbent pads are available which can be placed under the incontinent patient to help protect his bed and linen. Placing the urinal in position for the male patient helps to keep him dry. Occasionally a catheter is inserted and left in place to prevent the urine from irritating the skin. This is referred to as an indwelling catheter. It may cause serious irritation to the bladder and urethra. The physician may prescribe an enema for the incontinent patient. Giving a small enema daily helps to relieve rectal incontinence in some patients.

The patient's mouth should be kept clean and moist. A lubricating substance, such as mineral oil or glycerin, can be applied to the lips to prevent chapping.

### Convalescent Stage

Upon the patient's return to consciousness he becomes aware of his disabilities such as paralysis and speech disorder. The practical nurse can have a better understanding of the emotional shock experienced by the patient if she pauses for a moment and tries to imagine how she would feel if she awakened one morning and could not talk or move properly. When the patient becomes aware of his helplessness, he needs encouragement from the practical nurse. She should try to anticipate his needs, especially if he cannot talk. She can try to discover his wishes by identifying various objects. The nurse needs to realize that, although the patient cannot talk, this does not mean necessarily that he is unable to think or to reason. The family should have this explained to them.

The practical nurse who understands that this patient is likely to be emotionally unstable at first is more capable of paying little attention to unusual outbursts of emotion. The patient is likely to start crying or laughing suddenly. This may also be upsetting to the patient's family. The nurse can often ease their concern over this unusual reaction by explaining to them that this frequently occurs following a stroke.

The practical nurse should point out to the patient improvements that are being made. For example, when the patient is first able to do such a minor thing as holding his bread, or helping turn himself, the nurse should encourage the patient by calling this to his attention. He needs genuine praise from the nurse. Short-term goals, such as accomplishments which are likely to be made in the near future, should be stressed rather than long-term ones. For example, the goal of being able to feed himself is much more real and close than the final one of complete or maximal recovery.

Measures to prevent deformities which were started during the acute stage need to be continued. In addition to keeping the body in good alignment, the practical nurse may receive specific instructions regarding simple massage and exercises for the patient.

Although other members of the health team render an invaluable service to the patient, the practical nurse is often the one who is present during the patient's periods of discouragement. Her continued encouragement is an important factor in his return to maximal usefulness.

## VARICOSE VEINS

### Description

It is necessary for the practical nurse to recall certain important points about the veins if she is to have a clear understanding of varicose veins. Blood is returned to the heart through blood vessels called veins. She has only to look at her foot to realize that the blood is usually returning uphill. The squeezing action of muscles as well as the valves within the veins aid the blood in its upward climb.

The valve flaps close to keep the blood from flowing backward. Stretching of the vein walls causes the valve flaps to close improperly. Therefore, the valve leaks and blood flows backward. This increased amount of blood causes further dilation of the vein. Because of its elasticity, the vein becomes longer as well as larger. The vein appears tortuous, which means that it is twisted, when it can be seen beneath the skin. The practical nurse may find it helpful to think of a tortuous vein as being similar to a winding stream in appearance. Thus, a person with varicose veins has dilated and tortuous veins.

### Cause

An individual is most likely to develop varicosities in the surface veins of his legs. A tendency toward weakness of the vein walls and valves may be inherited. Varicose veins often occur during pregnancy because of pressure from the growing fetus on pelvic veins. They are also likely to develop in obese persons as a result of pressure from pads of fat on vessels in the pelvic area. Varicosities can result from long periods of standing and of wearing tight garments. Pressure from close-fitting clothes interferes with the return flow of blood which causes the vein to dilate.

### Symptoms

The person with varicose veins experiences a feeling of heaviness and tiredness in his legs. Aching and muscle cramps often occur. The vein becomes bluish, knotted, and tortuous. Bluish lumps are present which disappear slightly when the feet are elevated. Blood which should be going back to the lungs for oxygen stays in the vein longer than normal. This slowing down of venous blood interferes with the flow of oxygenated blood through capillaries. As a result the cells in that area are poorly nourished. This often results in varicose ulcers which are difficult to heal because of their underlying cause.

### Treatment

An important part of the treatment for varicose veins is prevention. Undergarments such as circular garters, tight girdles, and rolled hose should not be worn. It is best to avoid sitting for long periods of time while wearing a girdle. Activities which require a great deal of standing should be interrupted by regular rest periods during which the individual can elevate his feet as well as walk around. The pregnant woman should start her visits to the doctor early in an effort to prevent varicose veins and other complications of pregnancy.

The physician may prescribe an elastic stocking or an elastic bandage to relieve the discomfort from varicose veins. Pressure from these forces the blood into deeper veins which usually have healthier walls and valves. Injections of a sclerosing medication, such as sodium morrhuate, may be performed by the doctor. This substance blocks the blood vessel so that blood must return through other veins. Vein ligation is a surgical procedure in which the upper end of the vein is closed by tying; the blood vessel eventually dies. Stripping is another surgical procedure in which a portion of the vein is removed.

## THROMBOPHLEBITIS

Thrombophlebitis is the term used when there is a thrombus (clot) in the vein and the wall of that vein is inflamed. This condition most often affects the veins in the leg and pelvis. It may occur in any condition in which the return flow of blood to the heart is affected. For this reason it is often a complication of diseases which cause the patient to have long periods of bed rest. Thrombophlebitis is commonly seen in patients following lower abdominal surgery, delivery, and acute infections. The practical nurse may have heard this condition referred to as *milk leg*. It was called milk leg because it commonly followed childbirth. Injury and varicose veins may also cause thrombophlebitis.

A patient with thrombophlebitis can have varying degrees of the symptoms associated with an inflammation. When the vein affected is in the leg, the patient's extremity is swollen, warm, red, and painful. The patient experiences general symptoms of an inflammation, such as fever and malaise, depending upon the severity of the condition.

This patient is treated with bed rest. The affected limb should be elevated. In some cases the diseased vein is ligated above and below the thrombosed area. This is done mainly to prevent *embolism,* in which portions of the clot flow through the blood stream and lodge in other areas of the body. Embolism is the chief danger of thrombophlebitis since the embolus may lodge in a vital organ such as the lungs or brain. Heparin and bishydrocoumarin (Dicumarol) are examples of anticoagulants often prescribed by the physician to slow down further thrombosis.

## THROMBOANGIITIS OBLITERANS (BUERGER'S DISEASE)

The patient with thromboangiitis obliterans, or Buerger's disease, has a chronic inflammation of the blood vessels, especially in his legs. The cause is not known. It occurs most often in young men, is more common in heavy smokers, and is especially common among Jews.

Symptoms result from a deficient blood supply. Severe cramps in the calves of the legs occur with walking and are usually relieved by rest. The feet are cold, and may be red when hanging down and pale when elevated. The pulse in the affected extremity may be weak or absent. Gangrene is likely to occur.

Measures to improve circulation such as Buerger's exercises are often prescribed. In ordering these exercises, the physician designates the specific length of time for the patient to keep his feet and legs in various positions. The use of tobacco is prohibited. Since this patient is likely to develop gangrene, his feet and legs will need to be cared for in a manner similar to that of a diabetic patient which is discussed on pages 296 to 297. Amputation is often necessary.

## SUGGESTIONS FOR STUDY

1. Compare an old rubber hose with a new one to aid in understanding the changes occurring in the arteries of a person with arteriosclerosis.

2. With what diseases is arteriosclerosis often associated?

3. Why is a patient with arteriosclerosis likely to develop a thrombus?

*P. 140* 4. Why is a patient with hypertension likely to develop an enlarged heart?

*P. 142* 5. What are the three causes of a cerebral vascular accident?

*P. 143* 6. What two main factors determine the amount of paralysis in a person who has had a stroke? *location size of area*

*P. 144* 7. Why is this patient likely to have another stroke?

8. Discuss the nursing care of a patient with a cerebral vascular accident during the acute and convalescent stages.

*P. 148* 9. Discuss the cause, prevention, and treatment for varicose veins.

10. What is the difference between an embolus and a thrombus?

*P. 150* 11. What is thromboangiitis obliterans (Buerger's disease)? *inf. vessels*

12. Can arteriosclerosis cause hypertension? *yes*

13. What disease of the arteries in the feet and legs can cause a person to need special care of his extremities? Review the care of a diabetic person's feet and legs which is given on pages 296 to 297.

## REFERENCES FOR CHAPTER 10

Brooks, Stewart M.: *Basic Facts of Pharmacology*. W. B. Saunders Co., Philadelphia, 1957, pp. 116-20.

Brown, Amy F., *Medical Nursing*, 3rd ed. W. B. Saunders Co., Philadelphia, 1957, pp. 279-324 and 650-60.

Eliason, Eldridge; Ferguson, L. Kraeer; and Sholtis, Lillian A.: *Surgical Nursing*, 10th ed. J. B. Lippincott Co., Philadelphia, 1955, pp. 260-77.

Emerson, Charles P., Jr., and Bradgon, Jane S.: *Essentials of Medicine*, 17th ed. J. B. Lippincott Co., Philadelphia, 1955, pp. 253-72 and 626-32.

Faddis, Margene O., and Hayman, Joseph M.: *Care of the Medical Patient*. McGraw-Hill Book Co., New York, 1952, pp. 199-210 and 479-86.

Hull, Edgar, and Perrodin, Cecilia: *Medical Nursing*, 5th ed. F. A. Davis Co., Philadelphia, 1954, pp. 220-48.

"If You Ask Me—How Do You Establish Communication with Patients Who Are Aphasic?" *Am. J. Nursing*, 56:1415, (Nov.) 1956.

Jensen, Julius, and Jensen, Deborah: *Nursing in Clinical Medicine*, 4th ed. The Macmillan Company, New York, 1954, pp. 590-601.

Krause, Marie: *Nutrition and Diet Therapy*, 2nd ed. W. B. Saunders Co., Philadelphia, 1957, pp. 304-7.

Musser, Ruth D., and Bird, Joseph G.: *Modern Pharmacology and Therapeutics*. The Macmillan Company, New York, 1958, pp. 558-77.

Proudfit, Fairfax T., and Robinson, Corinne H.: *Nutrition and Diet*

*extra systolic*

*Therapy*, 11th ed. The Macmillan Company, New York, 1955, pp. 458-77.

Sensenig, David M., and Morson, Betty J.: "Buerger's Disease," *Am. J. Nursing*, **57**:337-40, (Mar.) 1957.

Smith, Genevieve W.: "A Stroke Is Not the End of the World," *Am. J. Nursing*, **57**:303-5, (Mar.) 1957.

Stanton, Joseph R.: "Venous Thrombosis and Pulmonary Embolism," *Am. J. Nursing*, **55**:709-11, (June) 1955.

Young, Helen, and Lee, Eleanor: *Lippincott's Quick Reference Book for Nurses*, 7th ed. J. B. Lippincott Co., Philadelphia, 1955, pp. 93-97.

# Chapter 11

*THE PATIENT*
*WITH A DISEASE OF*
*THE BLOOD*

| *Chapter* | STRUCTURE AND FUNCTION | HODGKIN'S DISEASE |
|---|---|---|
| *Outline* | ANEMIA | HEMOPHILIA |
| | LEUKEMIA | MALARIA |

## STRUCTURE AND FUNCTION

Blood is the fluid which flows through the circulatory system. It has the vital task of carrying oxygen and food to all cells in the body. Also, it removes waste material from the cells.

### Plasma

The liquid portion of blood is known as plasma. Over one-half of the total amount of blood is made of this straw-colored fluid. Body tissues receive water, food, hormones, and immune substances from plasma. Plasma also contains *fibrinogen*, which is a substance necessary for the clotting of blood.

### Blood Cells

Three types of blood cells are found in plasma. Almost one-half of the total amount of blood is composed of these cells. Blood cells are formed in the marrow of bones, in the lymph nodes, and in the spleen. The three kinds of cells are (1) red blood cells, which are known as erythrocytes or R.B.C.'s; (2) white blood cells, which are known as leukocytes or W.B.C.'s; and (3) platelets.

#### Red Blood Cells

The main function of red blood cells (erythrocytes) is to carry oxygen to the body's cells and to remove carbon dioxide. The transportation of oxygen is made possible by a substance in the red blood cells which is called *hemoglobin.* This is the coloring matter in the red blood cells which contains iron. Since hemoglobin mixes readily with oxygen, it is the agent within the red blood cell which picks up oxygen as blood is pumped through the lungs. After delivering oxygen to the body's tissues, the red blood cells remove carbon dioxide.

Red blood cells are produced in the red marrow of bones in adults. After spending approximately 120 days in the blood stream, they are destroyed in the liver and spleen.

The normal red blood cell count ranges from 4½ to 5 million in 1 cu mm of blood. In other words, this is the average number of red blood cells which would be found in a drop of blood the size of a small pinhead. The count is slightly higher in men than in women. The normal amount of hemoglobin is approximately 15 gm per 100 ml of blood, or 80 to 100 per cent.

### White Blood Cells

White blood cells (leukocytes) play an important part in protecting the body against inflammation. For example, leukocytes remove dead cells from an inflamed area and combat the invading bacteria. There are three main types of white blood cells. When the physician requests the laboratory to do a differential count, he is interested in knowing the (number of each type.) Often this is a valuable aid to him in diagnosing the patient's illness, as the normal count of different white blood cells varies with certain diseases.

The normal white blood cell count ranges from 5000 to 10,000 in 1 cu mm of blood (tiny drop). The count increases in a patient with an infection. The patient has *leukocytosis* when the white blood cell count is higher than 10,000. When the count is under 5000 he has *leukopenia*.

### Platelets

Platelets are minute particles in blood. They play an important part in stopping hemorrhage. Platelets collect in an injured area and give off a substance which is necessary for the clotting of blood.

### ANEMIA

### Definition

Anemia means a decrease in the number of red blood cells or in the amount of hemoglobin. Usually both are reduced.

### Cause

An individual develops anemia when (1) there is defective formation of red blood cells, (2) red blood cells are destroyed more rapidly
than they are formed, and (3) blood is lost from the body.

## Anemia due to Defective Formation of Red Blood Cells

An insufficient amount of blood is produced when the body does
not receive the substances necessary for blood formation. Vitamins
$B_{12}$ and C, liver, iron, and proteins are necessary for the production of red blood cells. An inadequate supply of these substances
results in anemia. Also, poor absorption of these essential factors
from the gastrointestinal tract can cause anemia. As red blood cells
are formed in bone marrow, disease of this area, such as cancer,
results in defective formation of blood.

### Pernicious Anemia

The patient with pernicious anemia has an inadequate production
of red blood cells and hemoglobin. His anemia continues to increase
unless treated. Persons developing this disease were doomed to die
until the treatment was discovered in 1926; now no one should die
from it. This is one of the many advances made in medical science
during the present century which was mentioned in Chapter 1.

Pernicious anemia occurs most often in an individual over 40
years of age. Normally the stomach secretes a substance needed for
the digestion and absorption of materials which are necessary for
the production of red blood cells. This gastric substance is lacking
in a person with pernicious anemia. It has been found that liver
extract and vitamin $B_{12}$ supply the missing factor.

SYMPTOMS. The patient with pernicious anemia complains of
tiredness, indigestion, and tingling or numbness in his hands and
feet. His tongue is sore and appears red and smooth. His skin has
a yellowish color. When the contents of his stomach are examined
in the test called a gastric analysis, no hydrochloric acid is found.
(It is interesting to note that the administration of hydrochloric
acid does not cure the anemia.) His red blood cell count and hemoglobin are low.

TREATMENT. The patient with pernicious anemia can be treated
successfully with liver extract or with vitamin $B_{12}$. At first large

doses are given. When the blood picture has returned to normal, liver extract or vitamin $B_{12}$ is given less often and in smaller doses. The doctor determines the amount of medication needed to keep the red blood count normal. It is necessary for the patient to continue this treatment for the rest of his life.

### Anemia due to Increased Destruction of Red Blood Cells

An individual develops anemia when his red blood cells and hemoglobin are destroyed faster than they can be replaced by the bone marrow. This abnormal destruction can occur in the bone marrow when it is exposed to sufficient amounts of x-ray and radium. As these radioactive substances check the growth of cells, red blood cells are destroyed before reaching the blood stream. Infections of the blood stream, such as malaria, cause anemia; also certain drugs, such as the sulfonamides, destroy red blood cells.

### Anemia due to Blood Loss

Anemia follows the loss of an excessive amount of blood from the body. It can occur after one large hemorrhage or after smaller amounts of blood are lost over a period of time. Symptoms of shock which are discussed on page 57 are present in the acutely hemorrhaging patient.

### Symptoms

Since the patient with anemia has fewer red blood cells and less hemoglobin, the ability of his blood to carry oxygen is lessened. His main symptoms result from an inadequate supply of oxygen to the tissues. Shortness of breath, weakness, dizziness, and nervousness are symptoms frequently felt by this patient. He tires easily and has a poor appetite, and his skin and mucous membranes are pale. He often notices *palpitation*, which is an awareness of his heartbeat. It may seem to be fast or fluttering.

### Treatment

The physician bases his treatment of a patient with anemia due to increased destruction of red blood cells upon its cause. Blood transfusions are used in treating a person for hemorrhage. This treatment is used also when the red blood cell count and hemoglobin are extremely low in patients who have not hemorrhaged. Iron is given when the individual's intake of this substance is inadequate. The physician usually prescribes a diet high in protein, iron, and vitamins B and C.

## LEUKEMIA

### Description

Different types of leukemia constitute a group of diseases in which there is an abnormal increase of white blood cells, or leukocytes. To date the cause of leukemia has not been discovered. This is a fatal disease for which no cure is known. The more acute forms affect children and young adults.

The practical nurse needs to know that there are different types of leukemia. For example, the physician may classify it according to the speed of its development and the type of white blood cell. In referring to its speed of development, the doctor may call it acute, subacute, or chronic leukemia. In order better to understand that leukemia is classified according to the type of white blood cell, the practical nurse needs to recall the fact that blood contains three main types of white cells. A marked increase of one kind of white blood cell is referred to as a specific type of leukemia. For example, the patient with monocytic leukemia has an increased number of a type of white blood cells known as monocytes.

### Symptoms

The symptoms of different types of leukemia are often similar. The patient with this disease usually has an increased white blood cell count. There is an enlargement of the tissue which produces that particular kind of leukocyte. For example, frequently the spleen is enlarged; in some types of leukemia the lymph nodes are larger than normal. The patient feels weak and has a fever during the active stage. He develops infections easily. Ulcers form in and around his mouth. He is likely to hemorrhage because of fewer platelets, which help to check bleeding. Frequently there is bleeding from the nose, the gums, and the stomach; also anemia is present.

### Treatment and Nursing Care

As the cure of leukemia has not yet been discovered, the treatment and nursing care of this patient are symptomatic (aimed toward relieving the symptoms). Often the patient with leukemia is treated with x-ray. The purpose of this is to slow down the tissues which are producing such large numbers of white blood cells. Nursing care of a patient receiving radiotherapy is discussed on pages 89 to 90.

Special efforts should be made to protect the patient against infections because of his lowered resistance. His skin should be kept clean by daily cleansing baths. Symptoms of skin irritation should be reported promptly and treated according to the doctor's orders. The practical nurse should give special care to this patient's mouth because of the likelihood of his developing ulcerations.

The patient's anemia is treated with iron and blood transfusions. During the acute stage when fever is present, the practical nurse can use nursing measures for the patient's comfort which are discussed on page 36.

## HODGKIN'S DISEASE

### Description

A patient with Hodgkin's disease has a disease of the lymph nodes. It was named for an English doctor who first described it. Hodgkin's disease occurs more often in men than in women. Its cause is not known, but it is thought to be either a malignancy or an infection. Usually this disease is fatal within three to four years.

### Symptoms

The lymph nodes in the neck are generally the first to become enlarged in a patient with Hodgkin's disease. Later the lymph nodes under his arm and in his groin and abdomen increase in size. Also, the spleen may become larger than normal. As the lymph nodes enlarge, they press on nearby organs; this pressure causes additional symptoms. For example, diseased nodes in the neck may press on the trachea causing dyspnea; enlarged nodes in the chest may cause symptoms of lung disease; and enlargement of lymph nodes in the abdomen may result in nausea, vomiting, and diarrhea.

As the disease progresses, the patient loses weight and energy, develops anemia, and may have an increased number of white blood cells. Also, *pruritis*, which is (itching of the skin,) develops. The patient has periods of fever which alternate with periods of normal temperature.

### Treatment

Since no specific cure for this disease has yet been found, the treatment of a patient with Hodgkin's disease is directed toward making him comfortable.

Radiation therapy is used to slow down the overgrowth of lymph nodes. This prolongs the patient's life and makes him more comfortable. Nitrogen mustard is given intravenously for the same purpose. Blood transfusions may be given to relieve the patient's anemia. When large masses of lymph nodes produce symptoms of pressure, this tissue can be removed by surgery.

## HEMOPHILIA

### Description

Hemophilia is a rare disease which is hereditary and occurs only in males. It is transmitted to the male through the female. Often a patient with hemophilia is referred to as a "bleeder."

### Symptoms

The blood of a patient with hemophilia takes longer than normal to clot. The clotting time may be an hour or more. The normal length of time required for blood to clot is 3 to 10 minutes. The patient with hemophilia bleeds longer than normal after a slight injury. The oozing may stop after a while, but eventually this disease is fatal. Often there is bleeding into his joints which results in deformity. Large bruises appear following hemorrhage under the skin.

### Treatment

Women who are known to transmit hemophilia may be advised to have no more children. Although a woman is of a hemophilic family, this does not mean necessarily that her sons will have this disease.

A child with hemophilia should be protected against injury. When bleeding occurs, he is treated with complete bed rest and blood transfusions.

## MALARIA

Many textbooks for nurses have a chapter dealing with infectious diseases in which the discussion of malaria is included. The major portion of this text deals with the care of patients having diseases of the various systems. Some of the more common infectious diseases are included in the discussion of the system which is often affected by that infection rather than in a separate chapter. For these reasons, malaria is included in this chapter which deals with the care of patients with a disease of the blood.

### Description

Malaria is a common infectious disease in many parts of the world. It is caused by protozoa, which are microorganisms belonging to the animal kingdom. The protozoa causing malaria are introduced into a person's body through the bite of an infected female Anopheles mosquito. As this insect is found more frequently in tropical and subtropical areas, malaria is more common in these regions.

Protozoa causing malaria are called parasites because it is necessary for them to obtain food from another living organism. After the parasite has been introduced into a person's body by the Anopheles mosquito, it enters a red blood cell. While there, it grows by dividing and subdividing until the red blood cell is filled with parasites. The wall of the red blood cell ruptures, allowing the young parasites to enter the blood stream. The patient has shaking chills followed by fever during this time. The protozoa enter more erythrocytes, and the process of growth and rupturing of the red blood cells is re-peated.

There are four types of malaria. Each is caused by a different kind of malarial parasite. The time required for each of these four parasites to reproduce and to cause the red blood cells to rupture varies. Thus the patient who has chills and fever every two days has a type of malaria caused by a parasite which differs from the parasite causing a patient to have chills and fever every three days.

### Symptoms

The patient with malaria has attacks of fever. Usually these bouts of fever occur at regular intervals. Frequently the patient experiences a shaking chill, headache, nausea, and vomiting at the beginning of this acute attack. After the temperature returns to normal, the patient usually feels well until he has a return of symptoms.

If the patient is not treated, his general health becomes affected. He develops anemia because the protozoa are destroying the red blood cells. The spleen may become enlarged since it is filled with blood pigment and red blood cells containing malarial parasites. The patient may become unconscious and die if he is not treated promptly and adequately.

### Treatment and Nursing Care

Fortunately drugs which kill the malarial parasite have been discovered. Chloroquine, quinacrine (Atabrine), and quinine are three examples of drugs which the physician may prescribe for this patient.

The nursing care of the patient having an acute attack of malaria is symptomatic. The care of a patient having a chill, fever, anorexia, nausea, and vomiting is discussed in Chapter 4.

Malaria can be prevented if the people living in areas where malaria is common avoid coming in contact with Anopheles mosquitoes. This can be done by draining pools of stagnant water where these insects breed. Pouring oil on stagnant water causes the mosquito larvae to die. This seemingly simple measure is effective because the larvae must come to the surface to obtain air, and when the water's surface is covered with oil, the larvae's supply of air is cut off and they die. Houses and beds should be screened in mosquito-infested areas. When it is not possible to avoid exposure to these mosquitoes, quinine or quinacrine (Atabrine) may be given to prevent the individuals from developing malaria.

## SUGGESTIONS FOR STUDY

1. Review the function of red blood cells, white blood cells, and hemoglobin.
2. What is the normal red blood cell count? The normal white blood cell count?
3. What are the three main causes of anemia?

4. In which type of anemia is it necessary for the patient to continue indefinitely taking either liver extract or vitamin B₁₂? *Pernicious*
5. Why is a patient who is having a massive hemorrhage likely to develop shortness of breath? *lack of O₂*
6. Review the symptoms of leukemia. *ulcers mouth, anemia, weak, fever*
7. Discuss the nursing care of a patient with leukemia. *x-ray · symptomatic*
8. Which sex is affected by hemophilia? *male*
9. How is malaria transmitted? *bus?*
10. What causes a patient with malaria to have chills?
11. How can malaria be prevented?

## REFERENCES FOR CHAPTER 11

Brown Amy F.: *Medical Nursing*, 3rd ed. W. B. Saunders Co., Philadelphia, 1957, pp. 340-79.

Carter, Charles F., and Smith, Alice L.: *Principles of Microbiology*, 3rd ed. C. V. Mosby Co., St. Louis, 1957, pp. 536-42.

Emerson, Charles P., Jr., and Bragdon, Jane S.: *Essentials of Medicine*, 17th ed. J. B. Lippincott Co., Philadelphia, 1955, pp. 203-44 and 852-57.

Faddis, Margene O., and Hayman, Joseph M.: *Care of the Medical Patient*. McGraw-Hill Book Co., New York, 1952, pp. 617-19.

Goodale, Raymond H.: *Nursing Pathology*, 2nd ed. W. B. Saunders Co., Philadelphia, 1956, pp. 243-64.

Hartmann, John R., and Bolduc, Rose A.: "Hemophilia," *Am. J. Nursing*, 56:169-74, (Feb.) 1956.

Hull, Edgar, and Perrodin, Cecilia: *Medical Nursing*, 5th ed. F. A. Davis Co., Philadelphia, 1954, pp. 254-91.

Jensen, Julius, and Jensen, Deborah: *Nursing in Clinical Medicine*, 4th ed. The Macmillan Company, New York, 1954, pp. 303-31.

Krause, Marie: *Nutrition and Diet Therapy*, 2nd ed. W. B. Saunders Co., Philadelphia, 1957, pp. 309-14.

Marple, Charles D., and McIntyre, Marie J.: "Anticoagulant Therapy," *Am. J. Nursing*, 56:875-79, (July) 1956.

Muller, Gulli L., and Dawes, Dorothy E.: *Introduction to Medical Science*, 4th ed. W. B. Saunders Co., Philadelphia, 1958, pp. 279-317.

Proudfit, Fairfax T., and Robinson, Corinne H.: *Nutrition and Diet Therapy*, 11th ed. The Macmillan Company, New York, 1955, pp. 491-98.

Solomon, Charles, and Gill, Elizabeth S.: *Pharmacology and Therapeutics*, 7th ed. J. B. Lippincott Co., Philadelphia, 1956, pp. 303-26.

Wilson, Henry E., and Price, Geraldine: "Leukemia," *Am. J. Nursing*, 56:601-5, (May) 1956.

*Nursing the Patient*

*with a Disease of*

*the Respiratory System*

PART IV

*Wednesday 2-23-66*

Chapter 12

# THE PATIENT
# WITH A DISEASE
# OF THE UPPER
# RESPIRATORY SYSTEM

## STRUCTURE AND FUNCTION

Every cell in the body must be supplied with oxygen and relieved of carbon dioxide. This exchange of gases is called *respiration* or breathing. Respiration consists of taking air into the lungs, which is known as *inspiration*, and forcing air out of the lungs, which is known as *expiration*. Breathing is controlled by the respiratory center in the brain. Inspiration of air is made possible by contraction of the muscles of the diaphragm and the chest. This enlarges the chest cavity, which contains the lungs, and allows air to enter. An elastic recoil action of the lungs and gravity normally force air from the lungs during expiration.

The respiratory system is a group of organs which make it possible for the blood to exchange gases with air. These organs are the nose, pharynx or throat, larynx or voice box, trachea or windpipe, bronchi, and lungs.

Usually air enters the body through the nose where it is filtered, warmed, and moistened. It also enters through the mouth. Air passes from the nose into the nasopharynx, which is the space between the nose and throat. As air is carried to the lungs, it passes from the nasopharynx into the pharynx or throat. It then goes through the larynx into the trachea. Air is carried from the trachea through the two main bronchi into the bronchial tubes and the bronchioles of the lungs. Tiny sacs called alveoli are located at the end of the bronchioles. Oxygen and carbon dioxide are exchanged between air and blood here in these minute sacs. Having lost much of its oxygen and picked up carbon dioxide from the blood stream, the air leaves the

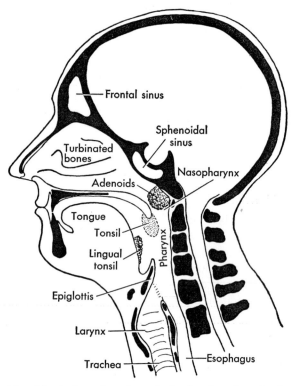

Frontal sinus

Sphenoidal sinus

Turbinated bones

Nasopharynx

Adenoids

Tongue

Tonsil

Lingual tonsil

Pharynx

Epiglottis

Larynx

Trachea

Esophagus

**Figure 22.** Vertical section through the head and neck, showing the principal anatomic features of the upper respiratory tract. (Burdon, Kenneth: *Textbook of Microbiology,* 4th ed. The Macmillan Company, New York, 1958.)

body through the same route. The blood containing a fresh supply of oxygen returns to the heart, which pumps it to all parts of the body.

The lower part of the respiratory system consists of the bronchi and their branches and the lungs, whereas the upper part of the respiratory system consists of the nose, pharynx, larynx, and trachea. Nursing patients with diseases commonly affecting the upper res-

*Also sinus*

piratory system is discussed in this chapter. The sinuses are included because of their relationship to the nose.

Four pairs of hollow cavities in the head drain directly into the nose. These cavities are called *sinuses*. They are the ethmoidal, sphenoidal, maxillary, and frontal sinuses.

## THE COMMON COLD

### Description

The common cold is an acute infection which most often affects the upper respiratory system: nose, pharynx, and larynx. It is caused by one or more viruses. Although fatigue, chilling of the body, and wet feet do not cause the common cold, these factors may lower an individual's resistance to the virus.

A cold is the most common infection of the respiratory system. The cold and its complications cause the loss of a larger number of working days than any other disease. Most people have one or more attacks of this infection every year. A person's immunity to the common cold varies with different individuals. Resistance seems to be increased for a short period of time following a cold.

The viruses are spread by an individual who is sneezing, coughing, and blowing his nose during the early stage of the cold. They may be spread also by direct contact, such as by kissing.

The mucous membranes lining the nose and throat become inflamed when a person develops a cold. His resistance to secondary invasion by bacteria present in these areas, such as streptococci and pneumococci, is lowered. Thus, colds can be complicated by pneumonia, infections of the ear, sinusitis, and bronchitis.

### Symptoms

Usually a person notices a burning or itching feeling in the back of his nose and throat when the cold begins. Within several hours he has a watery discharge from his nose. The mucous membranes are swollen, and the nasal passage may become closed. In a few days the clear mucous discharge gradually decreases and becomes slightly yellow.

The patient with a cold also has general symptoms of inflammation. He generally has malaise, a chilly feeling, generalized aches and pains, a headache, and a burning feeling in his eyes. His temperature may be elevated. If the infection spreads into the larynx and bronchi, the patient becomes hoarse and develops a cough. At first the cough is dry and hacking; then it becomes productive.

## Treatment and Nursing Care

Specific measures to prevent the common cold have not yet proved effective. The use of vaccine, vitamins, and outdoor exercise has not been successful in preventing a cold. The best safeguards against developing this disease are to avoid contact with persons suffering from a cold and to maintain the best possible health. A person should avoid excessive exposure and becoming overly tired.

After the cold has developed, the treatment is entirely symptomatic. The patient should avoid contact with others whenever possible to prevent spreading the disease. If the patient's temperature is 37.8° C (100° F) or over he should rest in bed. He should be encouraged to drink an adequate amount of fluids. Frequently aspirin and other similar drugs are prescribed to relieve the generalized aches and pains. Discomfort from nasal congestion is relieved by nasal spray or nose drops as ordered by the doctor. The inhalation of steam may be used to soothe the irritated mucous membrane. A cough mixture may be ordered to relieve a useless, dry, and irritating cough. Drugs, such as the sulfonamides, penicillin, and streptomycin, do not cure the common cold. They may be effective in preventing or curing a bacterial infection, such as sinusitis and pneumonia, when it is a complication of the common cold.

## SINUSITIS

### Description

The patient with sinusitis has an inflammation of the mucous membrane lining one or more of his sinuses. The opening which leads from the air-filled cavity to the nose has become narrowed or closed; this can be caused by congestion of the nasal mucosa and by a plug of pus or of mucus blocking the tiny passage.

Sinusitis often occurs with infections of the nose such as the common cold. Usually inflammation of the sinuses disappears when the nasal infection is cured. Also, nasal obstruction caused by an allergy may result in sinusitis (see Chap. 8). The maxillary sinuses of the cheek can become infected from an abscess of an upper tooth.

### Symptoms

Secretions from the mucous membrane lining the sinus do not drain properly when the opening which leads to the nose is obstructed. This causes pressure on the sinus wall and results in pain. The patient generally complains of a facial headache on the involved side. He may also have tenderness over the area.

Bacteria growing in the nonflowing secretions may cause an infection. In this case, the patient has *acute sinusitis.* In addition to having pain over the affected area, he has symptoms of an infection, such as fever and malaise.

Sinusitis which continues over a period of time may cause an inflammation of the lower respiratory tract. Infectious material drains from the sinus into the nose and throat. If it is aspirated into the bronchi and lungs over a period of time, the patient may develop chronic bronchitis.

### Treatment

Treatment of a patient with sinusitis is directed toward promoting drainage of the sinus. Infection, allergy, and other conditions causing nasal congestion are also treated. The use of sprays or drops of drugs, such as epinephrine (Adrenalin), ephedrine, and phenylephrine (Neo-synephrine), may be prescribed. These drugs cause the mucous membrane to shrink. Local application of heat is ordered frequently to relieve the pain. The physician may prescribe an antibiotic to combat infection. He may also irrigate the involved sinus to remove the secretions which have collected within the cavity.

If medical treatment does not cause the diseased sinus to drain, surgery may be necessary. In some cases it is necessary for the surgeon to provide external drainage of the cavity. An incision is made above the upper teeth to drain the maxillary sinus and in the eyebrow to drain the frontal sinus.

## PHARYNGITIS

### Description

The patient with pharyngitis has an inflamed pharynx or a sore throat. This condition may be caused by either irritation or infection. For example, irritation from excessive smoking, inhaling irritating substances such as dust and chemicals, and talking too much can result in a sore throat. Usually pharyngitis is associated with infections of the upper respiratory tract, such as the common cold and sinusitis. Discharge from the nose and sinuses drains into the throat causing it to become inflamed. Also pharyngitis may result from a direct infection by viruses and bacteria such as the streptococci.

A sore throat can be a symptom of other diseases, such as poliomyelitis and diphtheria, or it may be followed by rheumatic fever. As these infections occur more frequently in children, the practical nurse needs to understand the importance of reporting to the physician a sore throat especially in a child.

## Symptoms

A patient with pharyngitis can have both local and general symptoms of inflammation such as redness of the throat and fever. These symptoms vary according to the cause. The person who has been smoking excessively may have only a red or slightly scratchy throat, whereas a patient with an acute infection in the pharynx has an extremely sore throat and discomfort when swallowing. He also has general symptoms of inflammation, such as fever, malaise, and headache.

## Treatment and Nursing Care

After determining the cause of the patient's pharyngitis, the physician plans the treatment. If the condition is a result of irritation, he tries to remove the irritating factor. For example, the patient who is smoking excessively is advised to stop; the person who has been using his voice too much needs to reduce talking to a minimum.

The patient should have bed rest when an acute infection is the cause of his pharyngitis. In some cases the doctor orders isolation, which is separating the infected person from those not infected with the same disease. Drugs to combat the invading bacteria are prescribed. Application of either cold or heat may be ordered. Frequently heat is used in the form of gargles. An example of this is warm salt water (saline). The application of an ice collar to the neck is the method commonly used in applying cold to the area. Since it is painful for the patient to swallow, it is necessary for the practical nurse to encourage the patient to drink fluids. The principles of nursing a patient with an inflammation in Chapter 6 should be reviewed.

## TONSILLITIS

### Description

Tonsillitis is an inflammation of the lymphatic tissue in the throat known as tonsils. Frequently the adenoids, lymphatic tissue in the nasopharynx, are inflamed also.

The patient with tonsillitis has symptoms of pharyngitis. In addition, his tonsils are red and swollen, and may have whitish patches on them.

### Treatment and Nursing Care

The treatment and nursing care of a patient with an acute attack of tonsillitis are the same as those discussed under pharyngitis. After the acute infection has been cured, the physician may recommend surgery.

#### *Tonsillectomy*

##### *Description*

Surgical removal of the tonsils is known as *tonsillectomy*. The physician generally removes the adenoids in connection with the tonsillectomy, if he finds that the patient's adenoids are diseased also. Pieces of lymphatic tissue located in the nasopharynx are known as *adenoids.* Enlargement of the *adenoids* is present mainly in childhood, and may cause the child to be a mouth breather because it obstructs the nasopharynx. When a patient is scheduled for a tonsillectomy and adenoidectomy, the operation is referred to as a "T and A."

##### *Preoperative Care*

In addition to the care of a patient before surgery already discussed in Chapter 5, the physician orders the blood to be examined to determine whether or not it clots normally. Normally it takes the blood from 3 to 10 minutes to clot after being exposed to air. The length of time varies slightly with the technique used to determine the *clotting time.* The patient with a prolonged clotting time is a poor surgical risk because of the danger of hemorrhage; therefore, this condition is treated before surgery. Sometimes vitamin K is administered to hasten the clotting of blood. Some physicians order this drug for almost all of their patients posted for a "T and A" to prevent excess postoperative bleeding.

### Postoperative Care

The patient who has had a tonsillectomy done under a local anesthetic is awake when he is returned to his bed. He should be placed in a position which is most comfortable for him. Having the head of the bed and the knee rest slightly raised is the position most often chosen by the patient.

If the patient has had a general anesthetic (put to sleep for the surgery), he should be placed in bed on his side or his abdomen. The purpose of either of these positions is to allow mucus and blood to drain from the throat. This prevents the fluid from draining into the larynx and trachea. When the patient is turned on one side, a pillow should be placed under his lower chest and his knees flexed. If the patient is placed on his abdomen, his head is turned to one side.

The responsibility of the nurse caring for the patient while he is still unconscious from the anesthesia is to watch for bleeding and to prevent aspiration of mucus. A small amount of bright red blood can be expected for a short while after surgery. Excess fluid in the mouth should be removed by frequent wiping and with suction. In using a suction machine the nurse should keep the pressure low. Also, extreme care should be used to prevent the suction tip from injuring the operative area.

The patient should be checked frequently for signs of bleeding after he has reacted from the anesthesia. Blood coming from the throat is bright red. If blood has been swallowed, it is brownish when the patient vomits. The practical nurse should report frequent expectoration of bright red blood and a moderate to a large amount of brownish vomitus. Symptoms of hemorrhage, such as restlessness, paleness, and a fast pulse, should also be reported.

In the absence of complications, such as bleeding, the patient is given cracked ice, water, and other cold liquids as soon as desired. No fruit juices should be given because they irritate the throat. Soft foods are given when the patient can tolerate them.

An ice collar is ordered frequently to prevent or to check oozing of blood and to relieve soreness. Many physicians prescribe chewing gum the day after surgery to relieve dryness and soreness. Aspergum is an example of the gum which may be ordered. Usually the patient is discharged from the hospital the day following the operation.

## LARYNGITIS

### Description

The patient with laryngitis has an inflammation of his larynx or voice box. Usually it follows an infection of the upper respiratory tract, such as pharyngitis and the common cold. It may accompany infectious diseases, such as measles, diphtheria, and whooping cough. Laryngitis may result from excessive use of the voice, inhaling irritating fumes and dust, and smoking too much. Tuberculosis, syphilis, and a tumor may cause it. The practical nurse should remember that persistent hoarseness, which is the chief symptom of laryngitis, may be an early symptom of cancer of the larynx. When a person is hoarse for more than a few days, he should consult his physician.

### Symptoms

Hoarseness is the main symptom of laryngitis. In some cases the individual has *aphonia,* which means inability to speak or loss of voice. A slight elevation of temperature may be present when the laryngitis is a result of infection. The patient may also have a cough and a feeling of tightness in his throat.

### Treatment

The doctor recommends that the patient with laryngitis avoid using his voice. Inhalation of steam may be ordered to soothe the irritated mucous membrane. If the laryngitis is a result of another disease, such as infection or cancer, the doctor directs his treatment toward the underlying cause.

## OBSTRUCTION OF THE LARYNX

### Description

An obstruction of the larynx may be caused by a tumor, inhaling a foreign object such as a pea or a coin, paralysis of the vocal folds, and edema. Laryngeal obstruction may also occur during or after an operation on the neck, such as a thyroidectomy.

### Treatment and Nursing Care

The physician performs a tracheotomy on the patient with an obstruction of his larynx. A *tracheotomy* (known as a *tracheostomy* when the opening is to be permanent) is an artificial opening into the trachea which is made below the obstruction so that the patient can breathe. This is a lifesaving operation when the patient has an acute blockage of his larynx.

After making an incision into the trachea, the surgeon inserts a tube into the opening. This tube, which is called a *tracheotomy tube* is made of a tube within another tube. The tracheotomy tube may be made of silver as well as rubber and plastic. When inserting the tube, the physician uses an instrument known as a *tracheotomy spreader* (top of Fig. 23); he also uses a *pilot*, which is a curved rod with an end shaped like an olive. After he has it inserted properly, he removes the pilot and puts the inner tube into proper position. Tapes are attached to the larger tube, or cannula, and tied around the patient's neck to keep the tube in place.

After the tracheotomy tube has been inserted through an incision into the trachea, the patient needs close attention from the nurse. It is necessary for the practical nurse to know the responsibilities of the nursing team in the care of this patient, as she is often asked to assist with his care.

It is the nurse's responsibility to keep the newly made opening clear so that the patient can breathe. She must remember that this is his only life line for air. Another important aim of nursing care of this patient is to relieve his anxiety. Breathing through a tube in his throat instead of his nose or mouth can be a frightening experience. Frequently the patient is afraid of not being able to breathe through the little silver tube.

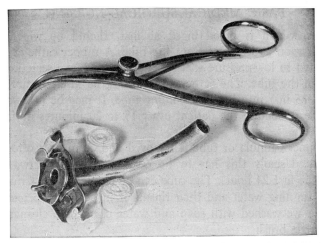

**Figure 23.** Tracheotomy spreader (*top*) and tube (*bottom*). (West, John P.; Keller, Manelva W.; and Harmon, Elizabeth H.: *Nursing Care of the Surgical Patient*, 6th ed. The Macmillan Company, New York, 1957.)

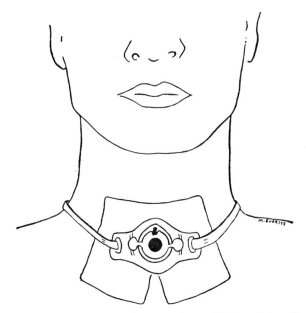

**Figure 24.** Tracheotomy tube in place (West, John P.; Keller, Manelva W.; and Harmon, Elizabeth H.: *Nursing Care of the Surgical Patient*. 6th ed. The Macmillan Company, New York, 1957.)

175

Mucus, which is blood-tinged at first, should be wiped away gently as soon as it comes from the tube. A rubber catheter which is attached to low-pressure suction is used to remove secretions collecting in the tube. The catheter should not be inserted more than 12.5 cm (5 in.) into the tracheotomy tube. It may be necessary for the nurse to suction the patient every 15 to 20 minutes during the first day.

The inner cannula or tube is removed and cleaned as often as is necessary. Usually this has to be done every one to two hours during the first 24 hours. The tube can be cleaned by first rinsing it in cold running water and then rinsing it in hydrogen peroxide. It can then we washed with soap and water using pipe cleaners or a small bottle brush.

The doctor usually changes the outer tube at least once each day. The inner and outer tubes and the pilot are cleaned thoroughly and sterilized. The package of sterilized equipment is returned to the patient's unit as quickly as possible.

The patient should be observed for signs of hemorrhage and difficulty in breathing. These should be reported immediately.

Paper and pencil should be provided for the patient to communicate with the nurse, since he usually cannot speak. He is generally unable to talk because his larynx or voice box is above the site of the tracheotomy. Air enters and leaves his respiratory tract without passing through the larynx.

The tracheotomy tube is removed before the patient leaves the hospital if the operation was a temporary measure. This removal usually is done gradually. One method which may be used for this purpose is the insertion of a small, sterile cork into the tracheotomy tube. The cork is left in place for short periods of time at first so that the patient becomes adjusted to normal breathing. The length of time is increased gradually. The physician removes the tracheotomy tube entirely when he believes that the patient needs it no longer. If the patient is to have a permanent tracheostomy, the physician and the professional nurse teach the patient or some member of his family how to care for it. He should be taught the danger of aspirating water through the tube. For example, he will need to be careful when taking a shower and prevent water getting into the tube.

## CANCER

### Introduction

Cancer may affect any part of the upper respiratory tract, but most often it affects the larynx. A malignancy of the larynx may occur in both men and women, but is more common in men during and after middle age. More than 90 per cent of the patients with cancer of the larynx can be cured if treatment is started early.

### Symptoms

An early symptom of cancer of the larynx is hoarseness. The patient may have difficulty in swallowing as the malignant tumor enlarges. Also, difficult breathing, coughing, and pain may occur as the disease progresses.

### Treatment and Nursing Care

The patient with cancer of the larynx is treated by surgery or by x-ray, or a combination of both. The affected part of the voice box may be removed, or the entire organ may be removed. When the entire larynx is removed, the trachea leading to the throat is closed, and the part of the trachea leading to the lungs opens permanently on the lower part of the neck. A silver tube similar to the tracheotomy tube is inserted into this permanent opening during the early post-operative period. This tube is called a *laryngectomy tube*. It is cared for in the same manner as the tracheotomy tube. The patient may be able to breathe through the artificial opening in his throat and do without the tube, after the edges of the wound have healed.

It is easy to understand why the patient who faces a laryngectomy is apprehensive. He probably has many questions in his mind, such as: Will I live? Do I have cancer? Will I be able to talk? The physician usually tells the patient before doing a laryngectomy that he will not be able to talk in the usual manner after surgery but that he will be able to carry on a conversation after a period of training.

After the patient has had his larynx removed, and a laryngectomy tube inserted, he needs, with a few variations, the same care as the patient having a tracheotomy. As his neck muscles are weak, the patient appreciates the nurse's supporting his head when he is moved. Following a laryngectomy, the patient is usually tube-fed. A tube is passed through the nose and esophagus into the stomach. After a specially prepared formula has been warmed to body temperature, it is poured through this tube into the patient's stomach. After the operative area has healed, the patient is allowed to eat his regular diet.

This patient is usually depressed. Therefore, he needs encouragement from all members of the nursing team. He can be taught to speak by a speech therapist or by another laryngectomized patient. Although the organ of voice is gone, this person can learn to speak by swallowing air and producing sounds when the air is forced back from the stomach. This is known as *esophageal speech*. Proper control of the muscles involved is essential.

## SUGGESTIONS FOR STUDY

1. Why is a person with a cold likely to develop secondary infections such as sinusitis and bronchitis?
2. Discuss frequently used home remedies for the common cold with some of your associates. How do they differ from those discussed in the text?
3. What complication may result from chronic sinusitis?
4. Review the nursing care of a patient following a tonsillectomy.
5. What are some of the causes of laryngitis?
6. What is the chief symptom of laryngitis?
7. What surgical procedure may be done for a patient with a laryngeal obstruction?
8. What are the responsibilities of the nursing team in caring for a patient with a tracheotomy?
9. What part of the upper respiratory system is most often affected by cancer? What percentage of these patients can be cured by early treatment? *90*
10. Can a person who has had his larynx or voice box removed talk again? *yes*

## REFERENCES FOR CHAPTER 12

Anthony, Catherine P.: *Textbook of Anatomy and Physiology*, 4th ed. C. V. Mosby Co., St. Louis, 1955, pp. 431-39.

Dakin, Florence; Thompson, Ella M.; and La Baron, Margaret: *Simplified Nursing*, 6th ed. J. B. Lippincott Co., Philadelphia, 1956, pp. 132-35.

Eliason, Eldridge; Ferguson, L. Kraeer; and Sholtis, Lillian A.: *Surgical Nursing*, 10th ed. J. B. Lippincott Co., Philadelphia, 1955, pp. 209-24.

Emerson, Charles P., Jr., and Bragdon, Jane S.: *Essentials of Medicine*, 17th ed. J. B. Lippincott Co., Philadelphia, 1955, pp. 149-67.

Faddis, Margene O., and Hayman, Joseph M.: *Care of the Medical Patient*. McGraw-Hill Book Co., New York, 1952, pp. 290-97.

Gill, Helen Z. (ed.): *Basic Nursing*, 4th ed. The Macmillan Company, New York, 1955, pp. 89-93 and 543-46.

Holinger, Paul H.; Johnston, Kenneth C.; Mansueto, Mario D.; and Jimison, Carmin: "Cancer of the Larynx," *Am. J. Nursing*, **57**:738-43, (June) 1957.

Hull, Edgar, and Perrodin, Cecilia: *Medical Nursing*, 5th ed. F. A. Davis Co., Philadelphia, 1954, pp. 104-11.

Shepard, Mary E.: *Nursing Care of Patients with Eye, Ear, Nose, and Throat Disorders*. The Macmillan Company, New York, 1958, pp. 159-219.

West, John P.; Keller, Manelva W.; and Harmon, Elizabeth H.: *Nursing Care of the Surgical Patient*, 6th ed. The Macmillan Company, New York, 1957, pp. 573-604.

Young, Helen, and Lee, Eleanor: *Lippincott's Quick Reference Book for Nurses*, 7th ed. J. B. Lippincott Co., Philadelphia, 1955, pp. 332-33.

*Read*
3 ·

Chapter 13

# THE PATIENT
# WITH A DISEASE
# OF THE LOWER
# RESPIRATORY SYSTEM

## STRUCTURE AND FUNCTION

*Know*

The lungs and the bronchi with their branches make up the lower respiratory system. The bronchi are two large tubes leading from the trachea to the lungs. One bronchus goes to each lung. There it branches into smaller tubes called *bronchial tubes*. These in turn divide into smaller tubes known as *bronchioles*. As described in Chapter 12, alveoli, minute sacs, are at the end of the tiny bronchioles. The trachea leading to the two bronchi with their many branches look like a tree turned upside down. Thus, it is spoken of as the *bronchial tree*.

Each of the two lungs is divided into lobes. The right lung contains three lobes, whereas the left lung has only two lobes. The lungs are covered by a serous membrane called *pleura*. This membrane consists of two layers which are separated by a lubricating substance. The layer covering the lungs is known as the *visceral pleura*, and the layer lining the chest wall is called the *parietal pleura*.

## ACUTE BRONCHITIS

### Description

The patient with acute bronchitis has an inflammation of the mucous membrane lining the bronchial tubes. Usually the trachea is also inflamed. Acute bronchitis commonly follows an infection of the upper respiratory tract, such as sinusitis, pharyngitis, and the common

180

cold. It may be associated with infectious diseases, such as measles and whooping cough.

## Symptoms

The patient's chief symptom is a cough. At first the cough is usually dry and unproductive. His fever may range from 37.8° to 38.3° C (100° to 101° F). He often complains of a feeling of discomfort

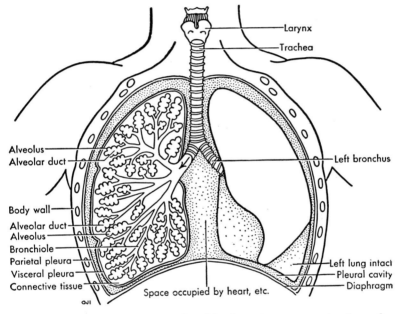

**Figure 25.** Lungs of man. The right lung is cut open to show the internal structure. (Hegner, Robert W., and Stiles, Karl A.: *College Zoology*, 6th ed. The Macmillan Company, New York, 1951.)

or burning beneath his sternum. The cough becomes productive after several days. The inflammation usually subsides in four or five days.

A dangerous complication of acute bronchitis is bronchopneumonia in which the infection spreads to the bronchioles and the alveoli. Infants, the aged, and individuals whose general health is poor are more likely to develop this type of pneumonia.

### Treatment and Nursing Care

The physician recommends bed rest if the patient's temperature is over 37.8° C (100° F). The room temperature should be comfortably warm since cold air may aggravate the cough. Steam inhalations are used frequently to soothe the irritated bronchi.

Expectorant drugs may be prescribed by the physician to relieve the dry and unproductive cough. Ammonium chloride and terpin hydrate elixir are two examples of expectorants. Frequently a drug, such as codeine, is added to the mixture to depress the cough reflex. The nursing care of a patient with a persistent cough is discussed more fully on pages 36 to 37.

## CHRONIC BRONCHITIS

### Description

Generally an individual develops chronic bronchitis as a result of another condition. A patient with chronic sinusitis may develop chronic bronchitis following the aspiration of infectious material. It may be caused by smoking too much, by bronchiectasis (dilatation of the bronchi), and by congestion in the lungs resulting from heart disease. Also, repeated attacks of acute bronchitis can develop into a chronic condition.

Chronic bronchitis is more common in older persons and is worse during the winter months. Coughing, which is the chief symptom of chronic bronchitis, is usually more troublesome at night. Spells of coughing frequently follow exercise. The patient's cough may be either productive or dry.

### Treatment

Treatment of a patient with chronic bronchitis is directed toward relieving the underlying cause. For example, the patient with chronic bronchitis resulting from chronic sinusitis would be treated for the sinus condition. Efforts are made to improve the patient's general health. In some cases the physician may suggest that the patient move to a dry warm climate.

## BRONCHIECTASIS

### Description

A patient with bronchiectasis has a chronic disease of the bronchial tree in which there is dilatation of one or more tubes. Bronchiectasis favors the formation of pus in the lower end of the diseased bronchial tube.

Bronchiectasis may result from chronic bronchitis, which weakens the bronchial wall. The inhalation of irritating substances, such as

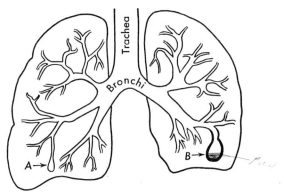

**Figure 26.**   Lungs affected by bronchiectasis. A small cavity is located at A, and a larger one containing pus is located at B.

dust containing sharp particles and harmful fumes, may cause bronchiectasis. Some individuals may have been born with a weakness in the bronchial wall which will lead to the development of bronchiectasis.

### Symptoms

The patient with bronchiectasis has a chronic productive cough. He expectorates a large amount of sputum which usually contains pus. His cough is frequently worse following a change of position. For example, going to bed and getting out of bed may cause him to cough more. Hemoptysis (expectoration of blood) occurs when a blood vessel is involved. After the patient has had this disease for some time, his finger tips may become flattened and widened. This is known as *clubbing of the fingers.* Fever, malaise, and other symptoms of an active infection are present during the acute stage of the disease.

### Treatment and Nursing Care

The practical nurse is asked to assist in preparing a patient suspected of having bronchiectasis for special procedures used in determining the diagnosis of this disease. For this reason she needs to understand their purpose. In addition to having an x-ray taken of the patient's chest, the physician may do a *bronchogram.* In this procedure he injects iodized oil through the pharynx and trachea into the bronchi. This substance makes the outline of the bronchial tree easier to see by x-ray. Thus, a bronchogram aids the doctor in making a definite diagnosis. A *bronchoscopy* is an examination of the bronchial walls. In order to do this, the doctor inserts an instrument called a *bronchoscope* through the patient's mouth, throat, and trachea into the bronchi. He can look directly through the bronchoscope into the bronchi for a closer examination.

If bronchiectasis is not treated, it develops into an incurable disease which shortens the patient's life. It may be complicated by pneumonia, lung abscess, and hemorrhage.

In treating a patient with bronchiectasis, the physician tries to improve the person's general health and to remove the cause if possible. For example, the patient who has this disease as a result of chronic bronchitis caused by chronic sinusitis is treated for both conditions. Antibiotics which are effective against the bacteria present are used during the acute stage of the disease.

The physician may aspirate fluid from the dilated bronchi through a bronchoscope. A small suction tube is passed through the bronchoscope into the dilated bronchus. The infectious material is then aspirated. Although this treatment does not cure the patient, it frequently gives him temporary relief.

*Postural drainage* may be prescribed. In this case the patient gets into a position in which his head is lower than his hips. The physician may recommend that the patient cough while in this position. This allows the fluid in the dilated bronchi to drain out by gravity. One method of having the patient assume a position for postural drainage is to use a bed available for this purpose. The postural drainage bed can be adjusted so that the patient's head is lower than his pelvis.

Another method of having the patient assume a position for postural drainage is to have him hang his head over the side of the bed. The patient can rest his arms on a padded footstool for support. Either a sputum cup or a small basin and tissues should be placed in a convenient position so that he can dispose of the expectoration. The patient may experience dizziness, headache, profuse perspiration, and other unpleasant symptoms when he is first learning how to do postural drainage. Because of this, the nurse should stay with the patient when he first begins these treatments. When the practical nurse observes such symptoms, she should help the patient back on the bed and report to her team leader. Usually, as the patient continues to practice postural drainage, he is able to increase the length of time that he can remain in this position. The physician orders the length of time the patient is to remain in this position and the number of times it is to be done each day. For example, he may prescribe postural drainage for 15 minutes three times a day.

With the perfection of lung surgery, new hope is offered to patients having bronchiectasis. Complete recovery is possible when the disease is localized in one or two lobes of the lung. The surgeon may do either a lobectomy or a pneumonectomy. Removal of a lobe of the lung is known as a *lobectomy*. Removal of an entire lung is known as a *pneumonectomy*.

## PNEUMONIA

### Description

A patient with pneumonia has an infection of his lungs. Normal lung tissue is spongy. When an inflammation is present, the tissue becomes more solid. This change in the lung tissue associated with pneumonia can be compared with a sponge. After the sponge is filled with water, it has fewer air spaces and is more solid.

Discovery of the sulfonamides and antibiotics, especially penicillin, has made a miraculous change in the possible outcome for a person with pneumonia. Although all individuals do not survive an attack of pneumonia, the drop in the death rate has been dramatic.

### Cause

Pneumonia can be caused by a number of bacteria and viruses. When this disease is caused by bacteria it is known as *bacterial pneumonia;* and when it is caused by a virus, it is known as *virus pneumonia.* The greatest number of cases of bacterial pneumonia is caused by the pneumococci.

Pneumonia is classified in this text according to its cause. As the practical nurse may hear of another classification based on the part diseased, it is mentioned here. *Lobar pneumonia* means that one or more of the lobes of the lung are affected. *Bronchopneumonia* means that the infection is of a patchy distribution around the bronchioles and alveoli.

Pneumonia is more likely to occur in persons who are poorly nourished, who are in a weakened condition from bad health habits, or who are in a debilitated condition from disease. For example, it may follow some of the communicable diseases, such as whooping cough and scarlet fever. It can follow surgery. A cardiac patient with poor circulation in his lungs will develop pneumonia when he stays in one position too long. This is known as *hypostatic pneumonia* and it occurs more often in older people. Pneumonia can follow the aspiration of material, such as vomitus into the lungs. Frequently it affects infants, aged individuals, alcoholics, and persons who have had a previous attack of pneumonia.

### Bacterial Pneumonia
#### Symptoms

As stated previously in this chapter, bacterial pneumonia is caused by bacteria which invade the lungs. After the lungs have been attacked by the microorganisms, an inflammatory process begins. Because of this, the patient has a fever, malaise, chest pain, and other symptoms of an inflammation. His respiration is rapid, difficult, and painful. Generally the cough is dry and hacking at first. Later it becomes productive, and the sputum is rusty in color. Cyanosis may be present.

#### Treatment and Nursing Care

Because the practical nurse often assists the professional nurse in caring for this patient, she needs to know the important points in his care. The treatment and nursing care are directed toward helping the patient's body overcome the infection. The physician prescribes either a sulfonamide or an antibiotic. If the drug is effective against the invading organism, the patient makes a dramatic recovery.

As in the care of patients with other types of infections, it is the responsibility of the nursing team to help the patient in securing the greatest amount of rest possible. The patient should be placed in the position which is most comfortable to him. His strength should be conserved so that his body has a better chance to overcome the infection. The thoughtful nurse can render an invaluable service by anticipating the patient's needs. For instance, articles such as water and the call bell should be placed within his reach so that it takes little effort for him to get them when he is thirsty or when he wants to call the nurse.

Measures to relieve the patient's pain, such as an icecap, a hot-water bottle, a mustard plaster, or drugs, are prescribed. Meperidine (Demerol), morphine, and codeine are examples of drugs which may be ordered to relieve pain.

The patient should be observed for symptoms which might indicate an unfavorable change in his condition. For example, a sudden elevation of temperature, an increased pulse rate, more difficulty in breathing, cyanosis, and disorientation should be reported promptly.

The patient should cough into a tissue to avoid spreading the bacteria to those around him. The soiled tissues are then placed into a paper bag and disposed of according to hospital procedure. Usually they are burned. The nursing care of a patient with a persistent cough is discussed on pages 36 to 37.

Oxygen therapy may be used for this patient. This is done to increase the amount of oxygen which the patient inhales. Thus, his cyanosis and dyspnea are relieved.

### Virus Pneumonia

#### Description

The patient with virus pneumonia has an inflammation in his lungs caused by a virus. The practical nurse may hear this disease referred to as either *virus pneumonia* or *primary atypical pneumonia.* Young adults seem to be affected most often by this type of pneumonia. Although the convalescent period is frequently prolonged, the outlook is good.

#### Symptoms

The onset of this infection is usually gradual. The patient complains of general aches and pains, malaise, and a cough. The cough is dry, hacking, and annoying. The patient also has a fever. The symptoms may last from one to six weeks.

### Treatment and Nursing Care

Rest is important for a patient with this infection. The nurse should try to prevent the patient from exerting himself until the doctor allows increased activity. A nourishing diet is important because of the long convalescence.

## PLEURISY AND EMPYEMA

### Definition

A patient with pleurisy has an inflammation of the pleura. When fluid collects between the two layers of the pleura (pleural cavity), the condition is known as "pleurisy with effusion." The patient has *empyema* if the fluid becomes purulent (contains pus).

### Cause

Usually pleurisy and empyema are secondary to another disease; that is, they follow or complicate another disease. They may result from a disease of the lungs, such as tuberculosis, pneumonia, cancer, and pulmonary embolism. Also, an infection of the pericardium and of the peritoneum may spread to the pleura.

### Symptoms

A person with pleurisy has a sharp pain in his side caused by the two layers of the inflamed pleura rubbing together. The pain is more severe when the patient breathes deeply. Thus his respirations are shallow and rapid. A dry, painful cough and a fever often occur. The patient's pain decreases if fluid collects in the pleural cavity. This fluid prevents the two layers of the pleura from rubbing together.

### Treatment and Nursing Care

The patient with either pleurisy or empyema needs bed rest. An icecap or a hot-water bottle may be ordered to relieve pain. In some cases the physician may limit the movement of the chest in an effort to relieve pain. This can be done by the use of a binder or by strapping with adhesive tape. When the physician straps the chest with adhesive tape, he may have the area shaved first in order to lessen discomfort when the tape is removed later. He may also want the area painted with tincture of benzoin because of its adhesive and antiseptic action. One of the sulfonamides or an antibiotic is ordered to combat the infection.

The practical nurse may be asked to assist the doctor in tapping the chest, a procedure known as a *thoracentesis*. He inserts a needle into the chest cavity and aspirates some of the fluid. This may be done for either diagnosis or treatment. If the purpose is for diagnosis, the fluid is examined to determine the infecting microorganism. The excess fluid is removed as a treatment measure when it causes the patient to have dyspnea.

In some cases, it is necessary for the purulent fluid in the pleural cavity to be drained by the use of *closed drainage*. In this type of drainage, fluid is removed from the pleural cavity without allowing air to enter it. Using sterile equipment, the surgeon inserts a small rubber tube through an incision into the cavity. This tube is clamped to prevent air from entering the pleural cavity. The tube is then attached to tubing which is connected with a long glass tube. This glass tube has its open end under water in a sealed drainage bottle. The amount of sterile water used is designated by the doctor. The purpose of the water is to prevent air entering the pleural cavity through the tubing. Pressure between the lung and the pleura is less than atmospheric pressure. If air enters the chest cavity through the tubing, it will cause the lung to collapse because of the difference in pressure.

When helping to care for the patient with closed drainage of the chest, the practical nurse needs to remember that the setup is actually closed. In other words, no air should be allowed to enter it. Thus, it is of extreme importance to keep the tubing connected. The equipment should be observed frequently for leakage. The open end of the glass tube in the drainage bottle should be below the water. This should also be checked often by members of the nursing team. The physician should be notified immediately when the drainage equipment is not working properly. The practical nurse needs to know that many hospitals have the policy that closed chest drainage is the physician's responsibility. That is, he is to insert, to remove, and to adjust the equipment. However, the nursing team is responsible for accurate observation and prompt reporting.

There should be no pressure on the tubing by pillows or the patient's body. Utmost care must be taken to prevent pulling the tube out of the incision. If the practical nurse observes that the tubing has become disconnected, she should clamp the tube leading to the patient's chest and summon help.

The physician may sometimes attach suction to the closed drainage system. This is known as closed drainage with suction. In this case, either two or three additional bottles may be used.

When the purulent fluid cannot be drained adequately by closed drainage and the cavity of pus has a protective wall around it so that the inflow of air through the incision cannot collapse the lung, the physician may do a _thoracotomy_. This is a surgical procedure in which the thoracic cavity is opened. The operation allows for freer drainage of the pus. Following the operation, the patient is placed in bed on his operative side until he reacts from the anesthetic. When he has reacted fully, he is allowed to assume the position which is most comfortable. The patient should be encouraged to take frequent deep breaths. The practical nurse may be asked to assist in changing the dressings as this has to be done frequently.

## PULMONARY TUBERCULOSIS

### Cause

Tuberculosis is an infectious disease caused by the tubercle bacillus. Two types of tubercle bacilli affecting people are the bovine and the human. The bovine type, which is spread by cow's milk, usually causes tuberculosis in parts of the body other than the lungs. The number of cases of bovine tuberculosis has been reduced greatly by testing cows for this disease and killing those found to be infected. Pasteurization of milk also has contributed to the decrease of this type of tuberculosis. The human type causes 95 per cent of the cases in this country. This type of tubercle bacillus is most likely to affect the lungs. A tuberculous infection of the lungs is known as _pulmonary tuberculosis_.

A person in poor physical condition is more likely to develop tuberculosis than his healthy neighbor. An inadequate diet, continuous overwork, and poor living conditions, such as overcrowding, can make a person more susceptible. Anemia, diabetes, and other chronic diseases can predispose to tuberculosis.

The tubercle bacillus is covered with mucoid material or capsule which makes it capable of living for long periods of time. It can live outside the body in both hot and cold weather. Knowing this characteristic, the practical nurse can readily understand the importance of preventing its spread through sputum and other body excreta. Although this microorganism can live for months in a dark area, it dies after a few hours of direct sunlight. The tubercle bacillus can also be killed by burning, boiling in water, and soaking in certain disinfectants, such as 5 per cent phenol.

### Transmission

Pulmonary tuberculosis is not inherited. It is transmitted or spread. Breathing air containing tubercle bacilli, kissing a person infected with the disease, and putting contaminated objects into the mouth, such as dishes, silver, and drinking glasses, are common ways in which this disease is spread. However, it is encouraging to note that once the tubercle bacilli have entered a person's body, they do not always cause tuberculosis. The body's defenses can overcome the invading microorganisms and prevent them from harming the body.

### Disease Process

After the tubercle bacilli reach the lungs, they find a suitable place to live. Then the battle begins between the invading microorganisms and the body's defenses. A wall of fibrous tissue begins to form around the colony of tubercle bacilli. Eventually, the wall surrounds the invaders forming a *tubercle* which is a small nodule. (The bacilli causing this disease are called tubercle bacilli since they cause small nodules or tubercles to form in the tissue.) This wall has two main functions: (1) it prevents the bacilli from spreading, and (2) it prevents the blood vessels from nourishing the bacilli. Cutting off the blood supply also causes the body's tissues within the affected area to die. The tissue breaks down into a cheese-like substance. This process is called *caseation*. The tubercle bacilli stop multiplying if the body's defenses are strong. Although the bacilli may remain alive within the wall or capsule for months or years, they eventually die. However, if the patient's resistance is lowered by such factors as overwork and poor health habits before the tubercle bacilli die, the infection may be renewed. If the body continues to win the battle, scar tissue is formed and lime salts are deposited. This area is known as a *healed calcified lesion*. The patient has recovered.

Unfortunately, the invader is not always killed so easily by the body. If the patient's resistance is not adequate, or if too many tubercle bacilli invade the lungs, his body may be the loser of the battle. Also, tubercle bacilli may penetrate the wall of the tubercle. Once on the outside, they seek other suitable places to live. The bacilli may invade a blood vessel and be carried to a distant part of the body. New infections are started. Ulceration occurs when the spreading infection reaches the surface of a bronchus wall. The cheese-like or caseous material within the infected area empties into the bronchus leaving a cavity in its place. The patient then expectorates sputum containing tubercle bacilli. If the patient's resistance is improved at this time, the cavity is surrounded by a wall.

### Incidence

It has been estimated that one-half of the people in the United States have had a tuberculous infection. However, only a small number of these have developed symptoms of tuberculosis. Individuals who have had this contact develop a degree of immunity to the tubercle bacilli. This can be observed when tuberculosis is carried into a community or group of people which has had no previous contact with the disease. For example, a large number of the American Indians died from tuberculosis when the white man came to this country bringing the disease with him. Nonwhite groups of people in the United States continue to have a higher mortality rate than white groups.

Pulmonary tuberculosis affects all age groups; however, it causes more deaths in our country in persons who are 15 years of age or over. The mortality rate in white people is highest in the older age groups. The highest death rate in nonwhite women is between 20 and 35 years of age. The highest death rate among nonwhite men is during the middle years.

Although the death rate from tuberculosis is still high, it has dropped 85 per cent in the last 50 years. This amazing decrease was primarily a result of concentrated efforts for early diagnosis and isolation of contagious patients. After the patient was placed in a hospital, he was able to obtain treatment. Also, he no longer served as a source of infection for people coming in contact with him. Other factors which have contributed to this decrease are better housing, improved working conditions, better nutrition, adequate facilities for diagnosis and treatment, advances in surgical treatment, new drugs, pasteurization of milk, and the testing of cattle for tuberculosis.

**Symptoms**

Frequently the patient with pulmonary tuberculosis notices no symptoms during the early stage of infection. Periodic chest x-rays of all adults and individuals in their late teens are encouraged in an effort to detect cases in the beginning stage. It is important to locate tuberculosis during this stage in order to start early treatment as well as to prevent its spread to other people. The *tuberculin test is* used for detection purposes, especially in children. In this test, an extract of the tubercle bacilli is either injected into the skin or placed on the skin. If the skin area tested becomes inflamed, it indicates a positive reaction. This means that the person has at one time had a tuberculous infection although it may have been a minor one. The active disease may be present at that time or it may have occurred some time before.

The patient generally develops vague symptoms as the tuberculous infection continues. He may notice that he tires easily, has a poor appetite, and is gradually losing weight. Indigestion may be present. In some cases, the patient awakens during the night and finds his bedclothes soaked with perspiration. This is known as a *night sweat.*

He develops a cough which frequently is nonproductive at first. His cough becomes increasingly productive as the disease progresses. The patient may have *hemoptysis, which is expectoration of* blood. The amount of blood lost may range from blood-streaked sputum to a massive hemorrhage of several pints.

The patient develops a fever. Usually, his temperature is slightly below normal in the morning and goes up in the afternoon. It frequently reaches 37.8° to 38.9° C (100° to 102° F) during the late afternoon.

### Diagnosis

When the physician suspects that a patient has pulmonary tuberculosis, he orders certain procedures to confirm his diagnosis. As an important member of the nursing team, the practical nurse is asked to assist with these diagnostic procedures. Because of this, she needs a basic understanding of them. The tuberculin test, chest x-ray, examination of the sputum, and examination of the stomach's contents are diagnostic procedures frequently used by the doctor.

Two types of the tuberculin test used frequently are the intradermal or Mantoux test and the Vollmer patch test. The dosage of tuberculin which is injected into the skin in the Mantoux test is a small part of 0.1 cc. A special tuberculin syringe is used to measure this minute amount. In the Vollmer patch test, a prepared patch is applied to the skin after it has been cleaned with either acetone or ether. If the patient's skin becomes reddened and swollen within 24 to 48 hours after the tuberculin has been either applied or injected, he has a positive reaction. As stated earlier in this chapter, a positive reaction indicates that the person has at one time had a tuberculous infection. It may not be actively present at the time of the test.

When the patient has a positive tuberculin reaction, he should then have a chest x-ray. The physician may use both the tuberculin test and the chest x-ray or he may use only the chest x-ray.

The doctor requests an examination of the patient's sputum for tubercle bacilli if the x-ray shows evidence of tuberculosis. The patient should be instructed to collect secretion which he coughs up from his chest and not saliva or drainage from the nose. The sputum should be collected in a clean wide-mouthed bottle or a special paraffined paper cup called a sputum cup. Frequently, the physician asks the nurse to collect the specimen when the patient first awakens in the morning because more sputum is usually raised at that time.

The practical nurse may be asked to assist either the physician or the professional nurse in doing a *gastric lavage*, which is washing out the stomach. This is done to obtain sputum from the patient's stomach which is then examined for tubercle bacilli. The stomach contains secretions from the lungs which have been swallowed during the night's rest. This procedure is used in children who are unable to follow the nurse's instructions and for patients who are unable to produce sputum from the bronchial tree. It is used also in patients who have had frequent sputum examinations which showed no tubercle bacilli. The practical nurse needs to remember that the patient should have no food or fluids for at least 8 to 10 hours before the test. The test is generally done before breakfast.

### Treatment and Nursing Care

After the physician has made a definite diagnosis of pulmonary tuberculosis, he outlines the course of treatment. Generally, the patient is admitted to a hospital or sanatorium which specializes in the care of patients with this disease. Members of the nursing team can expect the patient to have many adjustments to make in regard to having tuberculosis as well as to being in a strange place. Often, the patient is admitted to a hospital some distance from his home. Thus, he is cut off from his loved ones and familiar surroundings.

Financial worries may blacken his outlook. The patient's usual activities are discontinued or greatly reduced. Generally he is faced with a long illness. Another real concern of this patient may be whether or not he will get well. He may also dread the long months of hospitalization. This individual who has pulmonary tuberculosis finds that his way of life has suddenly been changed. He has to make innumerable adjustments—not as a well person but as a sick one. The nurse who understands the changes which the patient has to make can use this as a basis for giving nursing care at its best.

### *Rest*

The most important principle of treatment outlined by the doctor is rest. The patient will be kept on complete rest as long as there is evidence of activity in the tuberculous lesion. It is the nursing team's responsibility to help the patient obtain mental as well as physical rest. They physician determines the amount of activity which the patient is allowed while in bed. As the patient improves, his activity is increased gradually.

### *Drugs*

The use of drugs in connection with rest is brightening the outlook for many tuberculosis patients. Streptomycin, isonicotinic acid hydrazide (isoniazid), and para-aminosalicylic acid (PAS) are commonly used in the treatment of tuberculosis.

### Diet

The patient needs a well-balanced and appetizing diet. It should be high in protein, calcium, fat, and vitamins. Thus, milk is an important part of the patient's diet. The patient should be encouraged to take extra nourishment between meals. In general, most physicians want their patient to gain approximately 2.3 to 4.5 kg (5 to 10 lb) above their normal weight.

### Isolation

Measures to prevent the spread of tuberculosis are necessary. The physician requests that the patient be placed in *isolation*, which means separating the patient from those not infected with the disease. Frequently, an entire unit of patients with tuberculosis is isolated as a group. When the patient is no longer considered infectious by his doctor, he is removed from isolation.

When the nurse is caring for the patient with an infectious case of tuberculosis, she should wear a gown to protect her uniform. A mask which covers her nose and mouth should also be worn.

Dishes used by the patient should be sterilized by boiling. Soiled linen should be either boiled or soaked in disinfectant before it is sent to the laundry.

Much of the responsibility of teaching the patient how to avoid spreading his disease to others belongs to the nursing team. The patient needs to learn that he should not put into his mouth articles which are later handled by others. For example, tubercle bacilli can be spread by a simple object, such as a pencil, which has been placed in the patient's mouth. If a visitor uses the pencil and later puts food into his mouth before washing his hands, he may infect himself. The patient should be taught to moisten stamps and seal envolopes with clean water instead of saliva. He should be instructed to cough and to sneeze into tissues of several thicknesses. Soiled tissues should be placed into a paper bag and later burned. The patient's sputum should be collected in a covered container and disposed of by burning.

*Surgery*

In many cases of pulmonary tuberculosis, surgical treatment is indicated. Frequently, the surgeon performs surgery after the patient has been treated with antibiotics. Two main forms of surgery performed on these patients are *collapse therapy* and *resection*. When a patient is treated with collapse therapy, his lung is collapsed so that it may have additional rest. When a resection is done, the diseased part of the patient's lung is removed or resected. Resection as a method of treating the patient with tuberculosis seems to be used more often now than treatment with collapse therapy.

The practical nurse needs an understanding of the various methods used by the physician to collapse a patient's lung. She should know that these are measures used to rest the lung in addition to bed rest. Artificial pneumothorax, pneumoperitoneum, crushing the phrenic nerve, and thoracoplasty are procedures which the doctor may carry out to collapse the affected part of the lung.

When the physician does an *artificial pneumothorax*, he injects air into the pleural cavity. The air pressing against the lung causes it to collapse. This procedure has to be repeated periodically as the air is absorbed gradually from the pleural cavity.

The patient treated by *pneumoperitoneum* has air injected into the peritoneal cavity (abdominal cavity). The air pressing on his diaphragm pushes it upward into the chest. This pressure by the diaphragm on the lung causes it to collapse temporarily. The physician repeats this procedure as needed.

*Crushing the phrenic nerve*, which carries nerve impulses to the diaphragm, causes paralysis of one side of this muscular structure. The paralyzed portion of the diaphragm rises and presses against the lung, which subsequently collapses. The surgeon reaches the phrenic nerve through a small incision near the clavicle (collarbone). As the crushed nerve heals, the paralyzed part of the diaphragm resumes its function and the lung tissue expands.

Permanent collapse of a lung can be produced by a *thoracoplasty*. A portion of the ribs is removed over the part of the lungs which is diseased. This operation reduces the size of the chest wall causing it to press against the lung tissue. Thus, that part of the lung is permanently collapsed.

The physician may decide to do a pulmonary resection after careful evaluation of the patient's disease process. When an entire lung is removed, the procedure is known as a *pneumonectomy*. A *lobectomy* is the removal of a lobe of the lung.

### Convalescence

As the patient's body wins the battle being fought in his lungs, he is allowed to resume simple activities gradually. The physician gives specific instructions regarding the amount of rest and exercise which the patient needs. It is the responsibility of the nursing team to see that these directions are followed.

The patient now has to adjust to either a complete or a partial return to health. Although the idea of returning to his home is pleasant, the patient still has adjustments to make. He needs to change his thinking about himself and his disease. He was taught to think of himself as being sick when he entered the hospital; now he has the opportunity of learning to think in terms of becoming well again.

Often it is necessary for the nurse to stimulate the patient's interest in things other than himself and his immediate surroundings. The thoughtful nurse can help the patient to become interested in outside activities by encouraging him to read newspapers and magazines, to watch television, and to correspond with relatives and friends. If the hospital has an occupational therapist, she may be asked to guide the patient in diversional activities. In some instances the patient is taught a new way of making a living before being discharged from the hospital.

When the patient's tuberculous infection is considered to be arrested, he is removed from isolation as he is no longer likely to spread the disease. The patient should be given a tub bath and placed in a clean unit. Equipment in the isolated unit should be washed well with soap and water and then sunned and aired for at least two days. Mattress and pillows should be placed in direct sunlight for two days.

The patient has to learn what he can do without harming his health when he goes home. He should continue to use the good hygienic measures which he has learned in the hospital. These measures serve to protect him as well as others. The patient is given instructions by his doctor regarding follow-up visits.

## CANCER

### Incidence

A primary malignancy of the lungs (cancer which starts in the lungs) usually occurs in persons over 40 years of age. The practical nurse may want to review the general discussion of cancer in Chapter 7. Cancer of the lung most often occurs in one of the bronchi and is known as *bronchogenic carcinoma*. This type of malignancy causes 5 to 10 per cent of all deaths from cancer. It is more common in men than in women. The leading cause of death from cancer in men is bronchogenic carcinoma.

Research is being done to determine the relationship of smoking to lung cancer. Evidence is being accumulated which seems to indicate that the death rate from lung cancer is higher in smokers than in nonsmokers.

### Symptoms

Unfortunately the patient with cancer of the lungs has few, if any, symptoms during the early stage. He may be bothered by an irritating cough which gradually becomes worse. In some cases the patient has no symptoms until the malignant tumor has spread to the pleura. In this case, the patient complains of discomfort and pain in his chest. Hemoptysis (expectoration of blood), dyspnea (difficult breathing), and wheezing are seen frequently in the patient with lung cancer. The patient begins to lose weight as the disease progresses.

This patient may develop pleural effusion, which is discussed earlier in this chapter. He may also develop a severe infection in the lungs.

Usually a malignancy of the lungs has spread before the patient develops symptoms. Because of this, his prognosis is poor when the diagnosis is made. A ray of hope is being cast into this dark picture by the chest x-ray. Many cases of early lung cancer are being found by periodic chest x-rays. Of course, the physician must do a biopsy before he can make a definite diagnosis of malignancy. The practical nurse can understand from this discussion the importance of periodic chest x-rays, especially in men past 40 years of age.

Treatment

When the physician believes that the patient has a malignancy of the lungs, he does a biopsy (removal of a portion of the growth for examination with the microscope). This tissue is generally removed during a bronchoscopic examination.

The surgeon removes the diseased portion of the lung if the malignancy has not spread. In this case, a lobectomy or a pneumonectomy is done. The treatment of a patient with advanced cancer is directed toward making him comfortable. Although x-ray therapy cannot cure this patient, it is used frequently to slow the cancer's growth and to relieve discomfort. The nursing care of a person with cancer which is discussed in Chapter 7 is applicable to this patient.

SUGGESTIONS FOR STUDY

1. Review the nursing care of a patient with a persistent cough, which is discussed in Chapter 4.
2. What is bronchiectasis? What treatment is possible in some cases to cure the patient?
3. What causes pneumonia? Discuss the factors which predispose to pneumonia.
4. What is the difference between pleurisy and empyema?
5. What causes the patient with pleurisy to have pain? How can the practical nurse help to relieve his pain?
6. Discuss the factors which have contributed to the decrease in the death rate from tuberculosis in the last 50 years.
7. Discuss the responsibilities of the practical nurse in helping the doctor to diagnose pulmonary tuberculosis.
8. Review the nursing care of a patient with tuberculosis.
9. Why are periodic chest x-rays especially important for men past 40 years of age?

REFERENCES FOR CHAPTER 13

American Cancer Society, Inc.: A Cancer Source Book for Nurses. The Society, New York, 1956, pp. 82-84.
Anthony, Catherine P.: Textbook of Anatomy and Physiology, 4th ed. C. V. Mosby Co., St. Louis, 1955, pp. 439-68.

*Nursing care · oral hygiene*
*maybe tracheotomy*

Dakin, Florence; Thompson, Ella M.; and Le Baron, Margaret: *Simplified Nursing*, 6th ed. J. B. Lippincott Co., Philadelphia, 1956, pp. 356-69.

Eliason, Eldridge; Ferguson, L. Kraeer; and Sholtis, Lillian A.: *Surgical Nursing*, 10th ed. J. B. Lippincott Co., Philadelphia, 1955, pp. 225-54.

Emerson, Charles P., Jr., and Bragdon, Jane S.: *Essentials of Medicine*, 17th ed. J. B. Lippincott Co., Philadelphia, 1955, pp. 168-200 and 792-814.

Esau, Margaret C.; Fallon, Barbara R.; Frentzos, Kathryn S.; Phillips, Elisabeth C.; and Tourtillott, Eleanor A.: *Practical Nursing Today, Attitudes–Knowledge–Skills*. G. P. Putnam's Sons, New York, 1957, pp. 238-44.

Faddis, Margene O., and Hayman, Joseph M.: *Care of the Medical Patient*. McGraw-Hill Book Co., New York, 1952, pp. 297-331 and 580-90.

Goodale, Raymond: *Nursing Pathology*, 2nd ed. W. B. Saunders Co., Philadelphia, 1956, pp. 122-34.

Hull, Edgar, and Perrodin, Cecilia: *Medical Nursing*, 5th ed. F. A. Davis Co., Philadelphia, 1954, pp. 112-63 and 661-76.

Jensen, Julius, and Jensen, Deborah: *Nursing in Clinical Medicine*, 4th ed. The Macmillan Company, New York, 1954, pp. 342-82 and 759-79.

Parker, Lois: *The Calcified Cliffs*. National Tuberculosis Association, New York, 1954.

Sloan, Herbert, and Blackburn, Mary E.: "The Patient with Bronchiectasis," *Am. J. Nursing*, **55**:561-64, (May) 1955.

Solomon, Charles, and Gill, Elizabeth S.: *Pharmacology and Therapeutics*, 7th ed. J. B. Lippincott Co., Philadelphia, 1956, pp. 261-63 and 470-71.

South, Jean: *Tuberculosis Handbook for Public Health Nurses*. National Tuberculosis Association, New York, 1955.

Stafford, Edward S., and Diller, Doris: *Surgery and Surgical Nursing*, 3rd ed. W. B. Saunders Co., Philadelphia, 1958, pp. 172-201.

Steele, John D.: "Those Mysterious Drainage Bottles," *Am. J. Nursing*, **55**:1358-59, (Nov.) 1955.

West, John P.; Keller, Manelva W.; and Harmon, Elizabeth H.: *Nursing Care of the Surgical Patient*, 6th ed. The Macmillan Company, New York, 1957, pp. 203-27.

*Emphysema - blowing up of lungs*
*alveoli walls loose*
*elasticity & become dialated & descended*
*causes: Chronic Bronchitis - bronchiectasis*
*Complication of bronchial asthma*

R.S - Test MONDAY

P.184 Diagnostic test
  Pulmonary function
      vital capacity - maximum vol.
          expelled by forceful inspiration
      Residual volume - air't remaining in lungs
          after maximum exhalation
      Total capacity - total of above

      Tidal volume - air inspired normally

Bronchiograms - dye into bronchioles

Bronchoscopy

Esophagoscopy

_____

Pneumonectomy - back to operative side of d
    injection not drain to good lung
    other lung desired to expand
Lobectomy - pt. turn back to either side of d
    want both sides of lungs to expand

Wedge resection - back to unoperative side

Chest surgery - cough & deep breathe
                                        meth'care
 relieve of  O₂ therapy - Blood transfusion

# Nursing the Patient
# with a Disease of
# the Digestive System

*Test MENT. 3/14/96*

PART V

Test 4/17/66

3. 10 - 66

Chapter 14

# THE PATIENT
# WITH A DISEASE
# OF THE UPPER
# GASTROINTESTINAL SYSTEM

## STRUCTURE AND FUNCTION

The gastrointestinal tract may be referred to as the digestive system, or the alimentary canal. Its function is to change food into simpler substances which can be carried by the blood to the cells. In order to accomplish this function, the system must provide digestive juices. Food must also be transported through the canal. This movement is accomplished by *peristalsis*, which is a wormlike contraction of the intestines. After the food has been transformed into simple substances and absorbed, the waste products are carried to the lower part of the canal by peristalsis.

The digestive system consists of a tube approximately 7.8 to 9.4 meters (25 to 30 ft) in length. It begins with the mouth and ends with the anus. The mouth, the pharynx (throat), the esophagus, the stomach, the small intestine, and the large intestine are the organs of this system. The tongue, the teeth, the salivary glands, the pancreas, the liver, and the gallbladder aid the digestive system in its function. They are known as accessory organs.

The process of chewing food, which takes place in the mouth, makes digestion easier. Swallowing moves food from the mouth through the pharynx and esophagus into the stomach. The esophagus is a muscular tube approximately 22.5 cm (9 in.) in length.

Food remains for a while in the stomach, which is a dilatation of

205

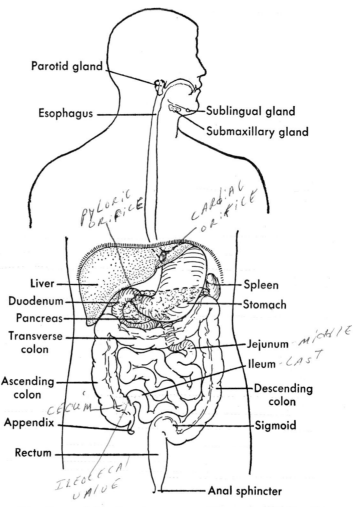

**Figure 27.** Parts of the digestive system. (Youmans, W. B.: *Human Physiology*. The Macmillan Company, New York, 1954.)

the alimentary canal resembling a pouch. The stomach is located in the upper left portion of the abdomen. The opening between the esophagus and the stomach is the cardiac orifice. The pyloric orifice is the opening between the stomach and the small intestine. The food is changed into a semiliquid condition in the stomach by its churning motion and by the secretion of gastric juice.

Peristalsis forces the partially digested food through the pylorus (lower part of the stomach) into the small intestine where absorption and further digestion take place. The upper portion of the small intestine is known as the duodenum. Substances to aid in digestion are usually emptied into the duodeum through a single opening known as the ampulla of Vater. The pancreatic duct and the common bile duct join to form this short tube. The pancreatic duct brings digestive juice from the pancreas. The common bile duct brings bile from both the liver and the gallbladder. The duodenum connects with the jejunum, which is the middle part of the small intestine. The jejunum leads to the ileum, which is the last portion of the small intestine. As the digested food is carried through the small intestine, the usable portion is absorbed into the lymph and blood vessels.

The waste products pass from the ileum into the large intestine. The four parts of the large intestine are the cecum, the colon, the rectum, and the anal canal. The first portion of the large intestine, which is the cecum, resembles a pouch. The ileocecal valve prevents the waste material from going back into the small intestine. The vermiform appendix is a small tube or wormlike projection attached to the cecum. The term vermiform means shaped like a worm.

Waste products are carried from the cecum into the colon, which is subdivided into the ascending, transverse, descending, and sigmoid colon. The ascending portion goes upward on the right side and the transverse goes across the abdomen. The descending colon goes downward on the left side. It leads into the sigmoid colon, which is shaped like the letter S; thus, it is called sigmoid which refers to the letter "S" in the Greek alphabet.

After waste material has been forced through the colon, it reaches the rectum. The rectum connects with the anal canal, which is the end portion of the large intestine. The anal canal is approximately 2.5 cm (1 in.) in length. It is closed by two sphincters (ringlike muscles) which open during defecation. The external opening is called the *anus*.

The *peritoneum* is a serous membrane which covers the abdominal organs. It consists of two layers which are in contact with each other. The inner layer of the peritoneum covers the abdominal organs and the outer layer lines the abdominal wall. A cavity may develop between the two layers when disease is present. This space, which may become a cavity, is referred to as the *peritoneal cavity*. The peritoneum secretes serum which lubricates the enclosed organs, and it also helps to hold these organs in place.

## STOMATITIS

A patient with stomatitis has an inflammation of the mouth. It may occur from one of many causes. The severity of stomatitis varies widely. A simple inflammation can be associated with a digestive disturbance and excessive smoking. Ulcerative stomatitis may occur in a person living in unsanitary conditions. Infections, such as thrush and Vincent's angina, which are caused by disease-producing microorganisms result in an inflamed mouth. Stomatitis may also be associated with a nutritional deficiency.

Treatment is directed toward relieving the underlying cause of stomatitis. For example, the patient with Vincent's angina is often given penicillin to combat the infection. The patient with a nutritional deficiency is treated by diet. The physician frequently prescribes a mouthwash for this patient. Good oral hygiene is of utmost importance.

## STRICTURE OF THE ESOPHAGUS

### Description

A stricture or narrowing of the esophagus may be present at birth. It can be caused by swallowing a substance, such as lye, which burns the tissues of the esophagus. The scar tissue which forms causes the esophagus to contract. This occurs most often in children. A mass near the esophagus, such as a tumor, may cause a stricture by pressure. A tumor growing within the esophagus will result in narrowing. Such a tumor is usually malignant.

## Treatment and Nursing Care

The patient with an esophageal stricture may be treated by dilatation. The physician inserts an instrument into the esophagus in an attempt to stretch the affected area. In some cases the surgeon can remove the narrowed portion. When the obstruction is complete and the above methods of treatment are not effective, a *gastrostomy* may be done. This is a surgical procedure in which a permanent, artificial opening is made into the stomach through the abdominal wall. A rubber tube is inserted into the opening. This makes it possible for nutrient liquids to be placed directly into the patient's stomach.

The nurse should attach a funnel to the rubber tube when she is responsible for feeding this patient. The prescribed fluid should be poured slowly into the funnel. Nausea and cramps may be prevented by first warming the liquid to body temperature. Water should be allowed to run through the funnel and tube after the feeding. This helps to remove the liquid food from the tube in addition to supplying part of the patient's daily water requirement. The tube should be clamped off after the feeding to prevent the fluid from escaping. The tube may be left in place or it may be removed after the feeding. The practical nurse should receive specific instructions from her team leader before removing the tube.

The patient's dressing needs to be changed frequently because of leakage from the stomach. Gastric juice tends to digest the skin. Because of this the operative area should be kept clean and dry. The nursing team should receive instructions for cleaning the area from the doctor.

This patient needs good oral hygiene. Because he is unable to take anything by mouth, he also needs to rinse his mouth frequently.

## GASTRITIS

### Description

A patient with gastritis has an inflammation of the mucous membrane lining the stomach. An acute case may be associated with an infectious disease, such as typhoid fever, measles, and influenza. An irritation of the mucous membrane caused by eating highly spiced foods, overeating, drinking too much alcohol, and taking too many aspirin results in gastritis. If a person continues with these irritating substances, he may develop chronic gastritis. A chronic case may also be associated with an ulcer, cancer, and liver disease.

Generally the patient with gastritis complains of abdominal dis-comfort, nausea, and eructation (burping). Hemorrhage may occur. Vomiting and abdominal distention are usually present. The symp-toms are more severe in an extremely acute case.

### Treatment

The physician prescribes a nonirritating diet to suit the individual patient's needs. The person with an extremely severe case of gastritis is generally given fluids intravenously. As his condition improves, he is able to take liquids by mouth and then a bland diet; later he is allowed to resume eating a regular diet gradually. However, the patient with a mild case may be treated from the beginning with a bland diet.

## PEPTIC ULCER

### Description

The patient with a peptic ulcer has an eroded area in the mucous membrane of either the stomach or the duodenum. It develops most often near the pylorus. The ulcer may penetrate muscle tissue under-lying the mucous membrane.

A peptic ulcer can affect all ages but is more common in persons between the ages of 20 and 50 years. Men are most likely to develop an ulcer between 30 and 50 years of age, and women between 20 and 30 years of age.

### Cause

The exact cause is not known. The patient with a peptic ulcer usually has an excessive amount of hydrochloric acid in his stomach. However, it does not occur in all individuals who have an excessive amount of this gastric juice. Peptic ulcer does not occur in a person who has no gastric hydrochloric acid.

Predisposing causes of a peptic ulcer can be emotional stress and strain, irregular hours of eating, and excessive smoking. Eating too rapidly may be a contributing factor.

## Symptoms

Although symptoms of a peptic ulcer vary, the patient generally has pain which has a relationship to the ingestion of food. He also has a history of dyspepsia (indigestion). The pain which is in the upper part of his abdomen results from irritation of the ulcer by gastric juice. This pain may be burning, boring, or gnawing in character. Frequently it occurs from one to three hours after meals. Relief from pain results from neutralization of the acid by food or an alkali such as sodium bicarbonate (baking soda). Vomiting, which rids the stomach of irritating gastric juice, may also relieve his pain.

## Diagnosis

The nursing team is responsible for assisting the physician in his diagnosis. The character of the patient's pain should be observed and reported. The nurse should also report any relationship of pain to either vomiting or eating. Symptoms of blood in either vomitus or feces should be noted. Frequently the practical nurse is assigned to collect specimens of vomitus and feces for examination.

Diagnostic procedures such as gastric analysis, gastrointestinal x-ray, and gastroscopy may be prescribed. In a gastric analysis, a small tube is passed by way of either the nose or the mouth through the throat and esophagus into the empty stomach. The contents are aspirated and examined. In an x-ray, the digestive tract is x-rayed after the patient receives a barium meal. A definite diagnosis can be made if the ulcer is shown by x-ray examination. In some cases the doctor examines the inside of the stomach with a gastroscope. This is an instrument which he inserts through the patient's mouth and esophagus into the stomach so that he can examine the stomach lining by looking at it.

The manner in which a patient is prepared for these diagnostic procedures varies in different institutions. In general, the patient is not allowed to eat or drink anything for a certain length of time before the procedure. The practical nurse should familiarize herself with the exact procedure in the hospital with which she is associated.

## Complications

Three serious complications of a peptic ulcer are perforation, obstruction, and hemorrhage. Perforation occurs when the ulcer becomes so deep that is goes through the entire wall of the diseased area. The patient with a perforated ulcer complains of sudden and severe abdominal pain. He becomes nauseated and vomits. He also develops symptoms of shock. Contents of the gastrointestinal tract leak through the hole into the peritoneal cavity. This is a cause of peritonitis which is discussed on pages 225 to 227.

The patient with excessive scar formation in and around the ulcerated area may develop an obstruction. Since scar tissue shrinks and is not elastic, it causes a narrowing of the passageway. If the pylorus is obstructed, it is known as *pyloric stenosis*. This patient vomits large amounts of food, and he often vomits undigested food which he ate the preceding day.

Hemorrhage occurs when the ulcer erodes the wall of a blood vessel. The amount of bleeding is determined by the size of the blood vessel. The patient develops hematemesis (vomiting of blood). The vomitus usually resembles coffee grounds. This change in the color of blood is due to the action of gastric juice. If the patient has a massive hemorrhage, he develops symptoms of shock which are discussed on page 57. Blood passing into the lower intestinal tract causes the stools to be black and tarry; this results from the action of digestive juices.

## Treatment and Nursing Care

### Medical Treatment

Medical treatment of the patient with a peptic ulcer is aimed toward protecting the raw area from further irritation by gastric juice and certain foods so that it can heal. This is accomplished by diet, rest, and drugs.

Bed rest is prescribed in acute cases. Most physicians advise their patients to stop smoking. Efforts are made to protect the patient from situations which produce stress and strain. Since emotional tension affects both peristalsis and digestive juices, it aggravates the ulcer. As the patient's condition improves, he is guided by the doctor and the nursing team in resuming his activities. He will continue to need to avoid becoming emotionally tense.

Although the diet is prescribed to suit each individual person, it is based on certain principles. In general, it consists of foods which are nonirritating and easily digested, and which supply the patient's nutritional requirements. The food is served at frequent and regular intervals and in small amounts. Alcohol is restricted as it stimulates the flow of digestive juices. This type of dietary regimen aids in protecting the ulcer from gastric juice and prevents further irritation.

Generally the patient is served a diet consisting of a mixture of milk and cream and cooked strained cereals during the acute phase of his illness. These are given frequently and in small amounts. It is important for the nurse to serve the correct amount at the hours specified. As the patient improves, he is given bland foods, such as soft-cooked eggs, custard, toast, puréed vegetables, and easily digested meats. He should avoid extremely hot or cold foods. When he is ready to assume a more regular diet, he is advised to avoid foods which irritate his stomach, such as highly seasoned foods and those which are difficult to digest. The patient should continue regular eating habits and avoid irritating foods after his ulcer has healed.

Antacids and antispasmodics are the two main types of drugs prescribed for this patient. An *antacid* neutralizes the acid in the stomach. An *antispasmodic* relaxes the muscles of the stomach and relieves the pain associated with spasms. Drugs, such as aluminum hydroxide gel, calcium carbonate, magnesium trisilicate, and magnesium oxide, are used in various combinations for their antacid effect. The practical nurse may hear these preparations referred to by their trade names, such as Amphojel, Creamalin, and Gelusil.* Tincture of belladonna and methantheline (Banthine) are examples of drugs which may be ordered for their antispasmodic effect.

### Surgical Treatment

Usually surgery is indicated when any one of the three complications (perforation, obstruction, or hemorrhage) occurs. It also may be necessary when the patient's pain is not relieved by medical treatment and when the ulcer does not heal properly. The surgical

---

* Amphojel and Creamalin are aluminum hydroxide gels; Gelusil contains both magnesium trisilicate and aluminum hydroxide gel.

procedure frequently performed is a *partial or subtotal gastrectomy*. In this operation, the lower two-thirds to three-fourths of the stomach is removed and the small intestine is attached to the remaining part of the stomach.

Gastric suction is used frequently to withdraw fluids and gas from the stomach either before or after surgery. This is accomplished by the insertion of a tube, such as the Levin tube, into the stomach. The tube is then attached to gentle suction. Gastric suction can be accomplished by a Wangensteen apparatus in which suction is obtained by the use of water flowing from one closed bottle to another. Electrical equipment to provide suction of the gastric contents is also available, and the practical nurse may hear the term "Wangensteen suction" used in reference to many types of equipment used for gastric suction.

It is the nursing team's responsibility to see that the equipment functions properly. The nurse should check it frequently to see that it is draining properly. Several ounces of water may be instilled into the tube with a syringe to remove such substances as mucus which can obstruct the free passage of fluid. Frequently the doctor leaves an order for the nurse to irrigate the tube every one or two hours to prevent clogging. The drainage should be measured and the amount reported. The practical nurse should also observe and report the color of the drainage.

In caring for the patient with gastric suction, the practical nurse should relieve the dryness of his mouth and throat. Use of mineral oil or glycerin mixed with a small amount of lemon juice should make the patient's dry lips more comfortable. Small amounts of cracked ice and sips of water may be given to the patient if permitted by the doctor. Generally the patient is given nourishment by infusion. In addition to its antiseptic effect, frequent use of a mouthwash helps to relieve dryness. The patient is usually given small frequent feedings after the tube is removed from his stomach.

## CANCER

### Mouth and Throat

Cancer of the mouth and throat is more common in older men. This is the fifth commonest site of cancer in men. Over 3 per cent of the men who die from cancer have the growth in either their mouth or throat. The prognosis for a patient having a malignancy in this area is good when he is diagnosed and treated early. Often the patient develops cancer in a portion of the mouth or throat which has been subjected to irritation over a long period of time.

Both surgery and radiotherapy are used in treating a malignancy in this area. Frequently the patient is undernourished when he reports for treatment. It may be difficult, uncomfortable, and even painful for him to eat. The nurse plays an essential role in encouraging the patient to eat. It is of great importance that the food be served in an appetizing manner. If the patient is unable to eat, he may have a tube inserted through his nose into his stomach so that he can be fed through the tube; the feeding is warmed to body temperature before it is given to the patient.

The nurse has only to remember her discomfort when she had a small ulcer (canker sore) in her mouth in order to imagine how this patient's mouth feels. Recalling this, she can easily understand the importance of scrupulous and frequent mouth care. This care adds to the patient's comfort and helps to prevent infection. The nurse may be assigned to irrigate the wound. The nature, treatment, and nursing care of a patient with cancer are discussed fully in Chapter 7.

### Esophagus

Cancer of the esophagus occurs most often in men. It causes 2 per cent of all deaths from cancer in the United States. The prognosis for a patient with cancer of the esophagus is poor. The average length of life after he has noticed the first symptom is approximately eight months.

The patient with a malignancy of the esophagus usually complains of *dysphagia,* which is difficult swallowing. He may be treated with surgery but the main treatment is radiotherapy.

### Stomach

Cancer of the stomach is common. It causes 10 per cent of all deaths from cancer. This disease is more common in men than in women. A malignancy of the stomach occurs most frequently during middle age but it may affect younger people. The prognosis is poor because the patient has few symptoms to warn himself or his doctor during the early stage of the tumor's growth.

Unfortunately, the symptoms of cancer in the stomach are indefinite during its early growth. One of the first symptoms experienced by the patient is dyspepsia (indigestion). Frequently the patient does not consult his doctor about this because he thinks it is of no importance. Remembering that people over 40 years of age are more susceptible to this disease helps the practical nurse realize the importance of encouraging friends and relatives to visit their doctor when indigestion persists. This seems to be of particular importance in an individual who is not accustomed to having indigestion.

The patient loses weight and strength as the disease progresses. He later becomes anemic. A gastric analysis shows that no hydrochloric acid is present. The patient may vomit blood and have blood in his stools. Pain is another late symptom.

A patient having cancer of the stomach is frequently treated with surgery. The surgeon does either a total or a partial gastrectomy whenever possible in an effort to cure the patient. Surgery is performed in some cases to make the patient more comfortable and to add a short time to his life if the malignancy has already spread. Radiotherapy is used on some patients.


## SUGGESTIONS FOR STUDY

1. Discuss safety measures for the home which should help to prevent stricture of the esophagus caused by swallowing substances which burn.

2. Why should water be instilled into the tube after the patient has been fed through a gastrostomy tube?

3. Discuss the types of food which the patient with gastritis would probably be allowed to eat. The patient with a peptic ulcer.

4. What are the predisposing causes of a peptic ulcer?

5. Review the responsibilities of the nursing team in assisting the doctor with his diagnosis of peptic ulcer.

6. What is the doctor's main aim in treating the patient with a peptic ulcer? What are the responsibilities of the nursing team in helping him to accomplish this aim?

7. Review the nursing care of a patient treated surgically for a peptic ulcer.

8. What are the early symptoms which an individual with cancer of the upper gastrointestinal system may have?

9. Review the nursing care of a patient with gastric suction.

## REFERENCES FOR CHAPTER 14

American Cancer Society, Inc.: *A Cancer Source Book for Nurses.* The Society, New York, 1956, pp. 70-78.

Brown, Amy F.: *Medical Nursing,* 3rd ed. W. B. Saunders Co., Philadelphia, 1957, pp. 380-403.

Eliason, Eldridge; Ferguson, L. Kraeer; and Sholtis, Lillian A.: *Surgical Nursing,* 10th ed. J. B. Lippincott Co., Philadelphia, 1955, pp. 287-315.

Emerson, Charles P., Jr., and Bragdon, Jane S.: *Essentials of Medicine,* 17th ed. J. B. Lippincott Co., Philadelphia, 1955, pp. 311-39.

Esau, Margaret; Fallon, Barbara R.; Frentzos, Kathryn G.; Phillips, Elisabeth C.; and Tourtillott, Eleanor A.: *Practical Nursing Today, Attitudes–Knowledge–Skills.* G. P. Putnam's Sons, New York, 1957, pp. 65-69 and 332-34.

Faddis, Margene O., and Hayman, Joseph M.: *Care of the Medical Patient.* McGraw-Hill Book Co., New York, 1952, pp. 333-59.

Gill, Helen Z. (ed.): *Basic Nursing,* 4th ed. The Macmillan Company, New York, 1955, pp. 79-88 and 535-41.

Jensen, Julius, and Jensen, Deborah: *Nursing in Clinical Medicine,* 4th ed. The Macmillan Company, New York, 1954, pp. 383-414.

Kimber, Diana; Gray, Carolyn E.; Stackpole, Caroline E.; and Leavell, Lutie C.: *Textbook of Anatomy and Physiology,* 13th ed. The Macmillan Company, New York, 1955, pp. 521-35.

Miller, Theodore R., and Cantwell, Agnes E.: "Gastric Cancer," *Am. J. Nursing,* 56:1420-23, (Nov.) 1956.

Musser, Ruth D., and Bird, Joseph G.: *Modern Pharmacology and Therapeutics.* The Macmillan Company, New York, 1958, pp. 581-95.

Proudfit, Fairfax T., and Robinson, Corinne H.: *Nutrition and Diet Therapy,* 11th ed. The Macmillan Company, New York, 1955, pp. 379-95.

West, John P.; Keller, Manelva W.; and Harmon, Elizabeth H.: *Nursing Care of the Surgical Patient,* 6th ed. The Macmillan Company, New York, 1957, pp. 262-88.

# Chapter 15

# THE PATIENT
# WITH A DISEASE
# OF THE LOWER
# GASTROINTESTINAL SYSTEM

## APPENDICITIS

### Description

The patient with appendicitis has an inflammation of the vermiform appendix, which is attached to the cecum. Since the appendix has only one opening, it is easily infected. Contents of the intestinal tract enter and leave the appendix through its one opening into the cecum. If the passageway is blocked by kinking or by fecal material, the appendix becomes infected by bacteria which are always present.

### Symptoms

Quite commonly a person who is developing appendicitis has generalized abdominal pain. It gradually becomes localized in the right lower portion of the abdomen. Fever, nausea, and vomiting frequently occur. He may be constipated although this symptom is not always present. The physician notices that the muscles in the right lower part of the abdomen are rigid. He also detects tenderness in this area. Leukocytosis, elevation of the white blood cell count, is found upon examination of the blood.

218

## Complications

A hole may develop in an inflamed appendix. In this case it is known as a *ruptured appendix* or a *perforated appendix*. The infected material seeps through the opening into the peritoneal cavity. This may cause either a localized or a generalized infection. When the patient has a localized infection, he develops an abscess. In this case, the inflammatory process is walled off by the body's defenses so that the infection is localized in that area. The patient with a generalized infection has peritonitis. This condition is discussed in more detail later in the chapter.

The patient's acute pain usually disappears suddenly when his appendix ruptures. He is comparatively comfortable for a few hours. Then he develops symptoms of a more acute infection and often of shock.

## Treatment and Nursing Care

The treatment of a patient with appendicitis is removal of the appendix, *appendectomy*. If the physician thinks the appendix has ruptured and peritonitis has developed, he may treat the patient medically with antibiotics, rest, and intravenous fluids. This is continued until the surgeon feels confident that the infection has become localized. Then he operates. If an abscess has formed, it may be drained before the appendix is removed.

The practical nurse should remember that a person with symptoms of appendicitis should not take a laxative or an enema. He should be advised to consult his physician. These self-prescribed remedies can cause the appendix to rupture. This information is so important for the general public to know that it is written on many labels of laxatives sold over the counter. Heat should not be applied to the abdomen of a person with these symptoms unless prescribed by the doctor because heat can hasten the formation of pus.

Since an appendectomy is frequently an emergency operation, the general preoperative care discussed in Chapter 5 is carried out within a shorter period of time. Two specific variations in the care of this patient are the use of an ice bag and the omission of an enema. Frequently the physician asks the nurse to place an ice bag on the right lower part of the patient's abdomen. In some cases a preoperative enema is not prescribed in order to prevent stimulation of peristalsis. The care of this patient after surgery is the same as that discussed in Chapter 5.

## COLITIS

### Description

The patient with colitis has an inflammation of the colon. There are many causes of this disease. It may be caused by conditions which produce diarrhea, such as typhoid fever, food poisoning, and dysentery) It may be associated with another disease of the gastrointestinal tract, such as cancer and *diverticulitis,* which is an inflammation of abnormal sacs or pouches in the bowel wall. Colitis may occur in connection with disease elsewhere in the body such as uremia and pneumonia. Emotional stress may be a causative factor.

### Symptoms

The patient affected with colitis has diarrhea and abdominal cramps. He may have alternating periods of constipation and diarrhea. Abdominal distention may be another symptom.

If a patient passes stringy mucus, he has a type of colitis known as *mucous colitis.* The mucus may be streaked with blood. The patient with ulcers in the colon has *ulcerative colitis.* His stools may contain blood, pus, and mucus. This is a serious type of colitis.

### Treatment and Nursing Care

The physician bases his treatment of this patient on the underlying cause. For example, the patient with dysentery is treated with either sulfonamides or antibiotics. A patient with diverticula may have them removed. The understanding physician attempts to help the patient with emotional problems. The nursing care of a patient with diarrhea, which has already been discussed on pages 30 to 31, is applicable to this patient.

Diet is one of the most important aspects of treatment. The doctor prescribes a low-residue, but nutritious diet. It should be high in proteins and vitamins. The purpose of the low-residue diet is to prevent roughage from entering the large intestine and causing further irritation.

The physician prescribes sedatives to relieve nervous tension when this is necessary. Antispasmodics, such as tincture of belladonna, may be ordered to relieve the pain from spasm.

## INTESTINAL OBSTRUCTION

### Description

The patient with an intestinal obstruction has a hindrance to the normal flow of the contents within the intestines. The obstruction may be either partial or complete, and it is a symptom and not a disease. Since the treatment of a patient with an intestinal obstruction is directed toward relieving this symptom first, the care of this patient is given special consideration. The obstructed portion of the intestine may become *strangulated.* This means that the blood supply to that area is decreased, and the tissue may become gangrenous. If the practical nurse remembers this complication, she understands the surgeon's reason for doing emergency surgery on a patient with intestinal obstruction.

### Cause

An intestinal obstruction can be caused by paralysis of the intestines which is known as *paralytic ileus*. In this condition the patient's intestinal muscles become paralyzed or lose their ability to contract. Frequently paralytic ileus is associated with peritonitis.

A growth, such as a tumor, pressing on the outside of the intestinal wall may obstruct the bowel. Also, obstruction can be caused by growths within the intestine, such as a malignancy and a polyp. An abnormal growth of tissue which appears to be growing on a stalk is known as a *polyp*. It can be thought of as tissue resembling a mushroom.

Swallowing an object which is large enough to obstruct the passageway can cause this condition. For example, a child may swallow a toy. *Intussusception*, which is the term used when one portion of the intestine slips into another part, results in an obstruction. This may be thought of as a telescoping of the intestine. Intussusception occurs more often in children. Bands of adhesions, which are masses of scar tissue resulting from an infection, may constrict the intestines. Also, an intestinal obstruction may be caused by *volvulus*, in which the intestine becomes twisted upon itself. (*Diverticulitis*) may cause an obstruction.

## Symptoms

The patient with an intestinal obstruction is constipated. At first he may pass small, loose stools. Constipation increases as the patient's condition becomes worse. For the most part, he passes neither gas nor feces when the canal is blocked completely. The patient complains of cramp-like pains in his abdomen which (come and go) The pain is spasmodic in nature because of the peristaltic waves hitting the obstruction. The patient's pain increases as his condition becomes more serious. Nausea and vomiting add to his discomfort. The vomitus may have a fecal odor. Abdominal distention develops. Frequently the patient has a fever, an increased pulse rate, and an increased respiratory rate.

## Treatment and Nursing Care

The physician's plan of treatment is directed toward relieving the obstruction as well as removing the underlying cause when possible. Both gastrointestinal suction and surgery may be used to accomplish this aim. In some cases one of these methods of treatment may be used without the other. For example, the patient with paralytic ileus resulting from peritonitis is generally treated with suction and not with surgery. The physician then directs his efforts toward treating the underlying cause, peritonitis.

### Gastrointestinal Suction

Since the practical nurse may be helping to care for the patient with gastrointestinal suction, she needs an understanding of it. A long catheter, such as either the Cantor tube or the Miller-Abbott tube, is inserted into the patient's stomach. The catheter is designed so that it passes through the stomach into the intestines. The Miller-Abbott tube has a rubber balloon on the end, and after the tube has been passed into the digestive tract, the balloon is inflated with air which is forced into it with a syringe. The Cantor tube has mercury (heavy metal) in a bag attached to the end which goes into the patient's stomach. The tube is carried into the intestines by the action of peristalsis on the balloon or the bag containing mercury. Since mercury is heavy, its downward passage is helped by gravity.

After the catheter has been inserted, it is attached to a suction apparatus such as that used for a patient with gastric suction.

The care needed by the patient with this type of suction is similar to that needed by the patient with gastric suction, which is discussed on page 214. Unlike the patient with a Levin tube in his stomach, this patient may be given liquid nourishment. In this case the physician prescribes the fluids after the tube has passed into the intestines. The nurse should keep an accurate record of the patient's intake and output.

The patient's symptoms of pain and distention are usually relieved by suction. The patient who has an obstruction caused by paralysis of the small intestine (paralytic ileus) can be expected to improve as he recovers from the condition which caused it.

### Surgery

The patient with an obstruction caused by diseases other than paralytic ileus usually requires surgery. In general, the physician performs surgery when he thinks the patient is capable of withstanding it. He may do surgery to relieve the obstruction or to remove the cause. When the patient has a temporary operation to relieve the obstruction, he needs a second operation to remove the cause.

When the surgeon does an *enterostomy,* he makes an artificial opening in the intestine through the abdominal wall. This opening is made above the obstruction so that the intestinal contents can flow through it. Thus, the condition is relieved. The surgeon may perform another operation to remove the cause, to make a permanent opening into the intestine, or to suture the intestine and close the abdomen.

The term *enterostomy* is a general term used in referring to the formation of an artificial opening in the intestine. Frequently the practical nurse hears other terms used which tell the site of this operation. The term *ileostomy* means the artificial opening was made in the ileum, *cecostomy* in the cecum, and *colostomy* in the colon.

As stated previously, surgery may be done to remove the cause of an obstruction. For example, tumors, polyps, bands of adhesions, and diverticula are removed by the surgeon in cases where this is possible. When the surgeon operates on a patient with an intussusception, he may be able to withdraw the telescoped portion of the intestine. If the intestine is affected by an inadequate blood supply, it is resected or removed. This type of operation is known as an *intestinal resection.* The patient with volvulus has the affected portion of his intestine untwisted; an intestinal resection is performed if the bowel has become gangrenous.

Generally the physician prescribes intravenous fluids, an antibiotic, and suction of either the stomach or intestines before surgery. Some surgeons have a Levin tube inserted in the patient's stomach before surgery. Frequently this treatment is continued for several days after operation. It is the responsibility of the nursing team to assist the surgeon in preparing the patient for surgery. The nursing care of a patient before and after surgery, which is discussed in Chapter 5, is applicable to this patient.

## DIVERTICULUM

### Description

The patient with a *diverticulum* has a sac or a pouch on the intestinal wall. It can be thought of as resembling the appendix. Although diverticula (plural for diverticulum) may occur in parts of the body other than the intestines (for example, diverticula may be found in the esophagus, stomach, and urinary bladder), this discussion deals with those in the lower gastrointestinal tract.

A person may be born with a diverticulum or he may develop it later in life. He may have more than one diverticulum. Frequently it occurs in a middle-aged person who is bothered with constipation. Diverticula occur most often in the colon. The patient with more than one diverticulum is said to have multiple diverticula.

### Symptoms

Usually the patient has no symptoms unless the diverticulum becomes infected. This is known as *diverticulitis.* Inflammation is encouraged by the collection of feces in the sac. In this case, the patient develops symptoms of an inflammation which resemble those of appendicitis. Diverticulitis may be complicated by an abscess.

### Treatment

The patient with a diverticulum who has no symptoms ordinarily requires no special treatment. A diverticulectomy (removal of di-

verticulum) is performed if an inflammation occurs. The patient
with multiple diverticula is frequently treated medically if he develops
diverticulitis. Measures such as low-residue diet, rest, and warm
applications to the abdomen may be ordered.

## PERITONITIS

### Description

The patient with peritonitis has an inflammation of the peritoneum. It may be localized, such as the inflammatory process around a
perforated ulcer, or it may be generalized. In this case, the entire
cavity is inflamed. Generalized peritonitis is a serious condition.

### Cause

Infection is the most common cause of peritonitis. Baceria spread
through a perforation in an abdominal organ. The infected contents
of that organ pour into the peritoneal cavity. For example, peritonitis
can be caused by a ruptured appendix or a perforated ulcer. Occasionally, peritonitis occurs in the absence of infection. Foreign substances
such as urine, bile, and digestive juices in the peritoneal cavity have
an irritating effect. These substances may escape from their normal
places during surgery; or the cavities in which they are contained may
be ruptured in an accident. The following discussion deals with
peritonitis resulting from infection.

### Symptoms

The symptoms of a patient with peritonitis vary with the amount
of infection present. He complains of abdominal pain. Frequently
the nurse notices the patient lying on his back. He tends to bring
his knees up toward his abdomen to relieve the pain. Nausea, vomiting, and constipation are present. The patient's abdomen becomes
distended and tender. He develops a fever and an increased pulse rate,
and later a weak pulse as the infection progresses. His respiration
becomes shallow and rapid because of abdominal distention and pain.
The patient also becomes thirsty.

### Complications

As stated earlier in this chapter, peritonitis may be complicated by
an intestinal obstruction. Another complication of an inflammation

in the abdominal cavity is _adhesions._ These are abnormal unions of surfaces which are normally separate. In other words, the surfaces of structures in the abdominal cavity stick together. This is a result of fibrous bands which form because of the inflammatory process. Adhesions can prevent smooth functioning of the organs. After the patient has recovered from the peritonitis, he may develop symptoms of adhesions, such as constipation, distention, abdominal pain, and vomiting. The adhesions sometimes cause an intestinal obstruction. The surgeon usually treats a patient with adhesions by cutting them so that the affected organs can once again function properly.

### Treatment and Nursing Care

Treatment of the patient with peritonitis is directed toward relieving the underlying cause if possible; it may be surgical, medical, or a combination of both. For example, surgery for a ruptured appendix or gallbladder may be performed. If the physician is not sure of the cause and he thinks an operation is necessary, he may do an _exploratory laparotomy._ This is a surgical procedure in which the abdomen is opened so that the doctor can search for the diseased area.

Rest, fluids, drugs to combat infection, and either gastric or gastrointestinal suction are important measures in the medical treatment of this patient. These factors may also be used in connection with surgery. It is the responsibility of the nursing team to make the patient as comfortable as possible so that he can rest. The physician prescribes a drug, such as morphine, when this is necessary to relieve the patient's pain. Fluids are given by infusion until the patient improves and nourishment can be given by mouth. A drug, such as penicillin, one of the sulfonamides, or streptomycin, is prescribed to combat the infection. Use of either gastric or gastrointestinal suction is continued as long as the patient's vomiting and distention are marked.

Following surgery, the physician may request that the patient be placed in Fowler's position. To carry out this order, the nurse should raise the head of the bed 45 to 50 cm (18 to 20 in.). It is believed that this position prevents the infection from spreading to the upper part of the abdomen, especially when the infection is in the lower abdomen. Frequently the surgeon leaves a drain in the incision. In this case the dressing needs to be changed frequently. The nature of the drainage should be observed and recorded.

_Analgesics & antibiotics given_

The patient's symptoms, such as (distention, pain, and fever) begin to decrease as the infection subsides. There is less drainage through the suction tube. The patient begins to pass flatus and feces as peristalsis and the muscle tone of his intestines return to normal.

## ABDOMINAL HERNIA

### Description

An individual with an abdominal hernia has a protrusion of a part of the contents of his abdomen through the abdominal wall. It may be congenital (present at birth) or it may be acquired later in life. Terms are used to indicate the location of the hernia. For example, an *inguinal hernia* is located in the inguinal canal in the groin. An *umbilical hernia* is in the umbilicus or navel. An *incisional* or *ventral* hernia is located in an operative scar. A hernia is *reducible* (when the abdominal contents can be forced back into the cavity by gentle pressure.) An *irreducible* hernia is one in which this is not possible.

Two complications of a hernia which may occur are strangulation and an intestinal obstruction. The hernia becomes strangulated when the abdominal contents which protrude through the opening receive an inadequate blood supply. An intestinal obstruction occurs when the intestinal contents are unable to pass through the bowel affected by the hernia. Emergency surgery is usually needed for both complications. *Hiatus hernia - stomach into diaphragm*

### Treatment     *N & U, digestive symptoms,*

The patient with an abdominal hernia is usually treated by surgery. A *herniorrhaphy* is done. This is an operation to repair the defect in the wall. The doctor advises the patient how long he should wait before resuming his normal activities. In some few cases, the physician may recommend a *truss*. This device is worn over the reduced hernia to keep it from slipping out again. *Sevin tube     Chest tube for hiatus!*

*Pre-op - prep                    F. catle*

## HEMORRHOIDS

### Description

The patient with hemorrhoids has dilated or varicose veins of the anal canal and the lower part of the rectum. Those which develop around the anal orifice are called *external hemorrhoids*. Dilated veins located in the area of the junction of the anal canal and the rectum are known as *internal hemorrhoids*.

Conditions which interfere with the flow of blood through the veins can cause a person to develop hemorrhoids. For example, chronic constipation and pressure by a tumor may result in this condition. They may occur during pregnancy as a result of pressure on the veins from the enlarging uterus. The vein walls in some individuals are weaker than in others; this predisposes to the development of hemorrhoids.

### Symptoms

Frequently the person with hemorrhoids passes bright red blood in his stools. He experiences varying degrees of discomfort when having a bowel movement. The pain is increased if the hemorrhoid becomes thrombosed. In this case, the blood within the dilated vein clots. Another symptom of hemorrhoids is itching around the anus.

### Treatment and Nursing Care

The usual treatment for hemorrhoids is their removal by surgery, hemorrhoidectomy. If the patient has a mild case, he may need only symptomatic treatment. For example, sitz baths to relieve discomfort, the local application of an ointment to shrink the mucous membrane, and a mild laxative, such as mineral oil, to soften the feces often bring relief to these patients. The physician sometimes injects sclerosing medication into the vein. This substance blocks the blood vessel so that blood has to leave the area through another vein. (Injecting a sclerosing medication into the vein may be used also for patients with varicose veins in the leg.)

The practical nurse is responsible for assisting other members of the nursing team in caring for the patient who has had a hemorrhoidectomy. Thus, she needs to know the special points which contribute to his comfort and welfare.

In addition to usual preoperative orders, the physician leaves specific instructions regarding the cleansing of the patient's rectum. Usually one or more enemas are ordered. Sometimes the practical nurse is instructed to give enemas until the solution returns clear. A thorough cleansing of the bowel is important so that the operative field is not contaminated by feces during surgery. The nurse should be sure that all of the enema solution is expelled.

In caring for the postoperative patient, the practical nurse should check the dressing frequently for blood. This should be reported promptly to her team leader or head nurse. It may be necessary to change the dressing frequently.

Some surgeons want to prevent the patient from having a bowel movement during the first few days after surgery. In this case, the the patient's diet consists of liquids. Paregoric may be prescribed to produce constipation. Generally the doctor orders a mild laxative and an oil retention enema several days after surgery. Following this, he allows the patient to have either a soft or a regular diet.

Other surgeons do not want to prevent the patient from having a bowel movement during his early postoperative days. The patient is given a regular diet soon after surgery. A laxative, such as mineral oil and psyllium hydrophilic mucilloid (Metamucil), is given as ordered so that the feces are soft. The area should be cleaned according to hospital procedure after the patient has had a bowel movement.

Many patients have severe pain after rectal surgery. The doctor prescribes narcotics, such as morphine and meperidine (Demerol), for its relief. Moist heat is also beneficial in relieving this patient's pain. It is used, as ordered, in the form of a sitz bath, compresses, and irrigations. These treatments help to relieve pain by relaxing muscle spasm. They also help to prevent infection because of their cleansing action.

Retention of urine is a frequent discomfort following rectal surgery. The patient should be checked for signs of retention. Nursing measures to stimulate voiding are discussed on page 43. If he is unable to void, the patient is catheterized.

## ANAL FISSURE

### Description

The patient with an anal fissure has an ulcerating crack or crevice in the mucous membrane of the anal wall. His main symptom is pain during and after a bowel movement. An anal fissure has a tendency to become chronic.

### Treatment

A mild case may be treated by a diet to correct constipation and by a laxative to soften the feces. Surgery is used in more extensive cases. The ulcer is removed, and the wound is allowed to heal from the bottom outward. The nursing care of this patient is the same as that discussed for the patient who has had a hemorrhoidectomy.

## ISCHIORECTAL ABSCESS

### Description

The patient with an ischiorectal abscess has an abscess in the fatty tissue near the anus. It results from an infection which started in the rectum and spread into the nearby soft tissue. The patient has throbbing pain around the rectum. He develops general symptoms of an infection, such as fever and malaise.

### Treatment

This condition is treated surgically. The surgeon makes an opening into the abscess to allow the pus to drain. This is known as incision and drainage. The patient has no further difficulty if the infected area heals completely. The nursing care of the patient who has had a hemorrhoidectomy also applies to this patient.

$(I \& D)$

## ANAL FISTULA

### Description

An anal fistula is an abnormal canal leading from either the anus or rectum. It may lead to the outside skin, another cavity such as the vagina, or the tissue of the buttocks. A person develops this condition following an ischiorectal abscess. The infected area heals incompletely, and a small draining canal or fistula develops and leads from the cavity left by the abscess to the rectum. Small particles of feces may enter the canal from the rectum and cause another infection. Another abscess is likely to form unless the opening into the rectum becomes closed.

Pilonidal cyst - located surface of lower sacrum means cyst of hair - may be congenital

## Treatment

The patient with an anal fistula is treated with surgery. The tract or canal is opened and excised completely so that healing can take place from the bottom upward.

## CANCER OF THE LARGE INTESTINE

### Incidence

Cancer of the large intestine is common. It may occur in any part of the large intestine. Men are affected most often by cancer of the rectum and women by cancer of the colon. Although this disease may affect young people, it is more common in older individuals. The prognosis for patients with a malignancy of the large intestine is good. Approximately 60 per cent of those with cancer of the colon get well. About 45 per cent of the patients with a malignancy of the rectum are cured.

### Symptoms

Usually the patient with a malignancy of the large intestine first notices a change in his bowel habits. Blood in his stools is frequently the symptom which sends him to his doctor. The patient begins to lose weight and becomes anemic as the disease continues. He develops symptoms of an intestinal obstruction if the malignancy blocks the bowel.

### Treatment and Nursing Care

There is a variety of surgical procedures for treating the patient with cancer of the large bowel. The malignancy and the surrounding tissue may be removed if the tumor is in the cecum, or in the ascending, transverse, or descending colon. Cancer of the lower part of the sigmoid colon generally requires an *abdominoperineal operation*. In this procedure, usually the entire rectum, anus, and part of the colon are removed. Part of the operation is done through an abdominal incision and part through a perineal incision. Thus, the term (abdominoperineal) operation is used. A permanent colostomy is done. In this case the colon is brought through the abdominal wall and an artificial anus is made.

Preparation of the patient for surgery of the large intestine may take from several days to a week. This time is necessary in order to clean the intestinal tract and to improve the patient's general state of health. In addition to knowing the general nursing care of a pre-operative patient discussed in Chapter 5, the practical nurse needs an understanding of the special care required by this patient. She can expect the physician to order a low-residue but nourishing diet, enemas, and drugs to combat or to prevent infection. The purpose of the low-residue diet is to avoid the presence of waste material after the operation. Enemas are given to clean the colon. Drugs, such as a sulfonamide or an antibiotic, are used to reduce the number of bacteria in the intestines before surgery. Thus, the possibility of postoperative infection is lessened.

The discussion which follows deals with the special needs of this patient after surgery. This is in addition to the general postoperative care discussed on pages 53 to 56. The physician usually does not allow the patient to have fluids or food by mouth for the first day or two after surgery. Frequently the practical nurse is asked to assist in giving the patient fluids intravenously or by hypodermoclysis (into the tissue beneath the skin). The physician may find it necessary to give the patient blood transfusions. Following an abdominoperineal resection, the patient usually has a retention (indwelling) catheter. It is the responsibility of the nursing team to measure and record the amount of urine every six to eight hours. The doctor may order a periodic irrigation of the catheter.

### Colostomy

As an important member of the nursing team, the practical nurse is frequently responsible for assisting in the care of a patient with a colostomy. The attitude of members of the nursing team toward this patient is of great importance. The practical nurse needs to know that a colostomy can be regulated. Many individuals return to their places in society and lead useful, satisfying lives. It is necessary for those who care for this patient to help him develop this attitude.

After the surgeon has done the colostomy, he may insert a large catheter into the colon for drainage or he may apply dressings. The catheter is inserted to allow the fecal material to drain through it. This prevents the wound in the colostomy site from becoming contaminated until it has healed. If a large catheter is used, it is attached to a drainage tube and bottle. When dressings are used to absorb the drainage, they must be changed frequently. This is necessary in order to prevent fecal drainage from irritating the wound, to make the patient more comfortable, and to prevent offensive odors. The skin around the area should be cleaned thoroughly with soap and water. Both the wound and the skin around the colostomy must be protected from the action of the intestinal contents. Petrolatum gauze, aluminum paste, or zinc oxide ointment may be prescribed for this purpose. Loose and absorbent dressings are used.

The care of this patient is aimed toward helping him to control his bowel movements through the colostomy by the proper diet and regular irrigations. The physician specifies the types of foods the patient is to receive. The diet usually progresses from semisoft to a low-residue one. The nurse should observe and report changes in the patient's bowel movements which seem to have a relationship to food. For example, if the practical nurse notices that the patient has loose stools the day after a new food was added to his diet, she should report it. The patient is guided by the doctor in regulating his diet according to his bowel movements.

The practical nurse may be responsible for assisting either the doctor or the professional nurse with the colostomy irrigation during the early postoperative period. The colostomy is irrigated with small amounts of solution at first. If two loops of the intestine are attached to the outside abdominal wall, generally both are irrigated. The practical nurse should understand that one opening leads from the upper intestinal tract. This is known as the *proximal loop*. The lower opening which is known as the *distal loop* leads to the rectum. This portion of the intestine is removed later when a colostomy is to be permanent.

The practical nurse may be assigned to do the colostomy irrigation when the patient has improved. She needs to obtain specific instructions from her team leader or head nurse before doing this procedure. The irrigation should be done at approximately the same time each day in order to help the patient establish regular habits of elimination.

The physician may suggest that the patient wear a *colostomy bag*. This is a plastic or rubber pouch which is placed over the colostomy

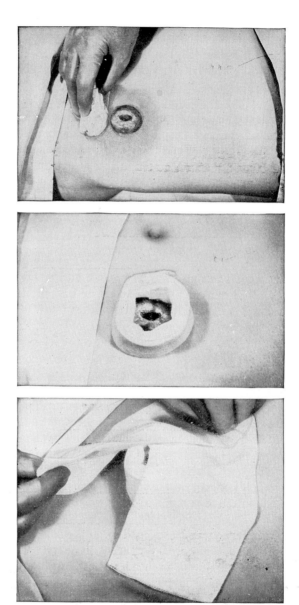

**Figure 28.** *Top,* preparation of area around colostomy stoma. *Center,* first step in dressing: colostomy doughnut. *Bottom,* additional gauze applied to absorb drainage. (Courtesy of Johnson & Johnson, New Brunswick, N.J.)

234

and held in position with a belt. It helps the patient to avoid embarrassment from an unexpected bowel movement. He needs to wear the colostomy bag until regular habits have been established or he may wear it indefinitely. He can learn to control his bowel movements by adjusting his diet and by daily irrigations. After he has established regular habits, he may need only a piece of gauze over the colostomy. A piece of waxed paper may be placed on top of the gauze for added protection. A man can hold this in place with a comfortable elastic belt and the woman with her girdle.

There are various types of irrigating sets available which allow the patient to care for himself in the bathroom. He is often taught to use one of these sets before going home. In general, they are designed so that the returning fluid is directed through a tube into the commode or toilet bowl. The manufacturer's instructions should be consulted regarding the use of a specific irrigator.

## SUGGESTIONS FOR STUDY

1. Define the following: diverticulum, leukocytosis, paralytic ileus, intussusception, volvulus, strangulated hernia, herniorrhaphy, hemorrhoids, anal fissure, ischiorectal abscess, and anal fistula.
2. What are some of the causes of colitis?
3. What kind of diet is usually prescribed for the patient with colitis? Why?
4. What may cause an intestinal obstruction?
5. Review the symptoms of an intestinal obstruction.
6. How does the care of a patient with gastrointestinal suction differ from that of a patient with gastric suction which is discussed in Chapter 14?
7. What symptoms are frequently caused by hemorrhoids?
8. Discuss the nursing care of a patient having rectal surgery.
9. What early symptoms may the person notice which indicate cancer of the colon?
10. Discuss the problems of adjustment which the person with a permanent colostomy is likely to have. How can the practical nurse help the patient in his adjustment?
11. Review the nursing care needed by the patient with a colostomy.

REFERENCES FOR CHAPTER 15

American Cancer Society, Inc.: A *Cancer Source Book for Nurses.* The Society, New York, 1956, pp. 78-82.
Brown, Amy F.: *Medical Nursing,* 3rd ed. W. B. Saunders Co., Philadelphia, 1957, pp. 435-42.
Dakin, Florence; Thompson, Ella M.; and Le Baron, Margaret: *Simplified Nursing,* 6th ed. J. B. Lippincott Co., Philadelphia, 1956, pp. 124-31 and 349-54.
Dubois, Eoline C.: "Hints on the Management of a Colostomy," *Am. J. Nursing,* **55:**71-72, (Jan.) 1955.
Eliason, Eldridge; Ferguson, L. Kraeer; and Sholtis, Lillian A.: *Surgical Nursing,* 10th ed. J. B. Lippincott Co., Philadelphia, 1955, pp. 315-45.
Emerson, Charles P., Jr., and Bragdon, Jane S.: *Essentials of Medicine,* 17th ed. J. B. Lippincott Co., Philadelphia, 1955, pp. 339-60.
Faddis, Margene O., and Hayman, Joseph M.: *Care of the Medical Patient.* McGraw-Hill Book Co., New York, 1952, pp. 360-71.
Jensen, Julius, and Jensen, Deborah: *Nursing in Clinical Medicine,* 4th ed. The Macmillan Company, New York, 1954, pp. 415-42.
Kimber, Diana; Gray, Carolyn E.; Stackpole, Caroline E.; and Leavell, Lutie C.: *Textbook of Anatomy and Physiology,* 13th ed. The Macmillan Company, New York, 1955, pp. 535-44 and 559-606.
Knapp, Margaret F.: *Cancer Nursing: A Manual for Public Health Nurses.* National Cancer Institute, Public Health Service, Department of Health, Education, and Welfare, Washington, D.C., and the New York State Department of Health, Albany, 1955, pp. 44-47.
Krause, Marie: *Nutrition and Diet Therapy,* 2nd ed. W. B. Saunders Co., Philadelphia, 1957, pp. 206-18.
Palumbo, Louis T.; Burnside, Ruby; Mossholder, Irene; and Jensen, Bernice: "Ulcerative Colitis," *Am. J. Nursing,* **55:**311-15, (Mar.) 1955.
Proudfit, Fairfax T., and Robinson, Corinne H.: *Nutrition and Diet Therapy,* 11th ed. The Macmillan Company, New York, 1955, pp. 396-410.
Stafford, Edward S., and Diller, Doris: *Surgery and Surgical Nursing,* 3rd ed. W. B. Saunders Co., Philadelphia, 1958, pp. 102-70.
West, John P.; Keller, Manelva W.; and Harmon, Elizabeth H.: *Nursing Care of the Surgical Patient,* 6th ed. The Macmillan Company, New York, 1957, pp. 288-312 and 320-26.

*for Friday*

*Test Monday 4*

Chapter 16

# THE PATIENT WITH A DISEASE OF THE LIVER, BILIARY TRACT, AND PANCREAS

*Chapter Outline*

STRUCTURE AND FUNCTION
JAUNDICE
ACUTE HEPATITIS (VIRAL HEPATITIS)
CIRRHOSIS OF THE LIVER

CHOLECYSTITIS
CHOLELITHIASIS
PANCREATITIS

## STRUCTURE AND FUNCTION

### Liver

The liver is located in the right upper portion of the abdominal cavity. It is the body's largest gland and is necessary for life. A gland may be considered as a manufacturing plant. It takes material from the body and forms a new substance. Bile is one of the substances manufactured by the liver. It aids in the digestion and absorption of fats. Ordinarily bile is greenish yellow, brownish yellow, or olive green in color.

The liver has many additional functions. Some of its main duties are included in this discussion. It changes glucose into glycogen, which is a form of sugar stored in the liver cells. Glycogen remains there until the body calls for it. The liver then reconverts the glycogen into glucose when the body needs more than it is receiving from food. This simple form of sugar is picked up by the blood stream and carried to the cells. The liver stores copper, iron, and certain vitamins. The amount of amino acids in the blood is controlled by the liver. *Amino acids* are chemical compounds obtained from proteins. The liver also aids in the destruction of red blood cells.

237

### The Biliary Tract

Bile is delivered from the liver cells through a network of tiny ducts (tubes) into the *hepatic* duct. This is a large duct through which bile leaves the liver. The hepatic duct joins a tube from the gallbladder called the *cystic duct*. These two unite and form the

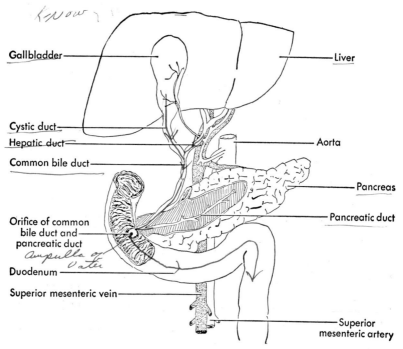

Figure 29.   Diagram showing relationships of the pancreatic and bile ducts and their entrance into the duodenum. (Stackpole, Caroline E., and Leavell, Lutie C.: *Textbook of Physiology.* The Macmillan Company, New York, 1953.)

*common bile duct* which joins the ampulla of Vater. This short duct leads to the duodenum. Normally bile may take one of two routes from the hepatic duct; it flows from the common bile duct into the duodenum when food is present in the intestine, or it flows through the cystic duct into the gallbladder when there is no food in the duodenum.

Bile is stored in the *gallbladder*. This organ is a sac similar to a pear in shape. It is located under the liver. The gallbladder is approximately 7.5 to 10 cm (3 to 4 in.) long and 2.5 cm (1 in.) wide. The storage of bile by the gallbladder is made possible by the closure of a sphincter muscle located at the end of the common bile duct. This circular muscle closes when the duodeum is empty. Thus, bile flows through the cystic duct into the gallbladder. The sphincter muscle opens and the gallbladder contracts, forcing bile through the cystic and common bile ducts into the duodeum during digestion.

### Pancreas

The pancreas is a gland located behind the stomach. It manufactures pancreatic fluid and insulin. Pancreatic fluid aids in digestion. It flows from the pancreas to the duodeum through the pancreatic duct. Insulin is produced by a special group of cells within the pancreas which are called the islands of Langerhans. This secretion is picked up by the blood stream. Insulin is necessary for the body tissues to utilize glucose which is their form of fuel.

## JAUNDICE

### Description

The patient with jaundice has a yellowish color. His skin, mucous membranes, and the whites of his eyes may become yellow. This is a result of bile pigments (coloring matter) in his blood. Jaundice is a symptom rather than a disease. It is usually a symptom of a disease affecting either the liver or the bile ducts. When bile does not flow normally from the liver through the bile ducts, it is picked up by the blood and carried throughout the body.

### Cause

Jaundice is frequently classified according to its cause. The three types are obstructive, nonobstructive, and hemolytic. Jaundice is referred to as *obstructive* when either the common bile duct or the hepatic duct are blocked. For example, a gallstone or a tumor may block one of these ducts. This prevents bile from flowing into the small intestine. Bile backs up into the liver and is absorbed in the blood. *Nonobstructive jaundice* occurs when the liver cells are damaged. Thus, they cannot eliminate bile pigments. For example, the liver cells may be damaged by an acute infection or by a poison such as arsenic. *Hemolytic jaundice* occurs when the destruction of red blood cells is abnormally fast. The normal liver is unable to remove the waste products of these destroyed red blood cells as fast as they are formed.

### Symptoms

In addition to having a yellowish color, this patient frequently complains of itching. His skin itches because of deposits of bile pigments. The stools are clay-colored because bile does not reach the intestinal tract. The urine may become darker in color as a result of the kidney's efforts to remove excess bile pigment from the blood. This patient often complains of dyspepsia because of poor digestion of fats. The clotting time of his blood may be lengthened because of the increased amount of bile pigment. This could result in a tendency to hemorrhage.

## ACUTE HEPATITIS (VIRAL HEPATITIS)

### Description

The patient with acute hepatitis or viral hepatitis has an inflammation of his liver caused by a virus. The infection quite commonly spreads into the bile ducts. The practical nurse may hear this disease called by other names, such as *infectious hepatitis* and *catarrhal jaundice*. Children and young adults are affected most often.

### Symptoms

Frequently the patient complains of anorexia during the early stage of this disease. As the disease progresses the patient develops other symptoms of an infection, such as a fever and malaise. Jaundice is an outstanding symptom. This develops because the flow of bile from the liver through the bile ducts is hindered by the infection. His urine may become darker and his stools clay-colored. The patient generally recovers within 3 to 12 weeks.

### Treatment and Nursing Care

The treatment and nursing care of the patient with acute hepatitis are mainly symptomatic. The physician prescribes bed rest until the acute infection has subsided. Frequently he orders a diet high in carbohydrate and low in fat.

Nursing care discussed in relation to the patient with an inflammation on pages 78 to 79 is applicable to this patient. This patient needs special care of his skin because of its itching and dryness. The practical nurse may be asked to apply an oil or a lotion to relieve these discomforts. Special ointments may be prescribed by the doctor. The practical nurse may also be responsible for disinfecting feces. She should receive specific instructions from the team leader or the head nurse regarding this.

## CIRRHOSIS OF THE LIVER

### Description

The patient with cirrhosis of the liver has a chronic disease of that gland. It usually takes him a period of years to develop this condition. Some of the liver cells grow more rapidly and others are destroyed and replaced by scar tissue. These changes can cause the patient's liver to become either larger or smaller. Contraction of the scar tissue can change the shape of this organ. Also, the scar tissue intereferes with the liver's function. The liver has a remarkable ability to compensate for the disease process. This compensation may keep the patient free from distressing symptoms for years.

### Cause

The cause of cirrhosis is not clearly understood. In the past it was believed to be caused by alcoholism as it occurs most often in heavy drinkers. Now it is thought to be caused by nutritional deficiency. Of course, the diet of many alcoholics is not well balanced.

### Symptoms

The patient with cirrhosis develops symptoms associated with a disturbance of blood flowing through the liver and inadequate functioning of the liver. Most of the blood from the digestive organs is carried through the liver. When this flow of blood through the liver is hindered, it collects in the gastrointestinal system. This causes the patient to develop symptoms of abdominal congestion. At first he is bothered with digestive disturbances such as (indigestion, flatulence (gas), loss of appetite, nausea, and vomiting.) Because of this change in the circulation within the liver, he may develop varicose veins in his esophagus. One of these may rupture and result in the vomiting of blood (hematemesis). The patient may also develop varicose veins of the rectum (hemorrhoids). As the disease progresses the patient may develop *ascites,* which is the (collection of fluid in the peritoneal cavity).

Functioning of the liver is affected as more of the cells are damaged. The patient may develop a slight or a moderate amount of jaundice. The doctor may be able to feel the enlarged liver. The patient loses weight, and he may not appear as alert mentally. He is likely to develop infections, such as (pneumonia and tuberculosis).

### Treatment

The main treatment of the patient with cirrhosis of the liver consists of diet and vitamins as it is believed to be a deficiency disease. The physician generally orders a diet which is low in fats and high in carbohydrates. He may also restrict the amount of salt in the patient's diet. It is important for the patient to eliminate the use of alcohol. Vitamins, especially vitamin B complex, are prescribed because of the patient's nutritional deficiency.

It may be necessary for the doctor to perform an *abdominal paracentesis* (tap the abdomen). This is a sterile procedure in which fluid is withdrawn from the peritoneal cavity. A *trocar*, which is a surgical instrument used to puncture a cavity to allow fluid to drain through it, is used.

4-4.6 6

### CHOLECYSTITIS

### Description

The patient with cholecystitis has an inflammation of the gallbladder. Frequently it is associated with gallstones. Cholecystitis may be complicated by the formation of pus in the gallbladder. Perforation often occurs if the wall becomes gangrenous. Contents of the gallbladder escape through the hole into the peritoneal cavity. This can result in peritonitis. Another complication of cholecystitis may be *cholangitis*. This is an inflammation of the bile ducts. Both those within the liver and those leading from the liver may be inflamed. The patient develops jaundice if the inflammation obstructs the flow of bile from the liver to the intestine.

## Symptoms

Symptoms of a patient with cholecystitis vary with the amount of inflammation. The person with a mild case has symptoms of digestive disturbances, such as indigestion especially after eating fatty foods. Flatulence is another discomfort. The person with an acute case has the above discomforts as well as more marked symptoms of an infection. He may have a feeling of malaise, fever, and vomiting. Pain in the right upper part of the abdomen is a common symptom. The pain may radiate to the right shoulder blade. The physician finds the area over the gallbladder to be rigid. Jaundice does not occur if the infection affects only the gallbladder. As stated earlier, the patient develops jaundice when the flow of bile from the liver to the small intestine is obstructed.

## Treatment and Nursing Care

The physician determines whether or not the patient actually has cholecystitis before the treatment is planned. Frequently he orders a gallbladder x-ray to aid him in diagnosis. An understanding of this type of x-ray helps the practical nurse in caring for this patient. A picture of the gallbladder cannot be taken by x-ray without special preparation. However, some gallstones are visible on the film. A special dye which is visible by x-ray is given to the patient. Usually it is given by mouth. This dye is picked up by the blood from the digestive system and carried to the liver. The liver puts the dye into the bile. Remembering that bile is stored in the gallbladder, the practical nurse can easily understand the dye being stored in the gallbladder. The patient is not allowed to eat fatty foods after he has taken the dye. It is important for members of the nursing team to see that the patient eats no fatty foods until allowed by the doctor. If the patient does eat foods containing fat, his gallbladder empties and loses the dye. Then the patient's preparation must be repeated. The drug may be lost from the stomach before reaching the blood stream if vomiting occurs soon after its administration. Remembering this, the practical nurse realizes the importance of observing and reporting promptly the occurrence of vomiting. The patient is given a fatty meal after the films are taken. Another x-ray is taken after he has eaten. This is done to check the emptying time of the gallbladder. The normal gallbladder releases the bile containing the dye when fatty food reaches the duodenum.

The usual treatment for the patient with cholecystitis is surgery. The surgeon may perform a *cholecystectomy* which is removal of the gallbladder, or he may do a *cholecystostomy*. In this latter operation, he makes an incision in the gallbladder. He frequently inserts a tube in the incision to allow for temporary drainage, and this tube is usually attached to a drainage bottle.

Following surgery the patient is frequently placed in Fowler's position. If a drainage tube is present, it should be attached to a drainage bottle. The amount of drainage should be measured and recorded. This is usually checked frequently for drainage and bleeding. The practical nurse should report the presence of either to her team leader or head nurse.

Members of the nursing team should make special efforts to prevent this patient from developing pulmonary complications. Remembering the closeness of the operation to the diaphragm, the practical nurse can easily understand why the patient avoids breathing deeply. She should encourage him to take frequent deep breaths. She should assist the patient in changing his position until he is able to do this alone. The practical nurse can expect to be asked to help in getting the patient out of bed soon after his surgery. This is another measure in the prevention of pulmonary complications.

The practical nurse should observe and report the color of the patient's stools. Knowing the color of the feces aids the doctor in determining when bile is reaching the intestines.

The above discussion deals with the nursing care needed especially by the patient having gallbladder surgery. The practical nurse who feels the need to review the care of a postoperative patient is referred to this discussion on pages 53 to 56.

## CHOLELITHIASIS

### Description

The patient with cholelithiasis has gallstones. They may occur either in connection with an infection of the gallbladder or in the absence of infection. Gallstones are more common in women, especially after 40 years of age. They are more likely to develop in an overweight person. The number of stones may vary from one to hundreds or more. Their size may range from that of a grain of sand to that of a lemon.

### Symptoms

Some individuals with cholelithiasis experience no symptoms; others have indigestion; and some have gallbladder colic. The patient has severe pain when the stone is being forced through the bile duct. The stone irritates the muscle of the duct which causes it to contract violently. This muscle spasm is known as *colic*. The severe pain spreads from the right upper part of the abdomen throughout the entire abdomen. It often radiates to the right shoulder blade. If the stone becomes lodged in either the hepatic or common bile duct, the patient develops jaundice.

### Treatment

The physician prescribes narcotics, such as morphine, to relieve the patient's excruciating pain during an attack of colic. Surgery is the usual treatment for a patient with cholelithiasis. The surgeon may perform a cholecystectomy in which the gallbladder with its stones are removed. He may do a *choledochostomy* which is opening the common bile duct to remove stones. Usually he inserts a tube into this duct to allow for temporary drainage.

## PANCREATITIS

### Description

The patient with pancreatitis has an inflammation of his pancreas. It may be acute or chronic. Oddly enough, the pancreatic juice which is secreted by this gland begins to digest the cells of its producer. A disturbance to the ducts draining the cells of the pancreas of its fluid allows this juice to come in contact with pancreatic tissue. Pancreatic juice is so strong that it digests the patient's own tissues when it comes into direct contact with them.

## Cause

Normally the pancreatic duct joins the common bile duct to form a short tube called the ampulla of Vater which leads to the duodenum. Pancreatic juice and bile enter the small intestine through this tube during digestion. Realizing the close association between the pancreas and the biliary tract helps the practical nurse to understand that pancreatitis frequently follows a chronic disease of the biliary tract. Because of this, it is more common in a middle-aged person who is overweight. Although disease of the biliary system is more common in women, pancreatitis is more common in men.

An acute case of pancreatitis may cause pus to form in this organ or the cells to die (which is referred to as gangrene). Another complication is hemorrhage. Bleeding occurs if a blood vessel is eroded by the pancreatic juice.

Patients having either a mild or a moderate case of pancreatitis have a better chance of recovery than those with a severe case.

## Symptoms

The patient with acute pancreatitis has severe pain around his umbilicus. Frequently the pain begins several hours after a large meal. Nausea and vomiting are also present. The patient may develop symptoms of shock.

The patient with chronic pancreatitis complains of indigestion and flatulence. His stools have a foul odor and are unusually large.

## Treatment

Bed rest is indicated for the patient with acute pancreatitis. The physician orders an analgesic, such as morphine, to relieve pain. Fluids are given intravenously because of the patient's nausea and vomiting. They also help to combat shock. Surgery is necessary in some cases to allow for drainage of the inflamed area.

The patient with chronic pancreatitis is usually given a diet low in fat and proteins. Since the patient frequently develops this condition as a result of biliary tract disease, he should be treated for the underlying cause such as gallstones.

## SUGGESTIONS FOR STUDY

1. What causes a person to develop jaundice?
2. Why does the patient with jaundice frequently complain of itching? What causes his stools to become clay-colored?
3. Why would a patient with acute hepatitis be likely to develop jaundice?
4. What causes cirrhosis of the liver?
5. Why is it important for a patient to eat no fatty foods when he is being prepared for a gallbladder x-ray?
6. Discuss the nursing care of a patient who has had a cholecystectomy.
7. Define the following: cholelithiasis, cholecystitis, and choledochostomy.

## REFERENCES FOR CHAPTER 16

Brown, Amy F.: *Medical Nursing*, 3rd ed. W. B. Saunders Co., Philadelphia, 1957, pp. 404-35.
Eliason, Eldridge; Ferguson, L. Kraeer; and Sholtis, Lillian A.: *Surgical Nursing*, 10th ed. J. B. Lippincott Co., Philadelphia, 1955, pp. 346-54.
Emerson, Charles P., Jr., and Bragdon, Jane S.: *Essentials of Medicine*, 17th ed. J. B. Lippincott Co., Philadelphia, 1955, pp. 361-90.
Gifford, Dolores: "Acute Pancreatitis," *Am. J. Nursing*, **56:**1584-85, (Dec.) 1956.
Hull, Edgar, and Perrodin, Cecilia: *Medical Nursing*, 5th ed. F. A. Davis Co., Philadelphia, 1954, pp. 333-47.
Jensen, Julius, and Jensen, Deborah: *Nursing in Clinical Medicine*, 4th ed. The Macmillan Company, New York, 1954, pp. 443-74.
Krause, Marie: *Nutrition and Diet Therapy*, 2nd ed. W. B. Saunders Co., Philadelphia, 1957, pp. 219-28.
Moroney, James: *Surgery for Nurses*, 5th ed. E. & S. Livingstone Ltd., Edinburgh and London, 1958, pp. 411-24.
Proudfit, Fairfax T., and Robinson, Corinne H.: *Nutrition and Diet Therapy*, 11th ed. The Macmillan Company, New York, 1955, pp. 411-23.
West, John P.; Keller, Manelva W.; and Harmon, Elizabeth H.: *Nursing Care of the Surgical Patient*, 6th ed. The Macmillan Company, New York, 1957, pp. 312-20.

*Nursing the Patient
with a Disease of
the Skeletal and
the Muscular Systems*

PART VI

Mr. & Mrs. J. J. Pope

Chapter 17

# THE PATIENT
# WITH A DISEASE OF
# THE SKELETAL AND
# THE MUSCULAR SYSTEMS

## STRUCTURE AND FUNCTION

The skeletal and the muscular systems work together in a team relationship so that man can move. The practical nurse may hear these two systems referred to as the *locomotor system* since their main function is movement. A brief review is given as a background for the discussion of the care of patients having diseases of the skeletal and the muscular systems.

The skeletal system is composed of the bones and the connective tissues, such as ligaments and tendons. These tissues bind the bones and muscles together. The skeletal system helps to support other organs, to move the body, and to protect certain organs of the body. Another function of the skeletal system is to manufacture blood cells. These are produced by red marrow of the bones.

*Joints* are formed when the bones come into close contact with each other. The area of a bone which comes into close contact with another bone is known as the *articular surface*. These surfaces are separated by a softer substance, such as cartilage, which helps to absorb the jars of body movement. Most of the joints are freely movable. In this case, the articular end of the bones is protected by a capsule in addition to the cartilage. This capsule is lined with *synovial membrane* which gives protection by secreting *synovia*

251

which acts as a lubricant. It is a clear fluid similar in appearance to egg white. Some joints are protected by *bursae*. These are small sacs made of synovial membrane and filled with fluid. Bursae help to prevent two bony surfaces from rubbing together. For example, a bursa is found over the kneecap and the elbow which protects these two joints from friction.

The main function of the mus-cular system is movement. This in-cludes movement of the bones as well as the internal organs, such as the intestines and the heart. Another function of the muscular system is the support of other organs of the body.

*Orthopedics* is the branch of sur-gery which specializes in the treat-ment of a patient with a disease of the locomotor system. The physician in this specialty is called an *ortho-bedist.*

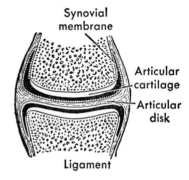

**Synovial membrane**
**Articular cartilage**
**Articular disk**
**Ligament**

Figure 30. Diagram of a section of a movable joint with an articular disk of cartilage. (After Gray's *Anatomy*.) (Kim-ber, Diana C.; Gray, Carolyn E.; Stackpole, Caroline E.; and Leavell, Lutie C.: *Textbook of Anatomy and Physiology,* 13th ed. The Macmillan Company, New York, 1955.)

## CONGENITAL DEFORMITIES

### Introduction

An individual may be born with a deformity of the locomotor system. Two kinds of congenital abnormalities of this system which the practical nurse is likely to see are clubfoot and dislocation of the hip. She may also see an infant who is born with parts missing, such as fingers, toes, and an entire limb. When caring for an infant or a child, the practical nurse should observe and report any seem-ingly abnormal body positions or missing parts.

### Clubfoot

The baby with clubfoot has a foot turned inward. Either one or both feet may be affected. If he learns to walk before this condi-tion is corrected, he walks so that his weight is carried on the outer part of his ankle.

Treatment should be started during early infancy. The chance of cure is lessened as the infant's bones begin to grow. The doctor manipulates the affected foot and ankle into a normal position in gradual stages. Each correction toward normal position is usually maintained by a plaster cast. For instance, the doctor generally removes the cast, further corrects the deformity, and applies another cast. This procedure may be repeated as often as once a week at first and less often as the deformity is corrected. The child is generally fitted with corrective shoes when allowed to walk. He may also have a splint or a brace applied at night to help in maintaining the proper position. Specific exercises may be ordered to strengthen the involved muscles.

## Dislocation of the Hip

The head of the femur (thigh bone) is not fixed firmly in its socket in a baby born with a dislocation of the hip. This deformity may not be noticed until the child begins to stand and to walk. The head of the femur slips out of its socket, causing the child to walk in a waddling or lurching manner.

The physician treats the child with a dislocation of his hip by placing the bone in correct position and then immobilizing it with either a splint or a cast. In some cases, surgery is necessary for the correct placement of the head of the femur into the joint.

## SPRAIN

### Description

*muscle to bones*

The patient with a sprain has an injury of the ligaments around the joint. The body responds to this injury by an inflammatory process. The blood vessels dilate so that more blood can be brought into the area. Small blood vessels are frequently ruptured. Localized swelling occurs as a result. The patient complains of pain, especially when he moves the joint.

### Treatment

*Prevent stagnation of blood in area*

The injured part should be elevated. This helps to relieve swelling and discomfort. Cold applications should be applied for the first 10 to 12 hours. This aids in checking the bleeding within the tissues as cold causes the blood vessels to constrict. Thus, swelling is also relieved by cold applications. The doctor may apply pressure by using a bandage, such as an elastic bandage. The physician may recommend that the patient rest the injured joint for several days and then to resume activity gradually.

## DISLOCATION

### Description

The patient with a dislocation has an abnormal condition of a joint. The ends of the bones which form the joint are not in their proper place. Dislocation frequently is caused by injury. However, dislocation of the hip, which was discussed earlier in this chapter, is usually congenital.

### Treatment

The doctor generally puts the bones in their proper position after the patient has been given a general anesthetic. He may immobilize the joint with either bandages or splints until it has healed.

## FRACTURE

### Description

The patient with a fracture has a broken bone which is caused usually by an accident. However, a fracture can result from a disease of the bone. For example, a malignant tumor can weaken the bone to such an extent that it may break during a normal activity such as turning in bed. The patient complains of pain after his bone has been fractured. Usually, he has a loss of normal function. The fracture may allow him to have unnatural movement. It may also appear deformed. The area soon becomes swollen. The patient may develop symptoms of shock.

An individual with a broken bone usually has an injury of other tissues in the area. His body responds by sending an increased amount of blood to the part. Recalling the process of inflammation, the practical nurse remembers that white blood cells and plasma go from the blood vessels into the tissues. This accounts for the localized swelling mentioned in the above paragraph. The white blood cells and plasma form a gluey substance called *callus*. This helps to hold the bone fragments together because of its sticky nature. As healing continues, lime salts and bone cells of the periosteum (membrane covering the bone) are deposited in the callus. These cells, which are deposited, gradually cause the callus to become hardened. Thus, new bone is formed and the fracture heals.

## Types

Because the practical nurse often hears of different types of fractures, she needs a basic understanding of them. A *simple fracture* is one in which the bone is broken, but the skin over the area is intact. When the patient has a wound leading to the broken bone, he has a *compound fracture*. He is likely to develop an infection

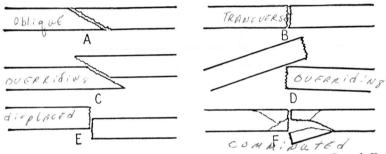

**Figure 31.** Types of fractures: A, oblique; B, transverse; C and D, overriding; E, displaced; F, comminuted. (West, John P.; Keller, Manelva W.; and Harmon, Elizabeth H.: *Nursing Care of the Surgical Patient*, 6th ed. The Macmillan Company, New York, 1957.)

because the opening allows bacteria to enter. Terms which may be used to describe the direction of the fracture are oblique and transverse. An *oblique fracture* is slanted, and a *transverse* one goes across the bone. Overlapping of the broken bone is present in an *overriding fracture*. In an *incomplete fracture*, the break extends part of the way through the bone. The *greenstick fracture* is an incomplete fracture which usually occurs in children because their bones are still somewhat flexible. It is known as a greenstick fracture because its break resembles the breaking of a young and green branch of a tree. When the bone is broken into at least three pieces, it is called a *comminuted fracture*. In an *impacted fracture*, the bone fragments are driven together.

## Treatment

When the physician suspects that the patient has a fracture, he usually has the part x-rayed. In addition to confirming his diagnosis, the x-rays guide him in reducing (setting) the fracture. Another x-ray may be required after the fracture has been reduced so that the doctor can determine whether or not the bone fragments are in the correct position.

The physician aims his treatment toward preventing further injury, placing the broken bone in good position, and holding the fractured bone in place until it has healed. He accomplishes the first two aims through careful handling and reduction. When he *reduces* a fracture, he restores the bone fragments to their normal position. This may be done by closed reduction, by open reduction, or by traction. In a *closed reduction,* the ends of the bone are placed in position by external manipulation. In other words, no incision is made. When the physician does an *open reduction,* he makes an incision which allows him to handle the bone fragments and place them in good position. In some cases, the doctor may have to secure the fragments with a special type of wire or screws. The fracture may be immobilized or held in place by a plaster cast, by a splint, or by traction. *Traction* means drawing or pulling. This is accomplished by the use of special equipment. Traction may be used also for reducing the fracture. For example, when the ends of the bone slip upon each other because of contractions of the muscles, a continuous amount of pull may be necessary to reduce and to immobilize the part.

The physician orders a diet to meet the individual patient's nutritional needs. In addition to containing the necessary food elements, the prescribed diet may be high in vitamins, calories, and proteins. When the patient is unable to eat a sufficient amount at mealtime, he may need special beverages high in proteins, calories, and vitamins between meals.

### Nursing Care

#### Emergency Care

Remembering that one of the aims in the care of the patient with a fracture is to prevent further injury to the area, the practical nurse can realize the importance of gentle handling. This should be a guiding principle in the emergency care of a person suspected of having a fracture. The fracture should be splinted if possible before the patient is moved. The purpose of this is to prevent additional damage to the area.

Movement of the patient with a suspected fracture of the spine should be done with utmost caution. If a vertebra is broken, the fragments may damage the spinal cord permanently when the patient is moved. He should be rolled over on his abdomen to avoid flexing his back. At least three people are required to lift him.

The patient with a possible fracture of the leg or thigh can have the part splinted with a long board, such as an ironing board. A small board can be used to immobilize the forearm. The upper arm may be bandaged to the chest with a blouse or a coat.

The person with a compound fracture should have a sterile dressing placed over the wound. The area may be covered with a clean cloth, such as a freshly laundered handkerchief if a sterile dressing is not available. No attempt should be made to reduce the fracture. This is the physician's responsibility.

### Admission to the Hospital

When helping to admit the patient with a possible fracture, the practical nurse should handle the patient gently. His clothing should be removed in such a manner that the fractured part is not moved. If movement is necessary, the injured area should be moved as little as possible. The practical nurse should not remove the temporary splint. She should keep the patient comfortably warm. Remembering that the patient with a fracture may go into shock, the practical nurse can realize the importance of observing him for symptoms of shock.

### The Patient in a Cast

A *cast* is usually made of plaster-of-Paris bandage. This consists of crinoline which has powdered plaster rubbed into the meshwork. A roll of plaster-of-Paris bandage is placed in warm water before being applied by the doctor. The area to be enclosed in a cast is usually covered first with glazed cotton and stockinette. The physician applies the wet plaster-of-Paris bandages to form the cast. This hardens or sets as it dries.

*Cold, clammy, pulse rapid*

The practical nurse may be asked to have a bedboard and a firm mattress placed on the patient's bed while he is out of his room having the cast applied. Also, she may be asked to put sandbags in his room. If pillows are to be used under the cast, they should be protected with either plastic or rubber covers. An overhead trapeze or crossbar, suspended from a Balkan frame, may be added to the bed to enable the patient to change his position.

The patient is returned to his room after the cast has been applied. The cast that is still wet should be protected from pressures which could cause a dent in it. The practical nurse may be asked to help place the patient in a body cast on pillows and to arrange the sandbags which are used to prevent pressure on the wet cast over bony prominences. Pressure on a cast which is still wet flattens it. This flattened area presses on the underlying tissue and can damage it after the cast has dried. Members of the nursing team should handle the wet cast with the palms of their hands instead of their fingers. Indentations made in the wet cast with fingers also may harm the patient's skin after the cast has dried.

The physician leaves either the fingers or toes exposed when he applies a cast on an extremity. Checking the circulation of an extremity enclosed in a cast is of vital importance. The practical nurse should check the circulation at frequent intervals by observing the color of the toes or fingers which are protruding from the cast. If she observes that they are pale or blue, she should report it immediately. Other symptoms of impaired circulation include swelling, coldness, numbness, and pain. If the practical nurse notices any of these symptoms, she should report them promptly to her team leader or head nurse. Complaints of a burning sensation should also be reported. The practical nurse may notice that a patient with an arm cast may have a hole cut in the cast over the radial artery. In general, the physician cuts this hole so the nurse can check the patient's pulse in that arm.* All members of the nursing team should remember that serious complications may result if the doctor is not notified immediately regarding symptoms of impaired circulation so that he can relieve the pressure.

---

* When both wrists are covered by dressings, a plaster cast, or a splint, arteries other than the radial (such as the temporal, facial, and carotid) can be used to determine the patient's pulse rate.

Usually the cast dries in approximately 24 hours. Members of the nursing team should keep the cast clean and dry. Sometimes this presents a real problem, especially if the patient is a baby or a child in a body cast. The cast around the perineum can be protected with dry waterproof material, such as plastic material or oiled silk. The material should be washed, dried, and powdered at frequent intervals. Care should be used in placing the patient on the bedpan to prevent soiling the cast.

The patient's position should be changed frequently. The practical nurse should receive specific instructions when helping to turn a patient in a body cast. The patient is practically helpless in such a cast, and adequate support is needed to prevent the weight of the cast from toppling him out of bed. The wise use of pillows and sandbags to support the patient in a cast adds to his comfort. Weight from linen on the patient's toes can be avoided by the use of a footboard or a cradle. Before leaving him the nurse should check to see that the patient's body is in good alignment.

Frequently the practical nurse is assigned to give the patient in a cast his daily bath. Parts of his body which are not in the cast should be bathed and dried thoroughly. The practical nurse should allow no moisture to get under the cast. This is an ideal time to observe the patient's skin for reddened areas which may be a symptom of pressure or other irritation. These observations should be reported. The practical nurse may be advised to wash the reddened area gently and to apply alcohol or baby oil. The patient's toes or fingers protruding from the cast need special attention. In addition to washing and drying them thoroughly, the practical nurse may find it helpful to apply either baby oil or lotion to them. The patient's nails should be trimmed properly and kept clean. The toenails should be cut straight across to help prevent ingrowing nails. Many patients prefer to have their fingernails filed instead of cut. The practical nurse should be careful to avoid injuring the surrounding tissue when cleaning, cutting, or filing the patient's nails. The practical nurse should keep the patient's bed free from crumbs of plaster and food as well as wrinkles.

As the patient improves, he should be encouraged to help himself as much as possible. The practical nurse should place the articles which he is likely to need within easy reach.

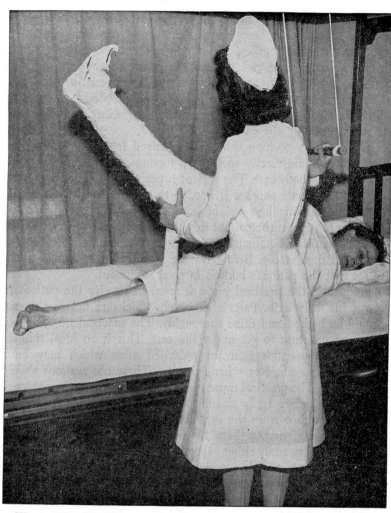

**Figure 32.** Turning a patient in a body cast. Patient assists by use of hand trapeze. (West, John P.; Keller, Manelva W.; and Harmon, Elizabeth H.: *Nursing Care of the Surgical Patient*, 6th ed. The Macmillan Company, New York, 1957.)

260

A long period of time is necessary for a bone to heal. Because of this, the patient may have a lengthy stay in the hospital. The physician frequently calls upon other members of the health team in the total rehabilitation of this patient. The physical therapist may be asked to give certain treatments, such as massage, exercises, and hydrotherapy (water baths). It may be the responsibility of the nursing team to see that the patient follows specific instructions. The occupational therapist may be asked to determine and to teach the patient activities which should help keep his mind and body active. It may be necessary for a child faced with a long convalescence to have a visiting teacher.

The cast is removed with either an electric cast cutter or a plaster knife and heavy scissors. After the patient's cast has been removed, he may feel insecure because of the sudden loss of support. The patient feels more comfortable if the part is supported for a while in the same position as it was in the cast. The patient's extremity which was enclosed in the cast usually feels weak and may appear smaller. Also, his joints may feel stiff. These symptoms result from lack of use. The patient may become depressed when he finds that his extremity has not regained its full usefulness with the removal of the cast. It takes a while for muscles and joints to regain their normal degree of usefulness. The patient should be encouraged to make gradual movements as outlined by the doctor.

The practical nurse may be asked to bathe the skin which was covered by the cast. Waste products have accumulated over the area. The skin should be bathed gently. The practical nurse should be careful not to injure the tender skin. Some doctors recommend the application of a lubricant such as oil to soften the crust before washing.

### The Patient in Traction

Traction may be obtained by the use of weights hung from cords which work from pulleys and other special equipment. The patient may be placed in traction for reduction and immobilization of a fracture. It may be used also to immobilize a joint which is infected, such as a joint infected with tuberculosis. Traction may be used to prevent or to correct a deformity caused by diseases, such as arthritis.

The patient with *skin* or *surface traction* has the traction equipment attached to the skin. For example, it may be attached to adhesive tape which has been applied to the patient's skin. If the physician uses adhesive tape, he may have the area shaved first in an effort to lessen discomfort when the tape is removed later. He may also paint the skin with tincture of benzoin which will help the tape to hold better. The patient with *skeletal traction* has the equipment connected with the bone. A metal pin, tongs, or a wire may be inserted into the bone and then connected with the traction apparatus. A greater amount of pull is possible with this setup.

The patient in traction should be observed for symptoms of impaired circulation in the affected part, which were discussed earlier in this chapter.

The care needed by this patient in regard to his skin and nails is similar to that described for the patient in a cast.

When the practical nurse assists in the care of a patient in traction, she should seek specific instructions regarding the patient's position. In some cases, the patient is not allowed to be turned. The part of his body which is in traction should be kept in the position designated by the doctor.

The pull of the weights on the rope should not be hindered by bedroom furnishings, such as linen or a misplaced bedside table. The rope should be kept on the pulley. The practical nurse should not remove the weights unless she has been given specific instructions by the doctor or the head nurse. If the practical nurse notices that a patient with head traction has his head resting against the headboard, she should report this to the head nurse. Also, if she notices that a patient with leg traction has his foot resting against the footboard, she should report it. A bandage which appears to be either too loose or too tight should be called to the head nurse's attention.

### The Patient on Crutches

The patient may need to use crutches after the fracture in his leg has healed. An individual who has had an amputation or one with a disease of his lower extremities such as arthritis may need to use crutches. The patient with paralysis of his lower extremities may need to use them also.

In many hospitals the physical therapist is responsible for teaching the patient to walk with crutches. In this instance, the nursing team is asked to assist. For example, the nurses may be responsible for specific practice exercises used to strengthen muscles prior to crutch walking as well as the actual practice with crutches. However, in some institutions the physician asks the nursing team to teach the

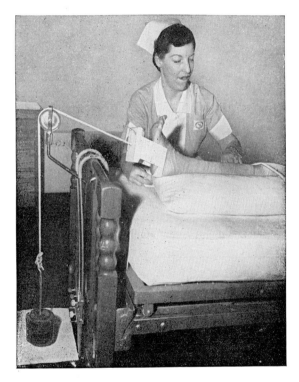

**Figure 33.** A patient in traction. The part of the patient's body in traction should be kept in the position designated by the doctor. The rope should remain on the pulley without touching other objects. The pre-scribed weights suspended from the rope should not be removed without specific instructions from the doctor or the head nurse. The affected part should be observed frequently for symptoms of impaired circulation.

The white area in the lower left of the picture is a foot stool placed under the weights to prevent persons from jarring the weights. In this instance, the foot stool was covered with white to help the weights to be seen more clearly in the picture.

patient how to use crutches, and the practical nurse may be asked to assist in the achievement of this goal.

The patient should be measured for his crutches. If the physician does not give specific instructions regarding the measurements, these can be obtained by measuring the patient while he is still in bed. The patient should be lying on his back with his arms at his sides. He should have on the shoes or the shoe which he will wear when he gets out of bed. The shoe should fit well and have a low and broad heel. Bedroom slippers should not be used for the patient learning to walk with crutches. The measurement should be taken from the axilla to a point approximately 15 cm (6 in.) to the side of the patient's heel. The hand bar should be adjusted to a level which permits the patient to hold his arm almost straight when leaning on the palms of his hands. This can be done when the patient is standing if an adjustable crutch is used. The top of the crutch should be padded with foam rubber to protect the patient's axillae. The crutch should have a firm rubber tip which fits snugly; this is an important part of the crutch which prevents slipping.

Exercises to strengthen the muscles of the arm, the hands, and the unaffected leg may be started while the patient is still in bed. He progresses from this to sitting on the side of the bed and then to standing on the unaffected side. He should learn to balance himself in an upright position before learning to use crutches. The patient should not be permitted to become overtired with these measures or when he is learning to walk.

The use of crutches should be demonstrated to the patient before he attempts to use them. The demonstrator should show the patient how to stand on crutches as this will be his first exercise with them. He should lean his body forward with the weight resting on the palms of the hands and his wrists, instead of on the axillae. There should be no pressure on the axillae as it may injure the nerves there and result in paralysis of muscles in the arm and hand. The demonstrator should show the patient how to shift his weight on the crutches. The crutches should be wide enough apart so that they support the patient but not too far apart to allow the crutches to slip. Important points of the gait which the patient is to use should be explained and demonstrated to him.

Various gaits have been worked out which can be adapted to an individual patient. The *four-point gait* may be used when the patient can bear some weight on each leg. In this gait, the person advances one crutch, the opposite foot; then the other crutch, and the opposite foot. For example, the patient may bring the left crutch forward, then his right foot; his right crutch forward, and then his left foot.

The *two-point gait* is used also when the patient can bear some weight on each limb. The patient learns to use the crutches by putting his weight on one crutch and the opposite leg at the same time. He brings the opposite limb and the crutch forward at the same time. The right foot and the left crutch are advanced at the same time. After shifting his weight to them, he should advance the left foot and the right crutch.

The *three-point gait* may be used when the patient can bear little, or no weight on one leg. He advances the weak limb and both crutches at the same time. After shifting his weight to them, he advances the good limb. The patient may be able to use only one crutch or a cane later. The crutch or the cane is placed on the good side. The weak limb and the crutch are advanced at the same time in order to give support to the affected limb.

Frequently the *swing-through or tripod gait* is used when the patient's lower extremities are paralyzed. The patient advances the crutches and then swings both legs forward.

After the patient has learned to balance himself on the crutches and has seen the gait which he is to learn demonstrated, he is ready for a short practice period. His path should be cleared of obstacles which might cause him to fall, such as loose rugs, chairs, flower petals, or wet spots on the floor. One person may stand behind the patient and one in front of him when he is learning to use crutches. The individuals assisting him should not be close enough to interfere with his movements or his crutches.

Frequently the patient slouches when he is learning to use crutches. He should be encouraged to maintain good posture. His shoulders should be back, his chin up, and his eyes looking forward. He may need to be reminded not to bear his weight on the ball of his foot.

## OSTEOMYELITIS

### Description

The patient with osteomyelitis has an inflammation of the bone which frequently involves the marrow. The infection may spread to surrounding tissue. The inflammation is caused by bacteria, such as staphylococci and streptococci. The bacteria are often brought to the bone by the blood stream. They may spread from an infection elsewhere in the body, such as tonsillitis. A person may also develop osteomyelitis following an injury, such as a fracture. Exposure in a wet, cold climate is a predisposing factor.

Osteomyelitis affects the long bones of the body most often. It is more frequent in children. The discovery of antibiotics, such as penicillin, has been helpful in reducing the long periods of illness experienced by these patients.

The patient with osteomyelitis has symptoms of an inflammation: malaise, fever, increased pulse rate, and an increased white cell count. The infected area becomes swollen, painful, and tender.

### Treatment and Nursing Care

The physician may prescribe one of the sulfonamides or one of the antibiotics to combat the infection. It may be necessary for the surgeon to perform a surgical drainage, especially if pus has formed. Frequently he applies a cast after the infected area has been opened. The cast immobilizes the bone so that it can have a maximum amount of rest. The physician leaves instructions regarding the changing of dressings. Sometimes the cast is split down each side so the nurse can change the dressing. However, when the physician leaves the cast intact the dressing cannot be changed.

The nurse should try to reduce the odor in the patient's room. Keeping the patient clean and providing good ventilation are helpful. A deodorizer may be used in the room. Soiled dressings should be removed promptly from the patient's room when they are changed.

This patient needs nursing care similar to the care needed by other patients with an infection. Measures of particular importance to this patient are rest, adequate fluids, and good skin care. When caring for this patient the practical nurse should handle the diseased part gently. His diet should be nourishing. A diet high in proteins and vitamins is often ordered to aid the healing process.

## ARTHRITIS

### Introduction

An individual with arthritis has an inflammation of his joints. It is a common disease and a frequent cause of disability. There are nearly eleven million individuals with some form of arthritis in the United States. The two main types of arthritis—rheumatoid arthritis and degenerative joint disease (osteoarthritis)—account for two-thirds of the total number of patients with this condition. Other types of arthritis which are less common are caused by an infection of the joint, an injury, or a metabolic disturbance, such as gout.

### Rheumatoid Arthritis

#### Description

Rheumatoid arthritis is a chronic disease which may affect many joints and result in deformity. It is more common between 20 and 50 years of age. Children may develop this disease also. Unfortunately rheumatoid arthritis causes a high percentage of disability. However, it is encouraging to note that approximately 70 per cent of the people with this disease recover from their first attack and have little or no disability as a result of it.

The course of this disease varies. The patient may recover after the first attack or he may continue to have the disease. The inflammation may smolder for years. During this time the patient frequently has periods in which the symptoms are acute. The disease may progress either rapidly or slowly or it may become arrested at any time.

The practical nurse needs an understanding of the changes within the patient's joints and how these changes result in deformities. Inflammation of the joint results in swelling of the synovial membrane and the tissues which surround it. Adhesions form and decrease the ability of the joint to move. Muscle spasms may occur around the joint and cause it to be painful, especially when moved. Cartilage may be destroyed. The amount of synovial fluid may be increased. The patient's joint may become immobilized (incapable of moving). After the patient's joint has become immobilized, the muscles around the joint atrophy, that is, they waste away or get smaller. This results from lack of use. The muscles surrounding the joint contract. The deformed joint appears much larger than the wasted and contracted muscles around it. The skin over the area usually appears thin and glossy.

### Cause

The cause of rheumatoid arthritis is unknown. Predisposing factors are conditions which lower the general resistance of the individual's body. For example, a person may develop rheumatoid arthritis after being exposed to a damp cold climate, overworking, or having an acute infectious disease, such as pneumonia. Also, a severe physical or an emotional shock may be a predisposing factor.

### Symptoms

The patient with rheumatoid arthritis has general symptoms of an inflammation, such as malaise and fever, during the acute phase of this disease. He may have a loss of weight. His main symptoms are the local ones which are associated with the inflamed joints. The severity of these symptoms vary. The joints may be stiff and sore or they may become painful and swollen. Frequently the joints of the fingers and knees are involved. As the disease progresses, it causes the joints to become deformed. The joints may become *ankylosed*, which means the ends of the bones are united firmly or have grown together and are no longer freely movable. Frequently the patient with an advanced case of rheumatoid arthritis becomes anemic.

### Treatment and Nursing Care

The physician directs his treatment toward improving the general health of the patient as well as caring for the involved joints. In order for the doctor to improve the patient's general level of good health, he may have to treat a chronic infection elsewhere in the body, such as tonsillitis. Adequate rest and a well-balanced diet help to improve the patient's general health.

*arthroplasy, surgery on ends of bones to restore motion*

### Rest and Prevention of Deformity

An important aim in the care of the patient's involved joints is the prevention of deformity. In addition to prescribing rest for the patient with acutely inflamed joints, the doctor wants the involved joint to have rest in a good position. Muscles which flex (bend) a part of the body are stronger than those which extend it. Because of this, the patient is likely to develop flexor deformities. The patient should be encouraged to keep the affected joint straight to help prevent a flexor deformity. The practical nurse should keep the patient in the position as directed by the doctor. In general, the patient should not remain for a long period of time in a position with the affected joint bent. For example, the patient with rheumatoid arthritis of the elbows should not remain in a position in which he has his elbow bent. The patient with affected knees should not use pillows under his knees as this encourages flexor deformity of these joints. The practical nurse may find that sandbags are helpful in keeping the extremities in good position. A footboard can be used to prevent foot drop. A cradle may be used over the patient's feet to keep bed clothing from pressing on his toes. A bedboard may be used under the mattress to prevent sagging.

The physician may immobilize the affected joint by the use of a cast or a splint. The use of these aids increases the amount of rest for the joint in an extended position so that flexor deformities do not develop. Frequently these orthopedic devices are applied so that they can be removed at specified times. The practical nurse should receive definite instructions regarding when and how to remove and to replace them. Traction is another type of treatment which may be used to prevent and/or correct arthritic deformities.

### Heat

The physician frequently prescribes the local application of heat. Heat applied to the joints increases the blood supply which aids in healing. It also relieves pain by relaxing the muscles around the involved joint. He may also select a method of applying heat which can be done by the practical nurse. For example, the doctor may recommend the use of an electric heating pad or a hot-water bottle. Precautions should be taken to prevent burning the patient (see

Chap. 6, pp. 75-76). The physical therapist may be requested to give heat treatments. For example, the physician may order either diathermy or paraffin-dip treatment. *Diathermy* is the use of a machine which sends an electric current into the tissues below the skin. This current produces heat in the arthritic joint. *Paraffin-dip treatment* is the use of melted paraffin for the application of heat. It is used mainly for an affected hand or arm. The patient's extremity is dipped a number of times into the warm paraffin until it is covered with a thick coat. The paraffin is usually removed by having the patient dip the part into the warm paraffin after approximately one hour.

### Exercise

As the patient's acutely inflamed joint begins to improve, he is encouraged to move the joint. Exercise is important in helping the patient to maintain and to improve the functioning of the joint. It also helps to prevent deformity. The physician tries to maintain a balance between rest and exercise which he believes to be necessary for that particular joint. The practical nurse should encourage the patient to move the joint as directed by the doctor. He commonly prescribes massage and specific exercises for the patient. The patient in a hospital which has a physical therapy department is usually referred to the physical therapist for treatment by exercise. This responsibility may be placed on members of the nursing team in institutions without a physical therapy department. In this case, the physician indicates the type of exercise he wants the patient to receive. Frequently the patient has certain exercises which he is to perform at specified times. The patient needs to be encouraged to carry out his exercises faithfully. He may be inclined to do them less often and for shorter periods of time because of the discomfort and the time involved.

### Occupational Therapy

Occupational therapy is an important aspect of the treatment of a patient with arthritis. The occupational therapist works with the doctor, the physical therapist, and other members of the health team in helping the patient to regain the function of his joints. Occupational therapy helps the patient spend time in a useful manner.

The practical nurse needs to realize that the patient is not necessarily learning a craft to be used later as a vocation. For instance, the patient with arthritis of his hands may not be learning to type as a means of livelihood but as a means of keeping his mind and body active during his convalescence. Another aim of the occupational therapist is to help the patient in becoming adjusted to a disability by emphasizing the things which he can do. Emphasis is focused on the patient's abilities rather than his disabilities. Genuine complimentary remarks by members of the nursing team help to encourage the patient in his efforts.

Frequently the practical nurse cares for the arthritic patient who is unable to receive guidance from an occupational therapist because of the hospital setup or because he is in his own home. The practical nurse with ingenuity can render an invaluable service to this patient. After determining his interests, she can stimulate and guide him in various projects. Activities which involve the use of affected joints are especially important.

### Skin Care

The patient with arthritis needs a warm cleansing bath daily. The practical nurse should give special care to the skin over areas subject to pressure to prevent decubitus ulcers. She should avoid exposure and chilling of the patient. This patient needs to be handled gently, especially his affected joints. The practical nurse should not rush or hurry in caring for him. Gentle and slow turning is greatly appreciated by this patient; however, he can often turn himself with more ease than when he is assisted by the nurse. In many cases he can tell the practical nurse how to turn him or how to help him to turn so that he has less discomfort. The practical nurse should remember that the patient is likely to choose the position which is most comfortable rather than the one most likely to prevent deformity. She should encourage him to assume the position which helps to prevent the development of a deformity.

### Drugs

The salicylates, gold preparations, and hormones may be prescribed for the patient with arthritis. (1) Salicylates, such as aspirin and Bufferin,* are used to relieve the patient's discomfort and pain. (2) Gold therapy may be used for the patient with a more active disease process. In caring for this patient, the practical nurse should observe and report toxic conditions caused by the drug, such as itching, hives, skin rash, soreness of the mouth or gums, digestive disturbances, and jaundice. (3) ACTH (adrenocorticotropic hormone) and cortisone are two hormones which may be prescribed to provide temporary relief. Frequently the patient has a recurrence after either ACTH or cortisone is discontinued. Both of these drugs can cause toxic effects. The practical nurse should observe and report symptoms of a toxic reaction which include mental changes, moon-faced appearance, edema, eruptions of the skin, high blood pressure, increased growth of hair, symptoms of digestive disturbance, and sugar in the urine. The physician may inject a form of cortisone into an acutely inflamed joint.

### Attitude of the Practical Nurse

The patient may undergo changes in his personality because of this chronic disabling disease. It is understandable that a person with arthritis may become irritable, impatient, and discouraged. His frequent bouts of pain and his concern over the crippling effect of the disease are two frequent causes of worry. Also, he may be concerned about returning to his job or wondering how he can earn his living.

The practical nurse is in a key position to help the patient in adjusting to his illness because of her close daily contact with him. It is important for the patient to learn to live within the limitations caused by arthritis. The practical nurse can be of great help to the patient by her understanding, optimistic, and thoughtful attitude. The patient needs to be encouraged to continue the treatment which the doctor has prescribed to aid in his recovery. His motivation is of vital importance in his rehabilitation.

Frequently the practical nurse spends many hours with the patient and his family. During this time she should develop an understanding of both. Having learned the patient's likes and dislikes, peculiarities, and problems, the practical nurse should report

* A trade-marked product; each tablet contains 0.3 gm (5 gr) of aspirin, aluminum glycinate, and magnesium carbonate.

information which she thinks the doctor might need to know. Such information can be of value to the physician when he makes plans for the patient's continued rehabilitation. Psychotherapy may be used to help the patient cope with problems of adjustment which result from his arthritic condition.

## Degenerative Joint Disease (Osteoarthritis)

### Description

An individual with degenerative joint disease has a chronic disease of the joints. The practical nurse may hear degenerative joint disease referred to as _osteoarthritis_ or _hypertrophic arthritis_. Unlike the patient with rheumatoid arthritis, this patient usually does not develop deformities. The practical nurse can expect the patient with rheumatoid arthritis to be younger than the person with degenerative joint disease, as the latter disease occurs most often in late middle life. She can expect to care for many patients with degenerative joint disease as it is the second main type of arthritis.

Degenerative joint disease progresses slowly. The changes in the joints of a patient with this disease are not as marked as those of a patient with rheumatoid arthritis. The bones in the affected joints of a patient with degenerative joint disease may become larger. Because of this, it is often called hypertrophic arthritis, since the term _hypertrophy_ means increase in size. Cartilage may be destroyed, but the joint usually does not become stiff, or ankylosed. For this reason, a person with hypertrophic arthritis is not as likely to develop deformities as is the patient with rheumatoid arthritis. _Spurs,_ which are outgrowths of tissue, may form in the joint. If a spur breaks loose, it may move around in the area, causing the patient acute pain.

### Cause

The exact cause of degenerative joint disease is not known. Injury, poor posture, and obesity (overweight) may be predisposing factors. An individual may develop hypertrophic arthritis following injury, such as that caused by constant and strenuous use of certain joints. Poor posture places a strain on certain joints, and over a period of years this may lead to degenerative joint disease. Usually an obese person has poor posture. His weight causes him to have more strain, especially on his weight-bearing joints. This may result in hypertrophic arthritis. An individual is most likely to develop this disease in the hips, knees, fingers, and lumbar spine.

### Symptoms

An individual with degenerative joint disease complains of pain in the affected joints. Frequently his discomfort is aggravated by changes in the weather. His joints gradually become enlarged. He notices stiffness in his joints, especially after resting.

### Treatment and Nursing Care

The physician directs his treatment toward relieving the conditions predisposing to hypertrophic arthritis and the patient's discomfort. For example, he treats the obese patient for this condition. The physician also helps the patient to correct his posture when it is faulty. He attempts to prevent further injury to the patient's joints when his occupation causes a constant strain on them. In order to accomplish this, he may recommend that the patient retire or change his work habits.

The physician usually recommends that the patient rest the affected joints when his pain is aggravated by exercise. He determines the amount of rest and exercise needed by each individual patient. The diseased joints should be protected from strain. The practical nurse can expect this patient to need frequent rest periods in order to avoid undue strain. Aspirin is often prescribed for the relief of pain. Physical therapy, such as heat, may be used to relieve the patient's discomfort. The patient should avoid becoming damp and cold.

## BURSITIS

### Description

A person with bursitis has an inflammation of a bursa which was described earlier in this chapter as a sac containing fluid. These sacs are located in and around joints to prevent friction. The patient with bursitis complains of pain in the region of the inflamed bursa. Movement increases his pain. A bursa may become inflamed because of injury or infection. Bursitis frequently occurs in the subdeltoid bursa, which is located in the shoulder.  *elbow* *patella*

## Treatment

The physician frequently prescribes rest of the inflamed part and the local application of heat. He may use x-ray therapy, or he may inject hydrocortisone into the area to hasten the patient's recovery. In some cases, the inflamed bursa is removed by surgery.

## SUGGESTIONS FOR STUDY

1. Why should a person with a sprained ankle have his foot and leg elevated? Why are cold applications used during the first 10 to 12 hours?

2. Why should an infant with a clubfoot have early treatment?

3. Break a stick or a chicken bone to illustrate the types of fractures.

4. Try to break a green branch from a tree. Compare this with the manner in which a dry stick breaks. How does the green branch break in comparison to the greenstick fracture described in this chapter?

5. Discuss the emergency care of the person with a fracture.

6. Review the treatment of a fracture. What is the difference between open reduction and closed reduction?

7. The patient who has been placed in either traction or a cast should have his toes or fingers examined frequently for impaired circulation. What are the symptoms of impaired circulation?

8. Discuss the nursing care of a patient in a cast.

9. Why is traction used?

10. Discuss the nursing care of a patient in traction.

11. Borrow a pair of crutches and practice the different types of crutch walking described in this chapter.

12. Review the nursing care of a patient with osteomyelitis.

13. What is the approximate number of individuals in the United States affected by arthritis?

14. Compare the differences between degenerative joint disease (osteo-arthritis) and rheumatoid arthritis in regard to the age group affected, deformities, and joint changes.

15. What is the meaning of ankylosis? In which type of arthritis is this more common?

16. Discuss the nursing care of a patient with arthritis.

17. What drugs have you heard discussed as a "cure" for arthritis? How do these compare with the information contained in this chapter?

## REFERENCES FOR CHAPTER 17

Brown, Amy F.: *Medical Nursing,* 3rd ed. W. B. Saunders Co., Phila delphia, 1957, pp. 687-708.

Eliason, Eldridge; Ferguson, L. Kraeer; and Sholtis, Lillian A.: *Surgical Nursing,* 10th ed. J. B. Lippincott Co., Philadelphia, 1955, pp. 527-96.

Emerson, Charles P., Jr., and Bragdon, Jane S.: *Essentials of Medicine,* 17th ed. J. B. Lippincott Co., Philadelphia, 1955, pp. 677-714.

Faddis, Margene O., and Hayman, Joseph M.: *Care of the Medical Patient.* McGraw-Hill Book Co., New York, 1952, pp. 414-33.

Hull, Edgar, and Perrodin, Cecilia: *Medical Nursing,* 5th ed. F. A. Davis Co., Philadelphia, 1954, pp. 397-414.

Jaschik, Eva, and Olsen, Catherine: "Nursing Care of the Arthritic Patient at Home," *Am. J. Nursing,* **55:**429-32, (Apr.) 1955.

Jensen, Julius, and Jensen, Deborah: *Nursing in Clinical Medicine,* 4th ed. The Macmillan Company, New York, 1954, pp. 513-41.

Jessar, Ralph A., and Hollander, Joseph L.: "Types of Arthritis and Their Medical Treatment," *Am. J. Nursing,* **55:**426-29, (Apr.) 1955.

Kitay, William: "The Practical Nurse and Arthritis," *Practical Nurses Digest,* **3:**3-5, (Mar.) 1956.

Krause, Marie: *Nutrition and Diet Therapy,* 2nd ed. W. B. Saunders Co., Philadelphia, 1957, pp. 355-58.

Larson, Carroll B., and Gould, Marjorie: *Calderwood's Orthopedic Nursing,* 4th ed. C. V. Mosby Co., St. Louis, 1957.

Proudfit, Fairfax T., and Robinson, Corinne H.: *Nutrition and Diet Therapy,* 11th ed. The Macmillan Company, New York, 1955, pp. 499-505.

Solomon, Charles, and Gill, Elizabeth S.: *Pharmacology and Therapeutics,* 7th ed. J. B. Lippincott Co., Philadelphia, 1956, pp. 387-95.

Stafford, Edward S., and Diller, Doris: *Surgery and Surgical Nursing,* 3rd ed. W. B. Saunders Co., Philadelphia, 1958, pp. 289-310.

Terry, Florence J.; Benz, Gladys S.; Mereness, Dorothy; and Kleffner, Frank R.: *Principles and Technics of Rehabilitation Nursing.* C. V. Mosby Co., St. Louis, 1957, pp. 129-35.

West, John P.; Keller, Manelva W.; and Harmon, Elizabeth H.: *Nursing Care of the Surgical Patient,* 6th ed. The Macmillan Company, New York, 1957, pp. 390-434.

*Nursing the Patient*

*with a Disorder of*

*the Endocrine System*

TEST MON. 9

PART VII

5 - 1 - 66

Chapter 18

# THE PATIENT
# WITH A DISORDER OF
# THE ENDOCRINE SYSTEM

Outline

STRUCTURE AND FUNCTION
GOITER: SIMPLE GOITER,
TOXIC GOITER

HYPOTHYROIDISM
ADDISON'S DISEASE
DIABETES MELLITUS

## STRUCTURE AND FUNCTION

The endocrine system is made of glands which help to coordinate and to regulate other systems of the body. These glands also have an influence upon each other. Glands of the endocrine system take certain materials from the blood, manufacture new substances called *hormones*, and secrete these substances into the blood stream. They are called *ductless glands* or *glands of internal secretion* because they secrete the hormones into the blood. Glands which secrete hormones are (1) the pituitary, located at the base of the skull; (2) the thyroid, located in the neck; (3) the parathyroids, located on the thyroid gland; (4) the adrenals, located above the kidneys; (5) the pineal, situated in the skull; (6) the gonads, or sex glands; (7) the thymus, situated in the chest; and (8) the pancreas, located behind the stomach. Special consideration is given to the thyroid, the adrenals, and the pancreas in this chapter as a background for discussing the care of patients with diseases of these glands.

The thyroid gland is located in the lower portion of the neck. The practical nurse can locate her thyroid gland by finding her Adam's apple. The soft tissue beneath this is the thyroid. It is made of two lobes which are situated on each side of the trachea. These two lobes are connected by a narrow band known as the isthmus. The thyroid gland secretes a substance called *thyroxin*, which contains iodine. The thyroid gland also stores iodine. Thyroxin plays an important part in controlling the metabolic rate of the body. It also controls the normal growth and development of young people.

279

There are two adrenal or suprarenal glands. One is located over each kidney. The inner portion of the adrenal gland is called the medulla. One of the hormones secreted by the medulla is epinephrine. This is secreted in response to stimulation from the nervous system to help the body cope with an emergency. The outer portion of the adrenal gland is called the cortex. It secretes a hormone called cortin

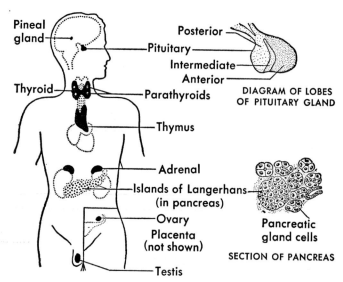

**Figure 34.** The *left* portion of the diagram shows the approximate location of the principal endocrine glands in man. Although the pineal gland and thymus are included, they are not known definitely to be endocrine glands. On the *right* is a section of a pituitary gland showing the lobes, as well as a diagram of the microscopic structure of the pancreas. (After Hegner and Stiles.) (Orr, Warren H.: *Hormones, Health, and Happiness.* The Macmillan Company, New York, 1954.)

and is necessary for life. Cortin regulates the water balance of the body. It also helps to control the metabolism of fats, proteins, and carbohydrates. The adrenal cortex is stimulated by the adrenocortico-tropic hormone (ACTH) which is secreted by the anterior pituitary gland.

The pancreas, which is behind the stomach, manufactures *insulin* and *pancreatic fluid.* Pancreatic fluid is carried to the small intestine by a duct. Insulin is manufactured by a special group of cells in the pancreas called the islands of Langerhans. This substance is picked up by the blood stream. Insulin is necessary for the body tissues to utilize glucose, which is their fuel.

## GOITER

### Introduction

The patient with a goiter has an enlargement of his thyroid gland. It is known as a *diffuse goiter* when the enlargement spreads throughout the thyroid gland. The term *nodular goiter* is used when one or more areas of the gland increase in size. The person with a goiter which produces no symptoms other than the enlargement itself has a *simple or nontoxic goiter*. The individual with symptoms of an overactive thyroid in addition to the enlargement has a *toxic goiter*.

Frequently the practical nurse is asked to help in preparing the patient for diagnostic tests to determine whether or not the goiter is toxic. The *basal metabolic rate* (B.M.R.) is done to determine the rate of metabolism when the patient is at rest. The patient needs to know that he should have no food or water for at least 12 hours before the test. The practical nurse can assure the anxious patient that no pain is associated with a B.M.R. The test is usually done in the early part of the morning following a good night's rest. The patient should not be disturbed for general nursing measures, such as a bed bath, until the test has been completed. A person with a basal metabolic rate within the range of a $+10$ to a $-10$ is considered to have normal metabolic rate. A B.M.R. higher than $+10$ may indicate an overactive thyroid, whereas a B.M.R. below $-10$ may indicate an underactive thyroid.

*Protein-bound iodine* is another diagnostic test. This is a laboratory test which is performed on the blood. Normally a person has 4 to 8 micrograms of protein-bound iodine in a specified amount of blood. The physician uses the report from this test in helping to determine whether or not the thyroid gland is functioning properly. A report of more than 8 micrograms leads him to assume that the patient has an overactive thyroid. A report of fewer than 4 micrograms indicates underactivity of the thyroid gland.

Another procedure which may be used to test the functioning of a patient's thyroid gland is the *radioactive iodine uptake study*. The thyroid gland normally stores some of the iodine which is taken into the body in foods. The remaining portion of the iodine is excreted in the urine. The amount of iodine taken up by the thyroid gland is affected by disease. This amount can be determined by giving the patient radioactive iodine, which means it gives off rays. A small amount of radioactive iodine is usually given in a glass of water by a specialist trained in this field. The amount of this substance taken up by the thyroid gland is measured 24 hours later by a special instrument, the Geiger counter. The amount of radioactive iodine passed in the urine may be measured also. The physician assumes that the patient has a toxic goiter when the report shows an increased uptake of radioactive iodine by the thyroid gland. This patient usually excretes less iodine in his urine. If the doctor finds that the patient's thyroid took up only a small amount of radioactive iodine and excreted more in his urine, he assumes that the patient has an underactive thyroid gland.

### Simple Goiter

#### Description

The patient with a simple goiter has an enlargement of his thyroid gland. It usually produces no symptoms other than the local swelling. However, an extremely large goiter may press on the trachea. The practical nurse may hear the simple goiter spoken of as a *nontoxic goiter* or a *colloid goiter.*

Simple goiter is more common in parts of the country in which the natural supply of iodine is insufficient. The area around the Great Lakes, the northwestern part of the United States, and the upper part of the Mississippi Valley are regions where the soil is poor in iodine. Although simple goiter is most likely to develop in persons living in these areas, it can develop in individuals living in other regions. The administration of iodine to children living in iodine-poor areas is important in preventing this condition. Frequently iodine is combined with table salt as a means of preventing simple goiter.

Simple goiter is more common in young individuals, especially girls. Frequently it appears during puberty and it may subside by the time the person reaches 25 or 30 years of age.

## Treatment

The person with a simple goiter may need no special treatment as the enlargement frequently subsides. In some cases the physician prescribes iodine preparations, such as Lugol's solution or potassium iodine. If the goiter does not become smaller in size, it may be removed by surgery.

## Toxic Goiter

### Description

The patient with a toxic goiter has an enlargement of his thyroid gland and symptoms of overactivity of this gland. This disease is also called *hyperthyroidism* and *Graves' disease.*

### Cause

The exact cause of a toxic goiter is not known. It is believed to be associated with a disturbance of the pituitary gland. This disease is more common in women. Toxic goiter often follows an acute infection, especially of the upper respiratory tract. It frequently follows a severe emotional shock or a nervous strain.

### Symptoms

The patient's overactive thyroid causes him to have symptoms of general hyperactivity. He becomes nervous, excitable, and apprehensive. Remembering that the thyroid gland regulates the body's metabolism, the practical nurse can readily understand why the patient loses weight. Although he eats an increasingly larger amount of food, he continues to lose weight because the overactive thyroid gland increases his metabolism. This may be compared with a fire burning rapidly in a stove. The faster the fire burns, the more wood it needs to keep it going. The faster the body uses its food for fuel, the more food it needs to keep it going. When the patient is unable to eat enough food, his body begins to use its own adipose tissues. Thus, the patient loses weight.

The patient's pulse rate increases. He develops a fine tremor of his hands and frequently complains of tiring easily. He cannot tolerate heat because of his increased metabolism. His skin feels warm and moist. The patient's eyes frequently appear bright and staring. They may also bulge or protrude. The disease is sometimes called exophthalmic goiter because of this symptom (ex means out, and ophthalmos means the eye). The basal metabolic rate, the protein-bound iodine, and radioactive iodine uptake study are higher than normal.

### Treatment and Nursing Care

The physician's aim in treating this patient is to relieve the hyperthyroidism. In order to accomplish this objective he may: (1) use drugs to reduce the activity of the thyroid gland, (2) destroy part of the gland by administering radioactive iodine, (3) remove part of the gland, or (4) use a combination of these methods of treatment. Propylthiouracil and iodine preparations, such as Lugol's solution and potassium iodide, are examples of drugs commonly used to reduce the activity of the thyroid gland. Frequently the patient's symptoms disappear with this treatment.

The physician may use radioactive iodine to destroy part of the thyroid gland. Radioactive iodine is given by mouth. Since iodine is usually localized in the thyroid gland, this type of iodine is also carried to this gland. Radioactive iodine destroys some of the cells of the thyroid gland. This type of treatment may cause the symptoms to disappear permanently.

The doctor may decide that surgical removal of part of the thyroid gland is necessary. Frequently the patient is treated before surgery with the drugs mentioned above: propylthiouracil and iodine preparations.

The patient with a toxic goiter needs both mental and physical rest. He should be placed in a room which is cool and quiet. The doctor may either restrict or limit visitors. The patient's surroundings should be conducive to relaxation. The practical nurse should avoid making sudden noises or movements around the patient. She should be patient and tactful with the patient since he is likely to be irritable and restless. It is often necessary for the physician to prescribe sedatives, such as phenobarbital, to relax the patient. Diversional activities approved by the doctor may help to relieve the patient's restlessness.

This patient needs good skin care as he usually perspires more than the average person. Alcohol back rubs often have a cooling and relaxing effect on this patient. The practical nurse may find it necessary to straighten the linen on the patient's bed frequently as his feeling of restlessness causes him to move around a great deal.

The doctor generally prescribes a diet high in calories, vitamins, and minerals. This is necessary in order to meet the increased nutritional needs of the body. Usually, the patient is not allowed to have stimulants such as tea and coffee. It may be necessary for the practical nurse to feed the patient or to help him with his meal if his hands are shaking excessively.

### Preoperative Care

In some cases surgical removal of part of the thyroid gland is necessary. The surgeon directs his treatment toward relieving the patient's symptoms and reducing the metabolism of his body before doing surgery. This patient needs the nursing measures which have been discussed in the preceding paragraphs. Drugs, rest, and a high-caloric diet are used to prepare the patient for surgery. The physician generally considers the patient ready for surgery when his B.M.R. is nearer normal, when his pulse rate is slower, and when he is beginning to gain weight. The patient should be less excitable than he was when admitted to the hospital.

### Postoperative Care

The practical nurse may be asked to help transfer the patient to his bed after surgery. The patient's head, neck, and shoulders should be supported so that his head does not turn to the side and put a strain on the incision. The patient is usually placed in semi-Fowler's position with pillows supporting his head and shoulders. The dressing should be checked frequently during the first 24 hours for bleeding. Blood on the dressing should be reported immediately.

The patient should be observed for symptoms of respiratory difficulty, such as noisy breathing, dyspnea, and cyanosis. The practical nurse should report these symptoms immediately to her head nurse or team leader. Respiratory difficulties may result from swelling within the larynx. Also, the nerves leading to the larynx may have been injured during the operation because of their closeness to the gland. This may result in paralysis of the vocal folds. It may be necessary for the doctor to insert a tracheotomy tube to relieve the patient's

*Near parathyroid - check for tetany*

difficult respiration. A tracheotomy tray is placed in this patient's room as a precautionary measure in many hospitals.

The patient should be observed for muscle spasms. The calcium in the patient's body becomes disturbed if the parathyroid glands are removed or injured during surgery. This can result in tetany, which is characterized by muscular spasms. This is a rare complication. The physician usually treats the patient with tetany with either parathyroid extract or calcium.

The practical nurse should report the following symptoms: an elevation of temperature, profuse perspiration, and restlessness. These symptoms may indicate a serious complication known as thyroid crisis. The patient may become delirious and die. Fortunately this is another rare complication. The condition is treated with cold applications, sedatives, the administration of intravenous fluids, and oxygen therapy.

This patient needs a longer period of time for convalescence in order to regain his strength. He continues to need a high-caloric diet and sufficient rest during this time.

## HYPOTHYROIDISM

### Description

An individual with hypothyroidism has a deficiency of the thyroid hormone. It is known as cretinism when it develops in the fetus or in early infancy. Hypothyroidism may occur in either a child or an adult who was previously normal. Women are more likely to be affected than men. An advanced form of hypothyroidism in adults is called myxedema.

### Symptoms

The symptoms vary with the amount of deficiency and the person's age when the condition started. The mental and physical growth of an infant with cretinism is stunted. In general, the patient with hypothyroidism gains weight and notices a gradual loss of energy. His basal metabolic rate is lower than normal. He becomes sensitive to cold, develops coarse dry hair, and may have a dry skin.

The patient with myxedema has the above-mentioned symptoms to a greater degree. As his condition progresses his temperature, pulse rate, and B.M.R. decrease. He develops a sallow, puffy facial appearance and becomes mentally sluggish. His skin becomes thick, and he suffers from cold weather.

### Treatment

This patient is treated with thyroid extract which is adjusted to his needs. Iodine is administered to pregnant women in iodine-poor regions to prevent cretinism in the fetus. Thyroid extract is used in treating an infant with cretinism.

## ADDISON'S DISEASE

A person with Addison's disease has a deficiency of the cortical hormone which is secreted by the cortex, or outer portion, of the adrenal glands. Addison's disease may be caused by atrophy (wasting away) of the cortex, and by tuberculosis of the adrenal glands. It is a rare disease.

The patient loses energy, weight, strength, and appetite. Frequently he develops nausea and vomiting and has a progressive drop in blood pressure. He develops areas of pigmentation which look like dark freckles. Brown spots may appear in his mouth.

This patient's condition can usually be controlled with either cortisone or an extract of the cortex of the adrenal gland. The physician may recommend a diet high in calories.

## DIABETES MELLITUS

### Description

The patient with diabetes mellitus is unable to utilize carbohydrates properly. A brief discussion of carbohydrates and other essential elements of food is given as a background for discussing this condition.

The body of man needs energy which is obtained from food. The three essential elements of food from which energy is produced are proteins, fats, and carbohydrates. Protein is necessary for the normal growth and the repair of tissues. It also supplies a portion of the body's energy. Lean meats and eggs are examples of foods high in protein. Fats are important for the normal functioning of the body tissue and serve as a reserve source of heat and energy. Milk, cream, butter, fatty meat, olive oil, and mayonnaise are examples of foods high in fat. The sugars and starches are known as carbohydrates. Foods such as cereals, breads, vegetables, fruits, macaroni, syrups, and sugars are high in carbohydrate. A large portion of the fuel needed for heat and energy is supplied by carbohydrates. It is necessary for the body to reduce carbohydrates to *glucose*, a simple form of sugar, before it can be used by the tissues in the production of energy.

A substance called *insulin* is necessary for the body to convert glucose into energy. Normally the body has its own supply of insulin from the islands of Langerhans in the pancreas. Insulin enables the body to produce energy from glucose. It also helps the body to store carbohydrates in the form of fat and as glycogen in the muscles and the liver. A person normally has 80 to 120 mg of sugar in 100 ml of blood. His blood sugar usually increases slightly after eating a meal containing a large amount of carbohydrates. The patient with diabetes has an insufficient amount of insulin, a condition which results in an accumulation of sugar in the blood. This increased blood sugar is known as *hyperglycemia.* He develops *glycosuria,* sugar in the urine. This is caused by the efforts of the kidneys to remove excess sugar from the blood stream. The patient's inability to utilize carbohydrates properly also affects his ability to use fats and proteins as these produce a small part of the body's glucose.

There seems to be a hereditary tendency for some persons to develop diabetes, although the individual may not develop it until later in life. It may affect any age group, but it is more common after middle life. The incidence is higher in women than in men. Diabetes may run a rapid course in young individuals unless they are treated promptly.

### Cause

Although it is known that diabetes is associated with an insufficient amount of insulin, the exact reason for this is not known.

Predisposing causes of diabetes are a hereditary tendency and obesity. Children born of parents who have diabetes are more likely to develop it than are children born of parents who do not have this disease. Diabetes is more common in obese individuals. However, a younger person with diabetes is likely to be underweight. Some physicians believe that a disorder of other endocrine glands, such as the adrenals or pituitary, may be a predisposing factor.

## Symptoms

An individual with diabetes usually has *polyuria*, which means that
he voids an excessive amount of urine. The kidneys take an increasing
amount of fluid from the blood stream in their efforts to rid the body
of excess sugar. Associated with polyuria is *polydipsia* (excessive thirst).
As his body tries to get rid of the excess amount of sugar through the
kidneys, it also increases his desire for water in an effort to dilute the
blood which is overloaded with sugar.

Since the patient with diabetes is unable to burn and to store carbohydrates, he suffers from poor nutrition. Although his cells are surrounded by an excess amount of sugar, they are unable to use it
properly because of insufficient insulin. It may be helpful to the
practical nurse to think of insulin as an important link in a chain
leading from food to energy. The link in this imaginary chain of a
diabetic patient is either inadequate or missing. As the patient's body
is not using food properly, he usually loses weight and feels weak
and hungry. The loss of some of his sugar through the urine also contributes to these symptoms of poor nutrition. Varying amounts of
sugar are found in the urine. The practical nurse should understand
that the presence of sugar in urine does not always indicate diabetes.
This symptom may occur in an entirely healthy person who has
eaten a large meal. In addition to having glycosuria, the person with
diabetes has an increased blood sugar.

The untreated patient is likely to develop infections which are
difficult to overcome. For example, he may complain of frequent colds
which last an unusually long time. His skin is particularly susceptible
to disturbances, such as frequent boils and pruritis (itching). Or he
may have a minor injury to the skin which heals slowly.

The diabetic individual may become constipated as the increased
amount of sugar in the blood favors the passage of water from the
intestinal tract into the blood stream. This lack of water causes his
stools to become hard.

The patient may complain of dimness of vision and various aches
and pains. He may experience a feeling of numbness and tingling.

## Diagnosis

After taking a complete history and doing a thorough physical
examination, the doctor usually requests various laboratory tests

which help him in diagnosing the patient's condition. A urinalysis shows whether or not sugar is present in the urine. A test to determine the amount of sugar in the blood is usually ordered; at times this is done in the early morning before the patient eats. If the practical nurse knows that the patient is to have a blood sugar test, she should check with the nurse in charge before giving the patient food.

The practical nurse may be asked to collect the patient's urine for a period of 24 hours. This is known as a 24-hour specimen. All of the urine is saved for this length of time. The practical nurse should find out whether the doctor wants part of the urine sent to the laboratory or whether he wants the entire amount sent. This type of specimen enables the doctor to know the total amount of sugar excreted in relation to the total amount of urine passed during a 24-hour period.

The physician may request a sugar (glucose) tolerance test. This is usually done in the morning before the patient eats. He is given by mouth or intravenously a specified amount of glucose, usually 50 to 100 gm. Specimens of his blood and urine are taken at intervals, usually one, two, and three hours after the glucose has been given. Both the blood and the urine are examined for sugar. When the practical nurse is asked to assist with a glucose tolerance test, she should collect the urine specimens at the intervals specified by a particular hospital or doctor. An increased blood sugar and the presence of sugar in the urine indicate diabetes; conversely, a normal blood sugar and the absence of sugar in the urine indicate that the patient does not have diabetes.

The practical nurse may be asked to check the patient's urine for sugar and acetone. Acetone is found in urine when the person's body is living on its own fats and proteins instead of carbohydrates. A number of commercial sets for testing urine are available. When using one of these, the practical nurse should follow the instructions which accompany the kit. Hospitals have various procedures for testing the urine for sugar and acetone. The practical nurse should familiarize herself with the method used in a particular hospital.

### Treatment and Nursing Care

Diet, exercise, and insulin are used in treating the patient with diabetes. The physician's main purpose in treating this patient is to enable him to use an adequate amount of food. This is done by regulating the patient's diet and exercise. Insulin is administered when regulation of the diet and exercise do not enable the patient to use enough food.

### Diet

The doctor prescribes a diet to suit the individual patient's needs. The purpose of diet therapy is to keep the patient healthy and strong as well as to prevent him from becoming either overweight or markedly underweight. The doctor specifies the total number of calories and the proportion of the three basic types of foods—carbohydrates, fats, and proteins—which the patient is to receive daily. Some of the factors which he takes into consideration before prescribing the diet are the patient's age, size, occupation, general state of health, appetite, food preferences, and ability to buy the recommended food. The physician must adjust the diet from time to time according to changes in the patient's food requirements. For example, he reduces the number of calories when the patient becomes overweight. Also, he adjusts the diet to meet the increased needs of the patient's body during an infection.

When the patient has a mild case of diabetes it may be controlled by regulation of his diet and exercise without having to take insulin. For example, he may have been in the habit of eating more than he needed. In this case the physician would prescribe a reduction in the amount of food eaten.

The dietitian calculates the hospitalized patient's diet after she receives the diet prescription from the doctor. It was stated earlier that the physician orders the total number of calories and the proportion of carbohydrate, protein, and fat which he wants the patient to receive daily. The dietitian takes this order and plans the type and amount of food which the patient should receive in order to have the prescribed amount of calories in their correct proportion each day.

In caring for the patient with diabetes, the practical nurse may be responsible for serving the patient's food. As it is important for the patient to eat at regular times, the practical nurse is asked to serve the tray at a definite time. This should be done promptly to prevent the patient from developing insulin shock. For example, the doctor may prescribe insulin 30 minutes before meals. In this case, the practical nurse may be asked to serve the patient's breakfast at 8:15 if he was given insulin at 7:45. It is her responsibility to serve the tray at the specified time. A forgetful nurse can cause the patient to develop insulin shock. The practical nurse should encourage the patient to eat all of his food. She should weigh or estimate the approximate amount of food which the patient does not eat. The type and the amount of food not eaten should be reported to her team leader or head nurse. She in turn notifies the dietitian so that supplementary food can be given. For example, the practical nurse has reported to her head nurse that the patient did not drink his milk and eat his meat and roll. This, in turn, was reported to the dietitian who determined the number of calories not received by the patient. She suggested that the nurse give the patient 240 ml (8 oz.) of orange juice in order to provide the patient with the number of calories prescribed by the doctor.

The practical nurse may be responsible for preparing the patient's diet. This is especially true when caring for the patient in his home. She should follow the diet list given by the doctor. The types of measures indicated on the list should be used.

Either the patient or some member of his family should have a thorough understanding of the prescribed diet. The physician, the dietitian, and members of the nursing team work together in teaching the patient and/or a member of his family about his disease and the role of his diet.

In planning the diet for the patient to follow in his home, the physician may ask the patient to weigh the food, to use simple household measures, or to use the food exchange plan. Weighing the food on scales is the most accurate method of determining the exact amount. Such measures as spoons, cups, and glasses are used when the doctor recommends simple household equipment. The food exchange plan is a simplified method of calculation developed by the Council of the American Diabetes Association, the American Dietetic Association, and the United States Public Health Service. This plan, which is based on the idea of food exchanges, consists of a list of seven groups of foods. The foods on the list of one group have approximately the same amounts of carbohydrates, protein, and fat. The patient is permitted to substitute a serving of food on that one list for another one on the same list. For example, one small, white potato can be substituted for one slice of bread since these two items are on the same list. Using the food exchange list allows for more flexibility of food selection and enables the patient to have a diet which is more like his earlier one. Sometimes the physician allows the patient to eat without following a specific diet plan. The doctor then regulates the insulin to take care of the carbohydrates which the patient's body is unable to handle.

### Exercise

Exercise is of particular importance to the person with diabetes. He needs exercise every day rather than on a week end or a holiday. Physical activity causes the body to use more carbohydrates. Thus, exercise decreases the amount of insulin needed by the patient. Another important effect of exercise is that it helps maintain an adequate circulation. Since the diabetic is prone to develop circulatory complications, he may be less likely to develop these if he exercises regularly. The patient should be consistent in the type of physical activity in which he engages. If he exercises vigorously one day and mildly another day, he may have undesirable changes in his blood sugar. Knowing that the blood sugar is decreased during strenuous exercise, the practical nurse can understand why the doctor recommends extra food for the patient before he participates in this activity.

### Insulin

The physician prescribes insulin when regulation of the diet and exercise do not control the patient's diabetes. Insulin is made from the pancreas of animals, such as hogs and cattle. The injection of insulin enables the body to change glucose into energy. Thus the patient's blood sugar is lowered. Insulin also restores the ability of the body to store carbohydrates.

Insulin is prepared in various strengths. The label is marked to indicate the number of units in each cubic centimeter of solution. The larger the unit written on the bottle, the stronger the insulin. The strong concentrations allow the patient to receive a large dose in a small amount of solution. For example, a bottle marked U-80 contains 80 units of insulin in 1 cc and is stronger than the bottle marked U-40 which contains 40 units of insulin in 1 cc.

The practical nurse needs to be familiar with the different types of insulin. *Regular* or *unmodified insulin* has nothing added to it to change its action. The action of regular insulin begins within a few minutes after it is injected and generally lasts for approximately 6 hours. Its peak action is reached in approximately 3 hours. Regular insulin is usually given 15 to 30 minutes before each meal. *Crystalline insulin* is a second type of insulin, which has the same action as regular insulin; it is a purified form of regular insulin. However, crystalline insulin is used more frequently than regular insulin because it is less likely to cause an allergic reaction. Either regular or crystal-

IS NEVER SHOOK - ROll IN HANDS
to PREVENT bubbles

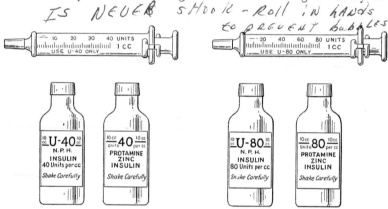

**Figure 35.**   The scale of the insulin syringe should correspond with the strength of insulin being used. The syringe with a U-40 scale should be used to measure U-40 insulin, and the syringe with a U-80 scale should be used to measure U-80 insulin.

line insulin may be used to reduce the patient's blood sugar rapidly because of their quick action.

*Protamine zinc insulin* is a third type of insulin. Insulin is mixed with a substance called protamine, which causes it to be slower in taking effect and makes the action last longer. A substance called zinc is added to make it more stable; thus its name—protamine zinc insulin. It usually reaches its peak action in 12 to 24 hours. Although the effect of protamine zinc insulin generally lasts for approximately 24 hours, it may last for 48 to 72 hours. This type of insulin is usually given once a day before breakfast. The practical nurse notices that it has a cloudy appearance. The bottle should be rolled in the hands gently to mix the protamine and the zinc with the insulin before it is measured in the syringe.

_Globin zinc insulin_ is a fourth type of insulin. Small amounts of globin and zinc have been added to regular insulin to make this preparation. It does not act so fast as regular insulin or so long as protamine zinc insulin. The practical nurse may hear it referred to as an insulin with an intermediate effect. Its peak action occurs approximately 8 to 16 hours after injection. The effect of globin zinc insulin may last for approximately 16 to 24 hours.

_Isophane insulin_ is a fifth type of insulin. It is commonly referred to as either NPH insulin* or _modified protamine zinc insulin._ It has an intermediate action. NPH insulin begins to take effect approximately 2 hours after injection and may last for as long as 28 to 30 hours.

_Lente insulin_ is the sixth type of insulin. It is intermediate in action. The effects of lente insulin are similar to those of NPH insulin. Since lente insulin contains no protein, it is used frequently for patients who have an allergy. There are other types of lente insulin available. _Semi-lente insulin_ is more rapidly absorbed and has a shorter action than lente insulin. _Ultra-lente insulin_ has a long action which is similar to that of protamine zinc insulin.

Insulin is administered by subcutaneous injection. The physician prescribes the type of insulin, the dosage in units, and the time of administration. Since the practical nurse may be responsible for administering insulin, she needs an understanding of the principles involved.

The bottle containing the type of insulin prescribed should be kept in a refrigerator or a cool place. However, insulin should not be injected while still cold. A special syringe is usually used to measure insulin. This syringe is marked in units as well as in cubic centimeters. The scale on a particular insulin syringe is intended for a specific strength of insulin. It is important that the strength of insulin being used correspond with the scale on the syringe. For example, the doctor has ordered 30 units of globin zinc insulin for the patient. The nurse should read the label on the bottle carefully to determine its strength and type. If she sees that it is marked globin zinc insulin

---

* Neutral protamine Hagedorn insulin; a preparation of isophane insulin developed by Dr. H. D. Hagedorn.

U-40, she should then select a sterile syringe with a U-40 scale on it. She would then fill the syringe to the mark indicating 30 units. If she sees that the bottle is marked globin-zinc insulin U-80, she should select a syringe with a U-80 scale on it. She would then fill the syringe to the mark indicating 30 units.

The insulin should be given subcutaneously (tissue under the skin) at the time specified by the doctor. The outer part of the patient's upper arm and either the front or the outer portion of his thigh may be used for the injections. The patient's abdomen may be used if he has sufficient subcutaneous tissue in that area. The site for injection should be rotated to prevent irritation of the tissues. For instance, the injections could be given in the patient's right arm, right side of his abdomen, right thigh, left thigh, left side of his abdomen, and left arm. This system of rotation could be started again in the right arm. However, an area approximately 2.5 to 5 cm (1 to 2 in.) from the previous site of injection should be used. By using a similar rotation scheme, the patient or the person giving the insulin can allow six to seven weeks to elapse before the same injection site is used again. The patient or some member of his family generally is taught to give insulin before the patient is discharged from the hospital.

### Skin Care

The person with diabetes needs special skin care because of his susceptibility to infections and delayed healing time. The patient needs a cleansing bath daily. The practical nurse should inspect the skin for symptoms of inflammation, such as redness. These should be reported promptly to the head nurse or team leader. Strong soap and antiseptics should not be used on his skin. The patient should be advised to consult his doctor about a suitable antiseptic. The feet of this patient also need special attention. They should be washed and dried thoroughly. The practical nurse may apply alcohol if the skin becomes too soft, or a lubricating substance, such as lanolin, may be needed to keep the skin soft. When cutting his toenails, the practical nurse should cut them straight across. She should be careful to avoid injuring the surrounding tissue. Ingrown toenails, calluses, corns, and bunions should not be cut by the nurse or the patient. The doctor may ask the nurse to soak the patient's feet and peel off the loose, soft outer layers of a corn or a callus. She can rub some of the dead tissue off gently with a bath towel. Further treatment is given by the doctor.

The patient should not wear circular garters because they interfere with the circulation of the feet and legs. Clean hose or socks are worn daily. Proper fitting shoes are also important to prevent irritation.

The practical nurse should use extreme caution when asked to apply heat, such as a hot-water bottle or an electric heating pad. There is real danger of burning the diabetic person because he may not feel heat so quickly as the person not affected with diabetes. His ability to feel cold may also be affected. A burn on a person with diabetes does not heal so quickly as it does on a healthy person.

The practical nurse should observe and report promptly symptoms of either diabetic coma or insulin shock. These are discussed later in this chapter.

### Preparation for Discharge

The physician, the dietitian, and members of the nursing team teach the patient and his family about diabetes and its control before the patient is discharged from the hospital. The patient or some member of his family needs to understand the diet, the method of giving insulin, the symptoms of insulin shock and diabetic coma, the care of the skin and feet, the importance of regular exercise, and the method of testing urine for sugar. The practical nurse with a thorough understanding of these factors can play an important role in helping the team leader or the head nurse in teaching the patient. For example, the nurse in charge may ask the practical nurse to explain to the patient how to care for his feet during the daily bath. The practical nurse can help the patient to understand the importance of following the doctor's orders. An individual with diabetes should carry a card containing this information which would aid in prompt and adequate care in the event that he loses consciousness from either insulin shock or diabetic coma.

### Complications

### Diabetic Coma

Diabetic coma is a serious complication of diabetes. The patient may develop diabetic coma after eating a large amount of food or after omitting his insulin. He may also develop diabetic coma when he has an infection since this condition exaggerates the severity of diabetes. The practical nurse may hear diabetic coma referred to as *diabetic acidosis*.

The patient with diabetic acidosis is unable to use the glucose in his body. This causes him to have an abnormally high blood sugar and an excessive amount of sugar in the urine. His inability to use carbohydrates properly results in a disturbance of his ability to use fats and proteins. This, in turn, causes an excess amount of fatty acids in the blood stream, which disturbs the acid-alkaline balance of the body. Thus, the condition is called diabetic acidosis. The body burns more fatty acids than usual, resulting in the formation of substances called *ketone bodies* (acetone). Because the kidneys try to remove these harmful substances, the presence of ketone bodies (acetone) in the urine is revealed by a laboratory test. Also, the patient's fluid balance is disturbed, resulting in dehydration.

Generally the patient becomes weak, thirsty, tired, and sleepy during the early stages of diabetic coma. He may develop a headache, anorexia, and abdominal discomfort, such as pain, nausea, and vomiting. He takes rapid and deep breaths. His lips appear red and his face flushed. His symptoms increase as the acidosis continues, and he may become unconscious. He appears dehydrated. His breath may have a sweet, fruity odor.

The patient in diabetic coma is considered to be a medical emergency. He should be placed in bed in a warm room and kept warm with the use of adequate covers. If the practical nurse is asked to apply a hot-water bottle or an electric heating pad, she should use extreme caution as this patient burns easily.

The physician prescribes fluids and insulin. The fluids may be given by either intravenous or subcutaneous injection. After he has regained consciousness, he may be given fluids orally. Either regular or crystalline insulin is frequently prescribed for this patient because of their rapid action. The doctor needs to know the patient's blood sugar and the amount of sugar in the urine before prescribing the dosage of insulin. The practical nurse may be asked to obtain a catheterized specimen of urine from the unconscious patient. The patient usually responds to the treatment of insulin, fluids, and rest. His return to the former dietary plan, exercise, and insulin is gradual.

## Insulin Shock

The patient in insulin shock has an abnormally low blood sugar. This condition is known as *hypoglycemia*. Hypoglycemia may develop if the patient takes an unusually large dose of insulin or misses a meal. It may also follow unusual exercise and the loss of partially digested food by vomiting and diarrhea.

Symptoms often experienced by the patient with hypoglycemia are hunger, weakness, tiredness, profuse perspiration, and nervousness. He feels cold and clammy and may have tremors. As his blood sugar becomes lower, he frequently develops symptoms of emotional and mental disturbances, such as anxiety, excessive laughing or crying, and dizziness. He may become disoriented, unconscious, and have convulsions.

As the patient has too much insulin and too little sugar, he is treated with some form of sugar. Many diabetics carry a few lumps of sugar or pieces of candy with them to take when symptoms of insulin shock first appear. The practical nurse may be asked to give the hospitalized patient a glass of sweetened orange juice if he is still conscious. A nasal tube may be passed through the nose into the stomach of an unconscious patient for the administration of glucose. Another method of treatment which the doctor may use for the unconscious patient is the intravenous administration of glucose.

## Arteriosclerosis

Frequently the person with diabetes develops arteriosclerosis, especially after reaching middle age. He is likely to develop arteriosclerosis at an earlier age than the person who does not have diabetes. The exact reason for this is not known. The presence of this disease of the arteries decreases the patient's ability to overcome infections, especially of the skin. Arteriosclerosis results in a decreased flow of blood through the diseased arteries. The diabetic person is already prone to develop infections of the skin, such as boils. Having an additional disease makes it doubly hard for him to overcome an infection. For these reasons he is likely to develop gangrene of an extremity if his feet and legs do not receive proper care. Knowing this should help the practical nurse to remember the importance of proper foot care, which was discussed earlier in this chapter.

The diabetic with arteriosclerosis may develop other complications of arteriosclerosis. These are hypertension, coronary heart disease, and cerebral vascular accident (stroke).

Other diseases which may occur as a result of diabetes are cataract, neuritis, and infection. The person with a cataract has an opacity (nontransparency) of the normally clear lens, which is behind the pupil. In other words, the clear lens becomes cloudy so that he cannot see through it. Of course, an individual who does not have diabetes may develop a cataract. Surgery for removing a cataract or for any other purpose can be undertaken in the well-managed diabetic patient. It requires close teamwork between the surgeon and the internist, who is a doctor specializing in internal medicine. The patient with *neuritis* has inflamed nerves, which cause numbness, pain along the course of the nerve, and tingling sensations. The patient may also lose the use of the muscles innervated by the affected nerves. It has been stated earlier that the diabetic is likely to develop both local and general infections. For this reason efforts to prevent these are especially important. He should avoid coming in contact with individuals who have an infectious disease, such as a cold. If he develops an infection he should notify his doctor. Usually the doctor recommends bed rest as well as other forms of treatment. Proper care of the patient's skin and feet, which was discussed earlier, is important in the prevention of infection.

*answer all for 5-4-66*

## SUGGESTIONS FOR STUDY

1. Discuss the difference between a simple goiter and a toxic goiter.
2. What parts of this country have an insufficient natural supply of iodine?
3. Review the symptoms of hyperthyroidism. How do these compare with the symptoms of hypothyroidism? Discuss the nursing care which is needed by a patient with each of these conditions.
4. Discuss the nursing care of a patient before and after a thyroidectomy. What symptoms are especially important to observe and to report?
5. What essential element of food supplies the body with a large portion of its fuel? This essential food element is reduced to what simple form before the tissues can use it? What hormone is necessary for the production of energy?

6. Define the terms: glycosuria, hyperglycemia, and hypoglycemia.

7. How does the doctor determine whether or not a patient has diabetes?

8. Discuss the predisposing causes of diabetes.

9. Is it always necessary for a person with diabetes to take insulin? Give the reason for your answer.

10. Discuss the responsibilities of the practical nurse in regard to diet therapy for the diabetic.

11. What effect does exercise have on the body's use of carbohydrates? Should you expect a diabetic to eat more food before taking strenuous exercise? Why?

12. What does U-80 on a bottle of insulin indicate? What type of insulin syringe would you use to measure insulin from this bottle?

13. Name two types of insulin which have a rapid action. When should a patient who received one of these at 7:00 A.M. be observed for symptoms of insulin shock?

14. When would you observe the patient who received protamine zinc insulin at 7:00 A.M. for symptoms of insulin shock?

15. Name three types of insulin which have an intermediate action. When should a patient who received one of these at 7:00 A.M. be observed for symptoms of insulin shock?

16. Discuss the care of a diabetic patient's skin and feet. Why is this care important?

17. Why should heat be applied with caution to a person with diabetes?

18. Review the symptoms of hypoglycemia. How is it treated?

19. Review the symptoms of diabetic coma. How is it treated?

20. What diseases may occur as a result of diabetes?

## REFERENCES FOR CHAPTER 18

Brooks, Stewart M.: *Basic Facts of Pharmacology.* W. B. Saunders Co., Philadelphia, 1957, pp. 199-217.

Brown, Amy F.: *Medical Nursing,* 3rd ed. W. B. Saunders Co., Philadelphia, 1957, pp. 541-609.

*Diabetes Mellitus,* 5th ed. Eli Lilly and Co., Indianapolis, 1955.

Goodman, Louis S., and Gilman, Alfred: *The Pharmacological Basis of Therapeutics,* 2nd ed. The Macmillan Company, New York, 1955, pp. 1620-36.

Gould, Gertrude, and Golden, Jean: "Teaching the Diabetic at Home," *Am. J. Nursing,* **57:**1170-71, (Sept.) 1957.

Jensen, Julius, and Jensen, Deborah: *Nursing in Clinical Medicine,* 4th ed. The Macmillan Company, New York, 1954, pp. 144-77 and 542-53.

Krause, Marie: *Nutrition and Diet Therapy*, 2nd ed. W. B. Saunders Co., Philadelphia, 1957, pp. 248-69.

Martin, Marguerite M.: "The Diabetic at Home," *Am. J. Nursing*, **56**: 1294-98, (Oct.) 1956.

Musser, Ruth D., and Bird, Joseph G.: *Modern Pharmacology and Therapeutics*. The Macmillan Company, New York, 1958, pp. 651-76.

Peyton, Alice B.: *Practical Nutrition*. J. B. Lippincott Co., Philadelphia, 1957, pp. 192-201.

Proudfit, Fairfax T., and Robinson, Corinne H.: *Nutrition and Diet Therapy*, 11th ed. The Macmillan Company, New York, 1955, pp. 310-46 and 424-49.

Soehren, Irene: "Diabetes," *Today's Health*, **33**:24-29, (Nov.) 1955.

Solomon, Charles, and Gill, Elizabeth S.: *Pharmacology and Therapeutics*, 7th ed. J. B. Lippincott Co., Philadelphia, 1956, pp. 489-99.

Turner, C. E.: *Personal and Community Health*, 10th ed. C. V. Mosby Co., St. Louis, 1956, pp. 177-90.

*Nursing the Patient*
*with a Disease of*
*the Genitourinary System*

*Test 5/25/66*

*Thru - P. 384*

PART VIII

Kidney
Uterus
Bladder
urethra

*5-6-66*

# Chapter 19

# THE PATIENT
# WITH A DISEASE OF
# THE URINARY SYSTEM

*removes*

## STRUCTURE AND FUNCTION

Blood removes waste products from our body cells in addition to carrying food and oxygen to them. These waste products are carried to appropriate places for disposal. The respiratory system, the intestinal tract, the skin, and the urinary system remove waste material from the body. The urinary system removes most of the waste products which can be dissolved in water. This system also helps to control the fluid balance in our body. *acid base balance*

Diseases of the urinary system and the circulatory system are closely related. Conditions which interfere with the normal flow of blood through the body can result in disturbances of the urinary system. As stated in Chapter 9, heart failure causes the patient to have a smaller output of urine. Diseases such as arteriosclerosis of the blood vessels in the kidney can cause damage to these organs of excretion. Likewise, kidney disease can cause the patient to develop high blood pressure. This is a common complication of kidney damage.

The normal urinary system is composed of two kidneys, two ureters, a bladder, and a urethra. The kidneys form urine from waste materials which are taken from the blood. Urine is carried to the bladder by the ureters. The urethra carries urine from the bladder to the outside of the body.

### Kidneys

The practical nurse needs an understanding of the structure and function of the kidneys as a basis for understanding diseases of these two organs. The kidneys which are shaped like beans are located in the back below the chest. There is one on each side of the spine. The front portion of each kidney is separated from the abdomen by the peritoneum. The posterior portion is protected by the wall of the back. The kidneys are continuously purifying all of the blood

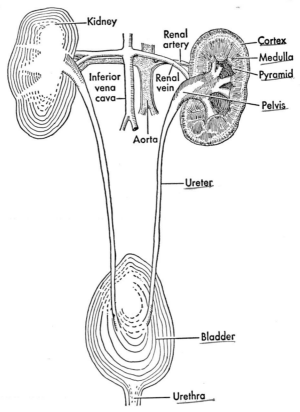

**Figure 36.** Dorsal view of kidneys, ureters, and bladder. (Stackpole, Caroline E., and Leavell, Lutie S.; *Textbook of Physiology*. The Macmillan Company, New York, 1953.)

in the body. Approximately 1 liter (1 qt) of blood goes through the kidneys every minute. The water and the waste products taken from the blood in the kidneys are known as *urine*.

Each kidney has a *pelvis*, which is a cavity shaped similar to a funnel. This cavity becomes smaller as it reaches the edge of the kidney. The narrow portion of the pelvis forms the ureter. The larger part of the pelvis is surrounded by tissue known as the *medullary substance* or *medulla*. This substance has cone-shaped projections called *pyramids* which project into cuplike divisions of the pelvis of the kidney known as *calyces*. The outer portion of the kidney is known as the *cortical substance* or *cortex*.

The cortex and the medulla contain many tiny units which serve as filters. Each of these units is made of cells which are arranged as *tubes* or *tubules*. The upper end of each tubule is shaped like a hollow ball. The top part of the hollow ball is pushed in by a knot of tiny blood vessels which is called a *glomerulus*. It is here that most of the waste products are taken from the blood. However, the glomeruli normally remove products which the body can use again. As the fluid flows from the glomerulus through the tubule, much of it is reabsorbed into the blood. For example, much of the water is returned to the blood stream. Additional waste products are added to the urine as it flows through the small tubule. The tiny tubules pour their contents into larger collecting tubes which in turn empty into the pelvis of the kidney.

## Ureters

A long, small tube called a *ureter* leads from the pelvis of each kidney. These two tubes are muscular and are lined with mucous membrane. Urine is carried down the ureters by peristalsis to the bladder.

## Bladder

The *bladder* is a hollow organ located in the pelvic cavity. This muscular sac is lined with mucous membrane like that which lines the ureters. The bladder serves as a reservoir for urine. After the bladder has collected a sufficient amount of urine, it contracts and forces the urine out of the body through the urethra.

## Urethra

The urethra is a small tube lined with mucous membrane which leads outward from the bladder. This tube is short in females and longer in males as it passes through the penis. The urethra has a sphincter muscle around it which prevents urine from flowing out of the bladder continuously. This sphincter muscle relaxes when the bladder contracts, and voiding takes place. The opening of the urethra is called the *meatus urethrae*.

## Urine

Urine is made of excess water, waste products which result from activities of the body's cells, and excess salts. The amount of solid waste products in the urine in relation to the amount of water determines the *specific gravity.* This is the comparison between the weight of urine and the weight of an equal amount of water. Normally the specific gravity of urine may range from 1.010 to 1.030. Thus, urine is heavier than water because of the solid waste products contained in the urine. The specific gravity of urine is normally regulated by the kidneys. An unusually high specific gravity or an unusually low one can indicate disease.

Normally the average amount of urine voided by an adult in 24 hours may range from approximately 1200 to 1500 ml (40 to 50 oz). Various factors, such as a change in the amount of perspiration, a change in the fluid intake, and a change in the environmental temperature can effect the daily output of urine. A variation in the urinary output can also be caused by disease. For example, diarrhea, vomiting, and hemorrhage, as well as a disease of the kidneys, heart, and blood vessels, may cause variations. The patient has *polyuria* when he passes large amounts of urine. Voiding small amounts is known as *oliguria*. If the patient's kidneys fail to excrete urine, he has *anuria.* This is known also as *suppression of urine.*

Urine generally has a slightly acid reaction and is clear yellow in appearance. The proportion of water and waste products in solution affects the color. For example, if the patient drinks an inadequate amount of fluids his urine is likely to be concentrated and deep yellow in color. When the patient drinks a large amount of fluid his urine is likely to be less concentrated and light in color.

Common abnormal substances in the urine which usually indicate disease of the urinary system are (albumin, pus, casts, and blood.) Albumin in the urine may indicate a disease of the tiny blood vessels in the glomeruli. Disease in this part of the kidney allows albumin to seep from the blood into the urine. The patient with albumin in his urine has *albuminuria*. Pus in the urine which is known as *pyuria* indicates an infection of the urinary tract. Casts indicate a disease of the tubules. Casts are formed when albumin or some other substance hardens in the tubules. The casts are then washed out of the tubules by the flow of urine. The presence of blood in the urine is known as *hematuria*, This may occur in the patient because of an injury, an inflammation, or a tumor of the urinary tract. An example of injury is seen in the patient with a kidney stone which has irritated the tissues. Injury may also result from the forceful insertion of a catheter. One example of an inflammation causing blood to appear in the urine is seen in the patient with nephritis. The inflammatory process causes the tiny blood vessels in the kidneys to bleed. A growing tumor can break down and bleed. Additional causes of hematuria are the ingestion of poisons such as carbolic acid and certain drugs such as the sulfonamides.

## ASSISTING WITH EXAMINATION

The nursing team frequently is responsible for assisting the physician with special types of procedures used in diagnosing diseases of the urinary system. As an important member of the nursing team, the practical nurse needs a basic understanding of these special methods of examination.

### Urinalysis

One of the most common methods used by the doctor to aid in determining whether or not the patient has a urinary disease is the *urinalysis*. This is an examination of the urine. A report of the urinalysis is helpful to the doctor in planning his treatment. The practical nurse is often asked to obtain a urine specimen. When getting a voided specimen from the female patient, the practical nurse needs to remember that the patient's vulva should be clean and that the specimen is collected in a clean container. However, the doctor may request a catheterized specimen from the female patient.

### Urine Culture

Another type of examination which the doctor may request is *urine culture*. This is a laboratory procedure used to determine which microorganisms are causing an infection of the urinary system. A small part of the urine specimen is placed on a substance, such as bouillon, agar, gelatin, or blood serum. This is kept warm so that bacteria will grow. The types of bacteria growing in the urine are reported to the doctor. Using this information, he can plan a more specific course of treatment. Remembering that bacteria present in urine can be grown in the laboratory, the practical nurse realizes the importance of obtaining an absolutely clean specimen. The female patient should be catheterized to obtain a specimen for culture. This is necessary to prevent the urine from picking up additional bacteria as it flows over the perineum. A specimen for culture may be collected from the male patient by having him void into a sterile bottle after the penis has been washed thoroughly.

### Sensitivity Test

Another laboratory procedure which the physician may request to aid him in treating the patient is the *sensitivity test*. This procedure is done in connection with the urine culture to determine which antibiotics will kill the bacteria. The laboratory technician places tiny pieces of paper which contain different antibiotics on the culture. Bacteria sensitive to a particular drug do not grow around the piece of paper containing that drug. The doctor uses this information in determining which drug to use in combating the infection.

### Cystoscopic Examination

The cystoscopic examination is a special procedure performed by the doctor. This may be done by a *urologist* who is a specialist in diagnosing and treating diseases of the urinary system in the female and of the genitourinary tract in the male. In this procedure he inserts an instrument called a *cystoscope* into the urinary bladder. The doctor looks through the cystoscope to examine the walls of the bladder and the urethra. He can also take urine specimens from the ureters which lead from each kidney. The physician can perform certain treatments of the bladder through the cystoscope. For example, he can remove small stones, obtain a specimen from a tumor, and remove small growths.

### Pyelogram

The patient scheduled for a *pyelogram* has x-rays made of his kidneys. The use of a special dye which is visible by x-ray examination is necessary. The patient may have either an intravenous pyelogram or a retrograde pyelogram. When doing an *intravenous pyelogram,* the doctor injects the special dye into the patient's veins. The kidneys remove the dye from the blood causing them to be visible by x-ray. Both kidneys are x-rayed soon after the dye is given. This type of examination helps the doctor to determine whether or not both kidneys are picking up the dye normally. A diseased kidney might remove little or no dye from the blood stream. When doing a *retrograde pyelogram,* the physician inserts a cystoscope into the bladder. He then passes small catheters through this instrument up each ureter into the kidneys. He injects a special dye through the catheters into the pelvis of each kidney. This dye causes the outline of the kidney to be visible by x-ray. The practical nurse should be familiar with the procedure used in the particular hopsital in which she is working for preparing the patient for a pyelogram.

### Kidney Function Tests

There are various types of tests designed to determine whether or not the kidneys are removing the proper amount of waste materials from the blood in the proper length of time. These tests are known as *kidney function tests.* The concentration test and the phenol-sulfonphthalein test are two examples of kidney function tests included in this discussion. The concentration test is done to determine whether or not the kidneys are concentrating the urine properly. One of the first functions to be lost by a diseased kidney is its ability to concentrate urine. Thus, the patient with kidney damage would be unable to concentrate urine normally. There are various types of concentration tests and different procedures for each. However, in general, there is a restriction of food and fluids for a certain length of time before the specimens of urine are collected. When caring for a patient who is having a concentration test, the practical nurse should seek specific instructions from the team leader, or head nurse, as to whether or not the patient may have fluids and food. Furthermore, she should know when the urine specimens are to be collected.

The second example of a kidney function test which the doctor may order is the *phenolsulfonphthalein test*, or P.S.P. test. A harmless red dye is injected intramuscularly or intravenously. This dye is removed mainly by the kidneys and colors the urine. The practical nurse may be asked to collect urine specimens at specific times during this test. She should collect these specimens promptly. If the patient is unable to void at a designated time, this should be reported to the head nurse. The amount of dye in the urine specimens is then estimated in the laboratory.

## ACUTE NEPHRITIS

### Description

The patient with acute nephritis has an inflammation of his kidneys which can result in serious damage to them. The practical nurse may hear this condition referred to as *acute glomerulonephritis* since the glomeruli are affected. It may also be called *acute hemorrhagic nephritis* because this patient usually has blood in his urine.

The exact cause of acute nephritis is not known at the present time. It is more common in children, especially boys. Acute nephritis frequently follows an acute infection of the respiratory system by streptococci. For example, a child may develop acute nephritis a week or two after having tonsillitis or sinusitis caused by streptococci. He may also develop this condition after having scarlet fever. However, acute nephritis may occur in a person who has no history of a recent streptococcal infection. It is believed that acute nephritis is an allergic reaction of the kidneys to the microorganism which caused an earlier infection elsewhere in the body.

Most patients recover from acute nephritis. The length of illness may vary from a few days to a few months. However, all patients may not be so fortunate. An individual may later develop chronic nephritis which is discussed on pages 314 to 315 in this chapter.

### Symptoms

Since the patient with acute nephritis has an inflammation of his kidneys, he can be expected to have urinary changes. The amount of urine generally is decreased. Thus, his blood would contain more waste products. The urine contains blood, albumin, and casts. The patient usually has edema or puffiness around his eyes, especially in the morning. Edema of his feet and ankles may develop later in the day; this is especially true if he has been in an upright position most of the day. The patient's blood pressure may become elevated. In general, this is considered an unfavorable development.

The patient with a severe case of acute nephritis may develop edema of the brain. This can result in visual disturbances, such as spots before the eyes, or even blindness, severe headache, convulsions, and coma. This patient would have a marked decrease in output of urine and an extremely high blood pressure. If his blood pressure remained high over a period of time, he could develop an enlargement of the heart. Also, he may have heart failure. The patient may develop edema of his lungs which is known as *pulmonary edema*. This would make him more likely to develop pneumonia.

### Treatment and Nursing Care

The physician generally prescribes bed rest for the patient with acute nephritis. It is the responsibility of the nursing team to help the patient obtain the greatest amount of rest possible.

Remembering that this patient is liable to develop respiratory infections, such as the common cold and pneumonia, the practical nurse readily understands the importance of keeping the patient comfortably warm. He should not be in a draft and should not become chilled. Those who have respiratory infections, such as the common cold, should not come in contact with this patient.

The doctor may prescribe penicillin. This is ordered because of the relationship of streptococcal infections and acute nephritis.

The patient needs a daily cleansing bath. He should not become chilled during the procedure. Members of the nursing team should give special attention to edematous areas to prevent decubitus ulcers. The care of a patient with edema is discussed in more detail on page 35.

The physician frequently orders a special diet for this patient. In general, the diet is low in salt. Varying amounts of protein may be ordered also.

The patient's intake and output of fluids should be measured and recorded. This information is of value to the doctor in planning treatment for the individual patient. He may request the nurse to keep a record of the patient's weight. The doctor may also indicate the amount of fluids which the patient is to receive daily. The practical nurse should be familiar with the tests commonly used in the hospital to determine functioning of the patient's kidneys. She should also know her responsibility in that particular institution regarding these tests.

## CHRONIC NEPHRITIS

### Description

A fairly small percentage of patients develop chronic nephritis as a result of acute nephritis. However, most individuals with chronic nephritis have not had acute nephritis. Their condition developed slowly for some unknown reason. Both groups have kidney damage.

The prognosis for a patient with chronic nephritis is poor. The progress of this disease varies. The patient may have long periods during which he is relatively free of symptoms.

### Symptoms

The patient with chronic nephritis may have a variety of symptoms. In general, he does not feel well and has headaches and edema during the early part of his illness. When examining the patient, the doctor usually finds that he has hypertension and albumin in the urine.

As the patient's condition progresses he has blood in his urine, a steady increase in blood pressure, and anemia. His kidneys eventually become unable to perform their functions. The patient may die of heart failure caused by hypertension, a secondary infection like pneumonia, or kidney failure (uremia).

### Treatment and Nursing Care

At the present time, physicians have been unable to determine an entirely satisfactory method of treating the patient with chronic nephritis. For this reason the treatment is directed mainly toward relieving the patient's symptoms. The patient is advised to avoid excesses in his daily activities, such as strenuous exercise, overwork, exposure, and overeating. In other words, while he is relatively free of symptoms, he should avoid activities which would increase the amount of waste products that the kidneys would have to remove. The patient may also be advised to limit or to eliminate tea, coffee, and alcohol.

During the acute phase of his illness, he needs the same kind of care which was discussed in the care of a patient with acute nephritis. The doctor adjusts the patient's diet to his symptoms. A low-salt diet is usually ordered for the patient with edema. The prescribed diet may be high in proteins to make up for proteins which are lost in the urine. However, the doctor may restrict the amount of protein if he finds that the patient is not excreting waste products formed from the metabolism of proteins. Highly seasoned foods should be avoided as these might irritate the kidney tissue.

## NEPHROSIS

### Description

The patient with nephrosis has a degeneration of the tubules of his kidneys. The exact cause of this condition is not known. Nephrosis usually occurs in children but it may affect young adults.

Edema is the main symptom of nephrosis. The patient may have albumin and casts in his urine. He may develop a fatal complication, such as kidney failure, heart failure, or an infection elsewhere in the body. Peritonitis and pneumonia are examples of complicating infections. It is encouraging to note that over half of the children affected by nephrosis do recover.

### Treatment

The physician generally directs his treatment toward relieving the patient's main symptom which is edema. He also attempts to prevent the complications which are likely to occur. Diuretics, drugs which increase the output of urine, may be prescribed in connection with a low-salt diet. Some physicians prescribe either adrenocorticotropic hormone (ACTH) or cortisone to aid in relieving edema.

The principles, discussed earlier in this chapter, of nursing care for a patient with acute and chronic nephritis apply likewise to the patient with nephrosis.

## UREMIA

### Description

The patient with uremia has kidney failure. His kidneys are unable
to remove waste products from the blood. This causes him to have
an increased amount of these waste products in his blood.

### Cause

An individual may develop uremia as a result of kidney disease
which damages the kidney tissue. For example, either acute or chronic
nephritis may produce this condition. Absorption of poisonous substances, such as mercury, can damage kidney tissue to such an extent
that the patient develops uremia. An obstruction in the urinary tract
which prevents urine from leaving the kidneys may cause this disorder. Also, conditions which interfere with the normal flow of
blood through the kidneys, such as shock, dehydration, and hemorrhage, can result in uremia.

### Symptoms

When a patient is developing uremia, he usually feels weak, loses
his appetite, and has a headache. Nausea and vomiting frequently
occur. These can result in loss of weight and dehydration. As the
patient's condition continues, he may complain of itching and is
likely to become anemic. He may develop an infection such as pneumonia, inflammation of the mouth, or pericarditis. As his condition
progresses, he is likely to have a foul breath, visual disturbances, and
muscle twitching; later the patient becomes confused and develops
Cheyne-Stokes breathing. He finally loses consciousness and may have
convulsions. *Uremic frost,* which is a white, powdery substance, may
appear on his skin. It may be helpful for the practical nurse to
recall the white streaks she has seen on a sweating horse in trying to
imagine how uremic frost looks.

### Treatment

If possible, the physician attempts to relieve the cause of this
patient's condition. When he is unable to do this, he prescribes
measures to relieve his discomfort. For instance, he might relieve

dehydration by ordering fluids to be given intravenously or sub-cutaneously, or at times by gavage.

## KIDNEY INFECTION

### Description

An individual may develop an infection in either one or both kidneys. The patient with an inflammation in the pelvis of either one or both kidneys has *pyelitis.* A person with an inflammation which involves the entire substance of either one or both kidneys has *pyelonephritis.* Remembering that the outer part of the kidney actually removes waste materials from the blood should help the practical nurse to understand that pyelonephritis can result in destruction of kidney tissue. This could eventually lead to hypertension.

### Cause

Kidney infection is caused by various pathogens. These microorganisms may reach the kidneys by way of the blood stream, or they may travel up the ureters to the kidneys. Pathogens which are carried to the kidneys by the blood usually come from some distant area of infection. For example, the patient with infected tonsils, teeth, or sinuses may develop a kidney infection. Microorganisms are more likely to spread upward to the kidney when a person has urinary stasis. In other words, the flow of urine through the urinary tract is slower than normal. For instance, a disease of the ureters, the bladder, or the urethra, such as an infection, a stone, or a tumor, may lead to kidney infection. A kidney which was formed abnormally in utero, a tumor pressing against a ureter, or the pressure of a growing fetus can cause urinary stasis which could result in kidney infection.

### Symptoms

The patient with a kidney infection generally has such symptoms as malaise, headache, chills, and fever. He may have pain and tenderness in the region of the infected kidney. Frequent and painful voiding may occur. An examination of his urine shows a combination of abnormal substances, such as pus, albumin, bacteria, and red blood cells.

### Treatment and Nursing Care

The doctor usually tries to determine which microorganism is causing the infection before prescribing a drug. The practical nurse may be asked to obtain a urine specimen for this purpose. The doctor frequently requests the laboratory to do a culture of the urine specimen. After the doctor knows the results of the laboratory examinations, he can select a drug which he knows is likely to kill the bacteria. For example, one patient with a kidney infection may be treated with penicillin, another with streptomycin, and another with one of the sulfonamides.

The patient with an acute infection needs rest in bed. Nursing measures important in the care of a patient with an infection, discussed in Chapter 6, are applicable to this patient unless the doctor orders otherwise. Usually forcing fluids is especially important in the care of this patient. *High protein*

## BLADDER INFECTION

### Description

The patient with an infection of the urinary bladder has cystitis. The microorganisms may enter the bladder by way of the urethra, or they may be brought down from the kidneys or ureters in the urine. An individual with a kidney infection is likely to develop cystitis.

### Symptoms

The patient with cystitis complains of frequent voiding which he describes as being painful and burning. He may also have a feeling of urgency to void. His urine generally contains pus and it may contain red blood cells. Usually the urine has a cloudy appearance. The patient may have an acute case of cystitis or he may have a chronic one. In an acute case, he may also have general symptoms of an inflammation such as fever and malaise.

### Treatment and Nursing Care

The doctor tries to remove the underlying cause of the cystitis. For example, the patient with this condition resulting from a kidney infection is treated for kidney disease. His cystitis usually clears up when the kidney infection is cured.

Nursing measures generally needed by a patient with an infection, such as rest, an adequate intake of fluids, and a nourishing diet, are needed by this patient. Bladder irrigation with urinary antiseptics may be prescribed; potassium permanganate and silver nitrate are two examples of urinary antiseptics. Instillation of an antiseptic, such as silver nitrate or mebromin (Mercurochrome) may be ordered also.

## NEPHROLITHIASIS

### Description

The patient with nephrolithiasis has kidney stones (renal calculi). One or more stones may be present in either one or both kidneys. The calculi (stones) may range from the size of a pinhead to one large enough to fill the entire pelvis of the kidney.

Stones are made of crystals of salts and organic material. Why a person develops kidney stones is not clearly understood. However, an individual who has a kidney infection, a slowing down in the flow of urine from his kidneys, or who excretes highly concentrated urine is likely to develop renal calculi. In addition, a person with an excessive amount of calcium in his body is likely to develop kidney stones.

### Symptoms

The patient may have no symptoms until the stone prevents urine from flowing normally or until it moves and causes local irritation. Sometimes the patient develops an infection as a result of the stone. The patient may also complain of a dull ache in the kidney region.

The patient frequently has an attack of *kidney colic or renal colic* when the stone becomes lodged in the ureter. Movement of the stone irritates the tissues around it. The patient suffers with excruciating pain in his back which goes to the lower part of his abdomen and into his genitalia. This severe pain may continue to the inner part of his thigh. The acute pain can cause the patient to perspire profusely, develop nausea and vomiting, or go into a mild state of shock. Blood is usually present in the urine because of local injury by the stone. In some cases the patient passes small stones. If the patient develops an infection, there is pus in his urine. Chills and fever may be present.

### Treatment and Nursing Care

The treatment of a patient with an attack of kidney colic is directed toward making him comfortable. Measures to relieve pain, such as heat to the area and analgesic drugs, are prescribed. Morphine is an example of an analgesic drug which is ordered commonly.

The doctor often asks the nursing team to force fluids on this patient. He may also leave an order for all of the urine to be strained through several layers of gauze. This is done to determine whether or not the patient has passed a stone.

The doctor may have the patient x-rayed to aid in determining the location and size of the stone. Some stones can be visualized by plain x-ray of the area and some cannot. The doctor usually has a pyelogram done, if the stones are not visible by the previous method.

The surgeon may decide that it is necessary to remove the stone from the kidney, the ureter, or the bladder. Removal of the stone through an incision into the kidney is known as a *nephrolithotomy*. The surgeon does a *ureterolithotomy* when he removes the stone through an incision into the ureter. Sometimes the physician can crush the stone in the bladder by inserting a special instrument through a cystoscope into the bladder. After crushing the stone, he washes its fragments out of the bladder.

With few exceptions, the patient having surgery of the urinary tract needs the same type of care which was discussed in Chapter 5. The nurse in attendance should observe the patient carefully for early symptoms of shock and hemorrhage after surgery. Remembering the large amount of blood which flows through the kidney and the close relationship between the circulatory and urinary systems should help the practical nurse to realize the importance of watching for early signs of these complications. The patient's dressing is checked frequently for bleeding and other drainage, and their presence reported at once to the team leader or head nurse.

## HYDRONEPHROSIS

### Description

An individual with hydronephrosis has a kidney which is distended with urine because of blockage. In other words, the urine does not flow normally from the kidney because of an obstruction elsewhere in the urinary tract. The urine usually fills the pelvis of the kidney slowly. This can cause the kidney tissue to be destroyed. The kidney eventually may become a fibrous sac filled with fluid. The normal flow of urine from the kidney through the ureter may be obstructed or blocked by a stone, a tumor, or a stricture of the ureter.

### Symptoms

The patient may have pain resulting from distention of the kidney. In some cases, the physician can feel the outline of the distended kidney. However, the patient may have no symptoms until he develops an infection. If he has hydronephrosis of both kidneys, he may develop uremia.

### Treatment

The physician attempts to remove the cause of the hydronephrosis. For example, he removes a stone which blocked the ureter. The surgeon usually removes the kidney, when he finds that the kidney has been damaged severely. This operation is known as a *nephrectomy*. In some cases he makes an incision into the kidney to allow it to drain. This is called a *nephrotomy*.

## TUMOR OF THE KIDNEY

### Description

Although tumors of the kidney are not common, they are frequently malignant. Men are more likely to develop cancer of the kidneys than women. A malignancy which affects the kidneys of young children is called Wilms' tumor.

### Symptoms

An individual with cancer of the kidney usually has blood in his urine. Frequently the tumor can be felt. The patient may complain of a dull, aching pain in the area. He loses weight as the condition progresses.

### Treatment

If possible, the physician removes the tumor. X-ray therapy is sometimes used.

## TUMOR OF THE BLADDER

### Description

An individual may have either a benign or a malignant tumor of of the bladder. The benign tumor may develop into a malignant one. Tumor of the bladder is more common in men than in women.

### Symptoms

One of the earliest symptoms experienced by the person with a tumor of the bladder is hematuria. The patient usually notices blood in his urine. The bleeding may come and go over a period of time. He may complain of frequent, painful voiding. The patient may develop kidney complications, if the tumor obstructs the opening of the ureter. Hydronephrosis and infection are examples of these complications. Symptoms of cystitis, such as frequent, painful voiding, occur also if the patient develops a bladder infection.

### Treatment

The surgeon removes the tumor if possible. He may do this by fulguration through the cystoscope. When doing a *fulguration*, he destroys the tissue by the use of electric sparks. The doctor may do a *cystotomy*, which is making an opening into the bladder, to remove the tumor. In some cases, the surgeon removes the bladder. This is called a *cystectomy*. He then places the ends of the ureters in the colon, or he brings them out through the skin. Radium and x-ray therapy may be used in treating the patient with a malignant tumor of the bladder.

## SUGGESTIONS FOR STUDY

1. Why should the female patient be catheterized when a specimen for urine culture is ordered?

2. What is the purpose of the following: urinalysis, urine culture, sensitivity test, cystoscopic examination, pyelogram, and kidney function tests?

3. What age group is most likely to be affected by acute nephritis?

4. Review the treatment and nursing care of a patient with acute nephritis.

5. What causes a person to develop chronic nephritis?

6. What causes a person to have kidney colic?

7. Describe the pain of a patient having kidney colic. What is usually done to relieve this pain?

8. Why would the practical nurse be asked to strain the urine of a patient with nephrolithiasis?

9. Why should the nurse caring for a patient who has recently had surgery of the urinary tract observe him closely for symptoms of shock and hemorrhage?

10. Define the following: hydronephrosis, nephrolithotomy, ureterolithotomy, nephrectomy, nephrotomy, fulguration, and cystotomy.

## REFERENCES FOR CHAPTER 19

American Cancer Society, Inc.: *A Cancer Source Book for Nurses.* The Society, New York, 1956, pp. 90-92.

Brown, Amy F.: *Medical Nursing,* 3rd ed. W. B. Saunders Co., Philadelphia, 1957, pp. 325-40.

Dakin, Florence; Thompson, Ella M.; and Le Baron, Margaret: *Simplified Nursing,* 6th ed. J. B. Lippincott Co., Philadelphia, 1956, pp. 136-38 and 370-78.

Eliason, Eldridge; Ferguson, L. Kraeer; and Sholtis, Lillian A.: *Surgical Nursing,* 10th ed. J. B. Lippincott Co., Philadelphia, 1955, pp. 363-80.

Emerson, Charles P., Jr., and Bragdon, Jane S.: *Essentials of Medicine,* 17th ed. J. B. Lippincott Co., Philadelphia, 1955, pp. 397-438.

Faddis, Margene O., and Hayman, Joseph M.: *Care of the Medical Patient.* McGraw-Hill Book Co., New York, 1952, pp. 391-412.

Gill, Helen Z. (ed.): *Basic Nursing,* 4th ed. The Macmillan Company, New York, 1955, pp. 94-97 and 552-58.

Hand, John R.: "Infections of the Urinary Tract," *Am. J. Nursing,* 57:1008-10, (Aug.) 1957.

Hull, Edgar, and Perrodin, Cecilia: *Medical Nursing,* 5th ed. F. A. Davis Co., Philadelphia, 1954, pp. 368-92.

Kaplan, Sol A., and Callison, Cornelia: "Nephrosis in Children," *Am. J. Nursing,* 56:300-303, (Mar.) 1956.

Kimber, Diana; Gray, Carolyn E.; Stackpole, Caroline E.; and Leavell, Lutie C.: *Textbook of Anatomy and Physiology,* 13th ed. The Macmillan Company, New York, 1955, pp. 646-69.

Jensen, Julius, and Jensen, Deborah: *Nursing in Clinical Medicine,* 4th ed. The Macmillan Company, New York, 1954, pp. 476-511.

Proudfit, Fairfax T., and Robinson, Corinne H.: *Nutrition and Diet Therapy,* 11th ed. The Macmillan Company, New York, 1955, pp. 478-90.

Turner, C. E.: *Personal and Community Health,* 10th ed. C. V. Mosby Co., St. Louis, 1956, pp. 150-58.

West, John P.; Keller, Manelva W.; and Harmon, Elizabeth H.: *Nursing Care of the Surgical Patient,* 6th ed. The Macmillan Company, New York, 1957, pp. 332-60.

*Chapter 20* THE PATIENT
WITH A DISEASE OF
THE REPRODUCTIVE SYSTEM

## THE MALE PATIENT

### Structure and Function

The male reproductive system consists of the scrotum and its contents, two seminal vesicles, the ducts through which the spermatozoa pass from the scrotum to the exterior, the prostate gland, and two bulbourethral glands. (Cowper's)

The *scrotum*, which is a pouch, normally contains two glands known as the *testes.* The glands produce the male sex hormones and spermatozoa (male germ cells). Each of the testes is made of two parts. The egg-shaped portion of the testes is called the *testis*, and the narrow part made of a long winding tubule is known as the *epididymis.* Spermatozoa formed in the testis are carried to the epididymis. These male germ cells leave the testes by way of a tube known as the *seminal duct.* The two seminal ducts, one from each of the testes, lead from the epididymis in the scrotum to the abdominal cav-

ity. There each joins another duct from the seminal vesicle to form an
*ejaculatory duct*. The two *seminal vesicles* are small sacs which store
the spermatozoa and add a fluid to them. The two ejaculatory ducts
pass through the prostate gland to the urethra.

The *prostate gland* is an organ made of muscular and glandular
tissue. This gland surrounds the lower end of the bladder and the
beginning of the urethra. The prostate gland secretes a fluid which is
added to the semen during ejaculation in sexual intercourse. Semen
is the fluid containing spermatozoa. This fluid is made of substances
produced by the two testes, the two seminal vesicles, the prostate
gland, and the two bulbourethral glands. The two small glands
located below the prostate gland are known as *bulbourethral glands*.
They produce a substance which is added to the semen through a
small duct opening into the urethra.

The *penis* is the male organ of copulation or sexual union. The
external opening of the urethra is located at the end of the penis
which has a slight enlargement known as the *glans penis*. The urethra
serves as a passageway for urine to leave the body during the act of
urination. It also serves as a passageway for seminal fluid which contains the male germ cells.

### Benign Prostatic Hypertrophy

#### Description

The patient with benign prostatic hypertrophy has an enlarged
prostate gland. This enlargement frequently is associated with benign
tumors which develop within the gland. The exact cause of the benign
prostatic hypertrophy is not known, but it is believed to be caused by
an endocrine disorder. This condition is more common in older men.

#### Symptoms

The patient with an enlarged prostate gland has difficulty in emptying his bladder because the enlarged gland presses on the urethra. His
symptoms may range from frequent, difficult voiding to an inability
to void. If the patient is unable to empty his bladder completely,
he has some urine left in his bladder, which is called *residual urine*.
This collection of urine may cause the patient to develop an infection of the bladder (cystitis). When there is a large amount of

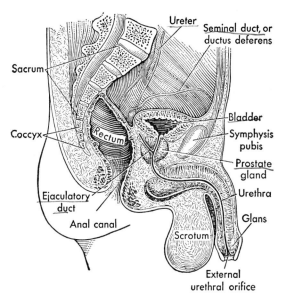

**Figure 37.** Median section of the male pelvis. (After Gray's *Anatomy*.) (Kimber, Diana C.; Gray, Carolyn E.; Stackpole, Caroline E.; and Leavell, Lutie C.: *Textbook of Anatomy and Physiology*, 13th ed. The Macmillan Company, New York, 1955.)

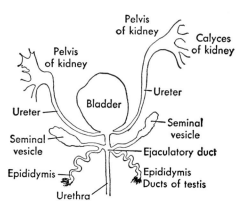

**Figure 38.** Diagram showing continuity of mucous membrane in the male genitourinary pathway. (Kimber, Diana C.; Gray, Carolyn E.; Stackpole, Caroline E.; and Leavell, Lutie C.: *Textbook of Anatomy and Physiology*, 13th ed. The Macmillan Company, New York, 1955.)

327

residual urine, it can cause pressure on the ureters and the kidneys. In extreme cases this back pressure upon the kidneys and ureters can result in damage to the kidneys. As the patient's condition continues, he may lose weight, develop digestive disturbances, and become depressed.

### Treatment and Nursing Care

The surgeon generally does a *prostatectomy*, which is removal of part or all of the prostate gland. The four main methods of doing a prostatectomy are suprapubic, transurethral, perineal, and retropubic. When doing a *suprapubic prostatectomy*, the urologist removes the prostate gland through an incision made into the bladder above the pubic region. In doing a *transurethral* prostatectomy, he inserts a special cystoscope into the urethra and removes the gland through this instrument. In a *perineal prostatectomy*, he removes the prostate gland through an incision made into the perineum. When doing a *retropubic prostatectomy*, the surgeon removes the prostate gland through an opening made into the lower part of the abdomen. He reaches the gland by going behind the bladder instead of through it.

### Preoperative Care

The preoperative nursing care which was discussed in Chapter 5 is applicable to this patient. However, he usually needs additional care because of his advanced age. In general, he is hospitalized for a longer period of time before surgery. Spending this time in the hospital helps him to become familiar with his new surroundings and with those who care for him. The physician may prescribe special measures, such as a nourishing diet, an increased intake of fluids, and rest in order to help the patient to attain the best possible physical condition before surgery. Suitable drugs may be ordered to combat infection.

The patient's output of urine should be measured and recorded. The doctor may order an indwelling catheter, such as the Foley catheter, for continous drainage of the bladder. This is used generally when the patient is unable to void or when he has residual urine. Caring for the patient with an indwelling catheter is discussed on page 43.

*Postoperative Care*

In addition to the nursing care of a postoperative patient which was discussed in Chapter 5, this patient needs special care from the nursing team. He should be observed frequently for symptoms of shock and hemorrhage. These should be reported promptly to the head nurse or the team leader.

The patient generally is returned to his bed with an indwelling catheter in place. The nurse should connect the catheter to the recommended drainage equipment. This equipment should be sterile in case there is a backflow of urine into the bladder.

Frequent bladder irrigations may be prescribed. The doctor may ask the nurse to carry out this procedure as often as every 10 to 15 minutes. Irrigation of the bladder helps to prevent small blood clots from plugging the catheter or the drainage tube. The procedure varies in different hospitals and with different surgeons. A small amount of the prescribed sterile solution generally is allowed to flow gently into the bladder. A syringe may be used to instill the solution through the catheter. Sometimes a bottle of solution is attached to the drainage system. In this case, the bottle of solution is usually hung on a standard. Tubing which leads from the bottle is connected to the drainage system by a glass connecting tube which is the shape of the letter Y. The nurse can irrigate the bladder as well as allow urine and solution to drain from the bladder by the proper adjusting of clamps on the drainage tube and the irrigation tube.

The patient with dressings should have these checked frequently for drainage and bleeding. The practical nurse should report either of these observations. It is important that soiled dressings should be changed frequently in order to prevent skin irritation and unpleasant odors.

The practical nurse should encourage the patient to drink liquids. The elderly person who is forgetful needs to be reminded frequently to do this. The patient's intake as well as his output of fluids should be measured and recorded.

Because of his age, the patient having a prostatectomy may become confused and disoriented in unfamiliar surroundings. This is especially true at night. Members of the nursing team responsible for his care should observe him closely to prevent injury. For example, he may fall out of the bed or pull his catheter out of place. Side rails should be attached to his bed in an effort to prevent him from falling.

This patient needs special skin care as his skin is likely to be thin and tender. It is the nursing team's responsibility to keep his skin clean and dry. The patient's position should be changed frequently to prevent pressure on any particular area. These measures are important in the prevention of decubitus ulcers. A frequent change of position also helps to prevent respiratory and circulatory complications. For these reasons the physician generally asks the nursing team to help the patient out of bed during the early postoperative period.

### Cancer of the Prostate Gland – *In notes under 4-14-66*

#### Description

Cancer of the prostate gland occurs frequently in older men. The patient with a malignancy which presses against the urethra has symptoms similar to those experienced by the patient with benign prostatic hypertrophy. In other words, he has difficulty in emptying his bladder which may range from frequent, difficult voiding to an inability to void.

#### Treatment

The physician usually removes the prostate gland if the diagnosis is made early enough to offer the patient a chance of recovery. He may treat the patient with an advanced malignancy by removing parts of the growth which interfere with voiding. Female sex hormones are sometimes prescribed in an effort to slow down the growth of the malignancy. In some cases, the surgeon may remove the testes (male sex glands) in an attempt to slow down the growth of the cancer.

### Hydrocele

#### Description

The patient with a hydrocele has a sac filled with fluid within the scrotum. It may occur in connection with an infection of the epididymis and the testes, or it may develop following an injury. However, an individual can develop a hydrocele even though he has no history of either infection or injury. This condition may also develop as a result of congenital malformation.

## Treatment

The physician may treat this patient by withdrawing the fluid through a large needle or by removing the sac of fluid. He sometimes injects a sclerosing substance into the sac after aspirating the fluid. The purpose of the sclerosing fluid is to cause the wall of the hydrocele to become inflamed and disappear eventually.

## Varicocele

An individual with a varicocele has varicose veins (enlarged veins) of the spermatic cord. A *spermatic cord* goes from each of the testes into the abdomen. Each cord is made of a seminal duct as well as the blood vessels and nerves which supply the testis. In an advanced case, the patient is treated by surgical removal of the varicose veins.

## THE FEMALE PATIENT

### Structure and Function

The practical nurse needs to be familiar with the normal structure and function of the female reproductive system. This knowledge serves as a basis for understanding the care needed by the patient with a gynecologic condition. *Gynecology* is a branch of medical science which deals with diseases of women, especially those of the reproductive organs. A specialist in this field is known as a *gynecologist*.

The female reproductive system is composed of the internal organs of reproduction (internal genitalia) and the external organs of reproduction (external genitalia). Two ovaries, two fallopian tubes, the uterus, and the vagina are the internal organs of reproduction. The mons pubis, the labia majora, the labia minora, and the clitoris make up the external genitalia. These are also called the *vulva*.

The *ovaries*, which are known as the female sex glands, are about the size of an almond. One ovary is located on each side of the uterus. The ovaries contain thousands of ova (egg cells). A single

ovum matures in the ovary periodically and is discharged. Another
function of the ovaries is to produce hormones which affect the
uterus.

The two *fallopian tubes* are muscular, small, hollow tubes which
are approximately 7.5 to 12.5 cm (3 to 5 in.) long. A tube is attached
to each side of the uterus. There is an opening from the uterus into
each tube. The outer part of each tube opens into the abdominal
cavity near an ovary. The outer end of each fallopian tube is *fimbriated*, which means that it appears to be fringed. The fallopian tubes
are lined with mucous membrane which is continuous with that of the
uterus, vagina, and urinary tract.

The *uterus* (womb) is the largest internal organ of reproduction.
This is a hollow, muscular organ which is similar to a pear in shape.
The uterus is approximately 7.5 cm (3 in.) long and 5 cm (2 in.) wide.
It is located within the pelvis between the urinary bladder and the
rectum. Ligaments help to hold the uterus in place. The upper
portion of the uterus is known as the *fundus*, and the lower portion
as the *cervix*. The cervix is smaller than the fundus and projects into
the vagina. In other words, the vagina surrounds the lower cervix.
The portion of the uterus between the cervix and the fundus is
known as the *body*. The upper part of the cavity within the uterus
connects with the hollow fallopian tubes, and the lower part connects with the vagina. Mucous membrane, known as *endometrium*,
lines the inside of the uterus.

The *vagina* is a canal which leads from the uterus to the outside
of the body. This canal is approximately 7.5 to 10 cm (3 to 4 in.)
long and is lined with mucous membrane. The urinary bladder and
the urethra are in front of the vagina, and the rectum is behind it.
The upper portion of the vagina surrounds the cervix. There is
normally a passageway from the vagina through the uterus and fallopian tubes into the abdominal cavity.

The *mons pubis* is a pad of fatty tissue covered with skin. It is
located over the front part of the pubic bones. The mons pubis
which is known also as the *mons veneris* is covered with hair after
puberty. *Puberty* is the period in which the individual's reproductive
organs mature and reproduction is possible.

The *labia majora* are two thick folds of tissue which begin at the
mons veneris and end at the perineum. The portion of the body
between the external genitalia and the anus is known as the *perineum*.

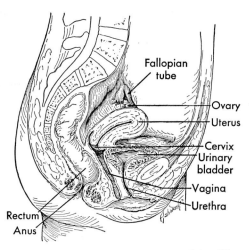

**Figure 39.** Median section of the female pelvis. (Youmans, W. B.: *Human Physiology*. The Macmillan Company, New York, 1954.)

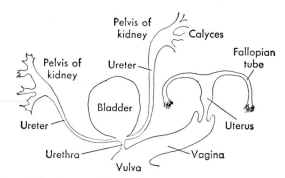

**Figure 40.** Diagram showing continuity of mucous membrane in the female genitourinary pathway. (Kimber, Diana C.; Gray, Carolyn E.; Stackpole, Caroline E.; and Leavell, Lutie C.: *Textbook of Anatomy and Physiology*, 13th ed. The Macmillan Company, New York, 1955.)

The outer surface of the labia majora is covered with hair after puberty.

The *labia minora* are two folds of tissue located within the labia majora. The *clitoris* is a small sensitive organ located at the top of the labia minora. The urinary meatus is located below the clitoris. The opening to the vagina is below the urinary meatus and above the perineum.

### Menstruation

Menstruation is a normal, periodic discharge of bloody fluid from the uterus. Menstruation is known also as *catamenia*. A girl begins to menstruate when she reaches puberty. This usually is between the twelfth and the fifteenth year of age. However, she may begin to menstruate at an earlier age or at a later one. The menstrual periods usually last from four to five days. Menstruation occurs approximately every 28 days, but there is considerable variation in different women. In general, each woman tends to have a constant schedule which is considered to be normal for her.

One of the many ova (eggs) begins to mature in the ovary before menstruation. The single ovum (egg) is enclosed in a sac known as a *graafian follicle*. A hormone known as the *follicle-stimulating hormone* is secreted by the anterior part of the pituitary gland. This hormone stimulates the graafian follicle to grow. It continues to grow until it reaches the surface of the ovary. The growing graafian follicle secretes a hormone, called *estrogen*. This is carried by the blood to the uterus and causes it to become more vascular in preparation for a fertilized ovum. The mature graafian follicle ruptures and throws the ovum into the peritoneal cavity. The ovum is picked up by the fimbriated ends of the fallopian tube. This single cell is carried down the tube by peristalsis and the movement of cilia, which are threadlike projections of the mucous membrane.

The graafian follicle is called the corpus luteum after it ruptures. A substance which is sent to it by the anterior lobe of the pituitary gland is called the *luteinizing hormone*. This substance stimulates the corpus luteum to develop and to produce a hormone called *progesterone*. This hormone is carried by the blood to the uterus. Progesterone stimulates the lining of the uterus to become thicker and more congested with blood in preparation for the fertilized ovum.

If the ovum is not fertilized soon after being picked up by the fallopian tube, it dies. Menstruation takes place approximately 12 to 14 days after the ovum leaves the graafian follicle and enters the fallopian tube. The mucous membrane, which has become thicker and filled with blood, begins to slough off and to bleed. The menstrual discharge leaves the body by way of the cervix and the vagina. Another ovum begins to mature soon after the menstrual period ends, and the same process is repeated again.

### Menopause

Menopause is the period in a woman's life when she stops menstruating. This period, which is also referred to as the *change of life* or as the *climacteric*, usually occurs between the ages of 45 and 50. Some women experience the menopause at an earlier age and some at a slightly later age. Artificial menopause occurs after both ovaries have been removed or have been treated by irradiation. A woman stops menstruating also after her uterus has been removed. She usually does not experience the general changes of menopause until later in life when her ovaries stop functioning.

Frequently the woman notices that the amount of flow with each menstrual period becomes less as she goes through the menopause. However, the periods end suddenly in some women. In either case, the ovaries stop functioning. The pituitary gland secretes more follicle-stimulating hormone in an effort to stimulate the ovaries. This may result in emotional excitability, hot flushes, periods of increased perspiration, and palpitation. The severity of these symptoms varies. Some women develop mental disturbances during this period. The reproductive organs and the breasts begin to atrophy, become smaller. The physician may prescribe estrogenic hormones and mild sedatives to relieve discomfort associated with the symptoms of menopause.

### Menstrual Disorders

#### Dysmenorrhea

#### Description

A woman with dysmenorrhea has painful menstruation. She usually complains of cramp-like pains in the lower part of her abdomen. She may also have a headache, backache, nausea, and vomiting.

### Cause

Dysmenorrhea can result from various factors. Unmarried women are affected more frequently than married ones. Painful menstruation may be caused by such factors as displacement of the uterus, a tumor of the uterus, an endocrine disturbance, an allergy, and an abnormally small opening in the cervix. Illness, fatigue, and emotional factors may be contributory causes of dysmenorrhea.

### Treatment

The usual treatment for a woman with dysmenorrhea is rest and the application of heat to the lower part of her abdomen. Drugs, such as aspirin, may be prescribed to relieve the pain. Proper diet, adequate rest, regular exercise, freedom from tension, and other good health habits are important factors in relieving painful menstruation. The person needs to understand that menstruation is a normal physiologic process.

The woman who continues to suffer with dysmenorrhea should consult her physician. Upon careful examination he may find a physical condition which needs correcting in order to relieve the dysmenorrhea. For instance, he may recommend surgery to correct a displaced uterus or a narrow opening in the cervix.

## Menorrhagia

### Description

The woman with menorrhagia has excessive menstruation. She may have a period which lasts too long or she may have a profuse flow. Anemia may result from the loss of blood.

### Cause

Menorrhagia may be caused by an abnormal condition of the reproductive system such as a tumor of the uterus; an infection of the uterus, tubes, or ovaries; and a tumor of the ovaries. A special type of tumor known as a polyp frequently causes this condition. A polyp is an abnormal growth of tissue which appears to be growing from a stalk. A disturbance of the endocrine glands, especially in young girls, may also cause excessive menstruation.

*Treatment and Nursing Care*

The doctor directs his treatment toward checking the flow, determining its cause, and relieving the cause. Measures which may be prescribed in an effort to check the excessive flow are bed rest and drugs, such as ergot, which cause the muscular uterus to contract. In contracting, the uterus clamps down on its blood vessels and makes them smaller. Thus the bleeding is lessened.

The physician may do surgery to determine the cause of bleeding or to relieve the cause. An operation, commonly performed for either of these purposes is a *curettage*. In this surgical procedure, he dilates the cervix and scrapes the lining of the uterus with an instrument called a *curette*. The practical nurse may hear this operation referred to as a *dilatation* and *curettage* (D and C). The uterine scrapings are examined carefully by the pathologist.

The patient's flow should be checked frequently following surgery. The practical nurse should report the amount to her team leader or head nurse. The surgeon generally allows the patient to get out of bed soon after surgery. Remembering that this patient has had surgery in addition to losing blood, the practical nurse can realize the importance of giving adequate assistance to the patient when she gets out of bed.

After determining the cause of the patient's bleeding, the gynecologist decides upon additional treatment when necessary. He may order hormones, such as thyroid, estrogen, and progesterone, if he decides that the menorrhagia is caused by an endocrine disturbance. Radiation therapy may be used, especially in older women. In general, the woman with a tumor is treated by surgery. Tumors of various parts of the reproductive system are discussed later in this chapter.

*Metrorrhagia*

The woman with metrorrhagia has bleeding between her menstrual periods. Spotting may occur when the ovum is discharged from the graafian follicle. Metrorrhagia can occur as a symptom of either a benign or malignant tumor of the uterus.

*Amenorrhea*

A woman who does not menstruate has amenorrhea. It normally occurs during pregnancy and the menopause. Amenorrhea can occur as a result of diseases of the endocrine glands, especially those of the thyroid, the pituitary, and the ovaries. Extreme anxiety can cause a woman to stop menstruating. Amenorrhea may also be associated with other diseases, such as tuberculosis and anemia. A change of climate or of activities can cause a woman to miss a number of menstrual periods.

After determining the cause of a patient's amenorrhea, the physician prescribes treatment when it is indicated.

## Ovarian Cyst

### Description

The patient with an ovarian cyst has a sac which contains fluid or some other material in her ovary. For example, the *dermoid cyst* is a sac containing different kinds of tissue, such as teeth and hair. A cyst can develop in either one or both ovaries. An ovarian cyst frequently is benign, but it may become malignant. The size of the cyst varies. It may be the size of a small pea or it may reach the size of a grapefruit or even a watermelon.

### Symptoms

A woman may have an ovarian cyst which causes no symptoms. This is true especially when it is small. She may develop irregular menstruation because of the cyst.

If the pedicle (stalk) to which the cyst is attached becomes twisted, it causes the person to have a sudden attack of acute pain. Twisting of the pedicle cuts off the blood supply to the tissues below it. This lack of blood to the area results in pain.

The patient with a large ovarian cyst may have symptoms caused by pressure on surrounding structures. For example, she may have constipation because of pressure on the rectum and edema of her legs because of pressure on the blood vessels. Her abdomen may become enlarged also.

### Treatment and Nursing Care

In general, the treatment of a patient with an ovarian cyst is surgical removal. The removal of an ovary is known as an *oophorec-*

*tomy.* Remembering that removal of both ovaries causes artificial menopause, the practical nurse can readily understand why the surgeon leaves a part of the ovary in place whenever possible.

The nursing care of a patient before and after surgery which was discussed in Chapter 5 applies to this patient. The practical nurse needs to understand that the patient who has surgery of the reproductive organs may have additional fears. For example, she may be afraid that she cannot have children or that she has cancer.

## Salpingitis

### Description

The woman with salpingitis has an inflammation of the fallopian tubes, which is commonly caused by bacteria. These invading microorganisms reach the tubes by way of the vagina and the uterus. Salpingitis is one of the causes of sterility, the inability to have children. When the fallopian tubes become closed as a result of infection, it means that the ovum and the spermatozoon cannot unite. Thus, the ovum is not fertilized and the patient is sterile.

Recalling that the fallopian tubes open into the abdominal cavity near the ovaries should help the practical nurse to realize that the infection may spread to the ovaries as well as the abdominal cavity. An infection that spreads to the ovaries is known as *oophoritis*. The condition is called *pelvic inflammatory disease* when the lower portion of the abdominal cavity is infected.

The patient with salpingitis may develop adhesions because of the infection. Adhesions, which were described earlier in the text (p. 226) as masses of scar tissue, can interfere with the normal functioning of the organs involved.

### Symptoms

The patient with an acute infection of the fallopian tubes has local symptoms of inflammation, such as swelling of the fallopian tubes. She usually complains of discomfort and pain in the lower part of her abdomen. Upon examination, the doctor finds that the abdomen is tender, especially over the inflamed area. This patient may have malaise, fever, and other general symptoms of an infection.

## Treatment and Nursing Care

The physician prescribes a suitable drug to combat the infection. One of the sulfonamides and penicillin are examples of drugs which he may order. The local application of either heat or cold may be ordered to relieve discomfort as well as to aid the body in overcoming infection.

Nursing measures, such as rest and an increased intake of fluids, needed by the patient with an infection which were discussed in Chapter 6 are indicated in caring for the woman with acute salpingitis. A nursing procedure commonly ordered by the doctor for this patient is a vaginal douche. The equipment used should be sterilized before and after doing a vaginal irrigation. This is necessary in order to prevent carrying an additional infection to the patient as well as carrying an infection to other individuals. The nurse should wash her hands thoroughly before and after doing this procedure for the same reasons. The practical nurse may be instructed to wear sterile rubber gloves when giving a douche to the patient with a highly infectious condition.

Surgery is necessary sometimes to free adhesions or to remove the damaged organs. Removal of either one or both fallopian tubes is known as a *salpingectomy*. When either one or both tubes and ovaries are removed, it is called a *salpingo-oophorectomy*.

## Fibroid Tumor of the Uterus

*Hysterecto Subtotal - body of uterus*

### Description

The woman with a fibroid tumor of the uterus has an abnormal growth of white fibers which are threadlike structures. Such a tumor is also known as a *fibromyoma*. A fibroid tumor can develop within the muscle wall, on the surface of the uterus, or beneath the endometrium. One or more of these abnormal growths may occur.

Fibroid tumors are the most common types of uterine tumors. These are benign and occur most frequently between the ages of 30 and 50. *90% of women have them that don't bother them*

### Symptoms

The most common symptom which the patient with a fibroid tumor is likely to experience is abnormal bleeding from the uterus. Ex-

*Hystersalpingram - X-Ray by dye into to determine sterility*

cessive bleeding can result in anemia. The woman may also complain of backache. However, fibroid tumors may cause no symptoms, especially if they are small. In some cases, a large tumor presses on the bladder and rectum. This results in symptoms associated with these organs, such as frequent voiding, diarrhea, or constipation.

### Treatment and Nursing Care

The gynecologist may not recommend treatment for the patient with small fibroids which cause no symptoms. The patient with a larger tumor which causes symptoms is generally treated by surgery. Removal of all or part of the uterus is known as a *hysterectomy*. The surgeon may not remove the cervix when doing this operation. The practical nurse may hear the term *panhysterectomy* used when the entire uterus is removed. The operative procedure is called an *abdominal hysterectomy* when the uterus is removed through an incision in the abdomen. Removal of the uterus through the vagina is known as a *vaginal hysterectomy*. The practical nurse should remember that the woman cannot menstruate after having her uterus removed.

In some cases, the surgeon can remove the tumor and leave the uterus. This is especially important for younger women who want to have children. The patient continues to menstruate if the uterus is not removed.

Radiation therapy is sometimes used to check the growth of a tumor. This can relieve the main symptom of a fibroid tumor, which is bleeding. Since radiotherapy stops the functioning of the ovaries as well as the uterus, this therapy causes the patient to have an artificial menopause.

Remembering that the uterus is close to the urinary bladder should help the practical nurse to remember that the patient's bladder should be emptied before she is transferred to the operating room. This is important to prevent injury to a filled bladder during surgery. The practical nurse can expect the patient to have a bloody vaginal discharge following surgery of the uterus. She should observe and report the amount of flow to the head nurse or team leader. The patient's pads should be changed as often as necessary, and her vulva should be kept clean. This makes the patient more comfortable and eliminates odors.

Pelvic pneumoperitoneum - X-Ray for cysts on ovaries - dye into pelvic cavity

## Displacement of the Uterus

### Retroversion

#### Description
Displacement of the uterus means that this organ is not in its normal place. A woman with *retroversion* or *retroflexion* of the uterus has a backward displacement of her uterus. In other words, the uterus is tilted backward.

#### Symptoms
The patient with retroversion of the uterus may have no symptoms or she may have dysmenorrhea, backache, and constipation. In some cases, sterility is believed to result from this condition.

#### Treatment
The patient may have surgery recommended by her physician, if she has symptoms caused by retroversion. Usually, no treatment is planned when she has no symptoms associated with this condition.

### Prolapse of the Uterus

#### Description
Prolapse of the uterus means that the uterus has slipped down below its normal level. A woman develops this condition if the tissues, such as the muscles and ligaments which hold the uterus in place, are stretched and torn during childbirth.

#### Symptoms
The woman may complain that she feels as if her insides were falling out. She has a mass protruding from the genitalia when her uterus has slipped through the vagina and hangs between her thighs. The prolapsed uterus may cause the patient to have constipation and difficulty in emptying her bladder.

#### Treatment
Surgery to correct prolapse of the uterus is generally recommended. Frequently the surgeon removes the uterus through the vagina and repairs the surrounding tissues.

The patient may be advised to wear a pessary to help hold the uterus in place if her condition is not suitable for surgery. A *pessary* is an appliance usually in the shape of a ring which is fitted around the part of the cervix which projects into the vagina.

## Cystocele

### Description

The patient with a cystocele has a prolapse of the urinary bladder into the vagina. It generally results from injury during childbirth.

### Symptoms

A cystocele can cause the woman to have partial urinary incontinence. She notices that she passes a small amount of urine especially when coughing or sneezing. She may also have difficulty in emptying her bladder.

### Treatment and Nursing Care

This patient is usually treated surgically. The surgeon repairs the defect in the pelvic floor which permitted the bladder to fall into the vagina and he returns the bladder to its normal place. The term used to describe this type of operation is *anterior colporrhaphy.*

The practical nurse may be asked to give special care to the vulva of this patient after surgery. This procedure frequently is called *perineal care.* The actual technique varies in different hospitals. In general, sterile equipment is used to clean the vulva. The patient should have perineal care after emptying her bladder or having a bowel movement. The practical nurse should learn the procedure used by the hospital in which she is nursing.

This patient should be encouraged to empty her bladder frequently. This prevents the full bladder from putting a strain on the operative area. In some cases, the patient may have an indwelling catheter for the first few days after surgery.

## Rectocele

### Description

A woman with a rectocele has a prolapse of the rectum into the vagina. This condition generally is caused by injury to the muscles of the perineum during childbirth.

### Symptoms

The patient with a rectocele may complain of a backache and constipation.

### Treatment

Surgical repair of the weakened tissues is the usual treatment for the patient with a rectocele. This operation is known as a *posterior colporrhaphy*. It may also be called a *perineorrhaphy*.

This patient, like the patient with an anterior colporrhaphy, should be encouraged to empty her bladder frequently. She should have perineal care also.

## Cervicitis

### Description

The woman with cervicitis has an inflammation of the cervix. It may be either acute or chronic. Chronic cervicitis is common. The practical nurse may hear this condition referred to as *endocervicitis*. This means that the mucous membrane which lines the cervix is inflamed.

### Cause

Bacteria may invade the cervix and cause cervicitis. A woman may also develop this condition following childbirth injury to the cervix which can result in an infection. An infection may cause the woman to develop *erosion of the cervix*. This means that some of the tissue covering the cervix is destroyed. Erosion of the cervix can also be pre-cancerous.

### Symptoms

The main symptom experienced by a woman with cervicitis is *leukorrhea*, which is a vaginal discharge. It may be white or yellow in color. The amount of leukorrhea varies. Sometimes the woman has a large amount.

### Treatment

The gynecologist directs his treatment toward controlling the infection in the cervix. The local application of an antiseptic in the

*hydAtidifoRN moIE - bEN'ga neoplasm*

*abnomal growth · occur in 1 f 2000*

*preg. embryonic tissues ah grape · cluster*

*symptom · early preg. bleeding, hemorhage*

form of vaginal suppositories may be prescribed. Vaginal douches to relieve discomfort from leukorrhea may be ordered. The physician may do a procedure known as a *cauterization*. This means that tissue is destroyed by applying a chemical or by using electricity which is passed through a thin blade or a wire loop. In this procedure, the doctor aims to destroy the infected areas. He may do a *conization*, which is removal of the eroded area by means of a fine, high-frequency electric current.

## Vaginitis

### Description

The woman with vaginitis has an inflammation of the vagina, which is frequently caused by microorganisms. *Senile vaginitis* is a special type of vaginitis which occurs in women who have been through the menopause. The woman's resistance to organisms found frequently in the vagina may become decreased after the menopause. These organisms can cause a mild inflammation of the mucous membrane lining the vagina which is greatly thinned because of a lack of estrogen.

### Symptoms

The main symptoms experienced by the woman with vaginitis are leukorrhea and itching. The elderly patient with senile vaginitis usually has very little vaginal discharge. She frequently complains of dryness in addition to the itching.

### Treatment

The physician generally prescribes vaginal irrigations for the patient with vaginitis. He specifies the type of solution to be used. For example, he may order a solution which acts as an antiseptic, one which changes the reaction of the vaginal mucosa from acid to alkaline, or one which changes the reaction of the vaginal mucosa from alkaline to acid. The local application of medicine in the form of a jelly or a vaginal suppository may be prescribed. The doctor may recommend suppositories containing estrogen for the patient with senile vaginitis.

## Cancer

### Description

Cancer may occur in any part of the female reproductive system. However, the uterus is the organ which is most likely to develop a malignancy. Uterine cancer is more common in women who are going through the menopause or who have already gone through it.

The cervix is the part of the uterus which is most often affected by cancer. The body of the uterus is another part of this organ which is affected fairly often by a malignancy. An older woman is more likely to have cancer in the body of the uterus.

### Symptoms

The woman with cancer of the uterus usually does not have symptoms during the early stage of this disease. For this reason, it is important for women to have a pelvic examination at least once a year. This is particularly important for women over 35 years of age. Use of the Papanicolaou smear to find cast-off cancer cells in the vagina is becoming increasingly popular as an aid in early detection. The physician does a biopsy of the patient's cervix if he finds cancer cells in the vaginal smear.

Cancer of the uterus can cause the patient to have a slight watery discharge. She may have a small amount of bloody discharge between her menstrual periods. Her menstrual periods may become longer than usual. The woman who has passed through the menopause may begin to have bloody discharge.

### Treatment

The physician attempts to eliminate all of the cancer cells, if he finds that the patient does not have an advanced malignancy. This destruction of the cancer cells may be done by radiation therapy with either x-ray or radium, by surgical removal, or by a combination of these two therapies. The practical nurse may find it helpful to review the discussion of these treatments, which is included in Chapter 7. The nursing care of a patient with cancer, which was discussed also in that chapter, is applicable to the woman with cancer of the uterus.

## VENEREAL DISEASE

An individual with a venereal disease has an infectious condition which is transmitted mainly by sexual intercourse. However, the practical nurse needs to understand that venereal disease is not always transmitted in this way. Syphilis and gonorrhea, which are two of the main venereal diseases, are included in this discussion.

### Syphilis

#### Description

Although syphilis may attack any part of the body, it frequently starts in the reproductive system. For this reason, it is included in this chapter which deals with the patient who has a disease of that system.

The person with syphilis has an infectious disease which is caused by the *Treponema pallidum*. This delicate organism is called a spirochete because it is similar to a corkscrew spiral in shape. These spirochetes may continue to live in the patient's body throughout his life. The *Treponema pallidum* lives only a short period of time outside the body and is killed in a short time by exposure to cold. Soap and water also destroy this spirochete.

Syphilis frequently is transmitted by sexual intercourse. However, it is not entirely a venereal disease since it can be transmitted by other types of direct contact, such as by kissing. Doctors and nurses have been known to develop this disease after examining and caring for patients with syphilis. A pregnant woman with untreated syphilis can transmit it to her unborn child. Because of this, many states require pregnant women to be tested for syphilis. Proper treatment started during the earlier part of pregnancy can prevent the child from developing this disease.

#### Symptoms

A person in the early stage of syphilis has a local lesion followed by generalized symptoms. Approximately three weeks after the individual becomes infected with syphilis, he develops a small inflamed area at the site where the spirochetes entered his body. This sore, which is usually painless and ulcerated, is called a *chancre*. Spirochetes in the chancre can be transmitted to another person by direct contact. This is especially true if they come in contact with a raw area, such as a tiny cut or a scratch on the well person. The chancre heals in three or four weeks.

Although the patient usually passes through a period during which he has few if any symptoms after the chancre heals, his body continues to be invaded by the spirochetes. These are spread throughout his entire body by the lymph and the blood. Approximately six weeks to six months after the chancre has healed, he usually develops a combination of symptoms. These include a skin rash, swollen lymph nodes, a sore throat, a slight fever, and sore places in his mouth. If the patient's bones are affected by the spirochetes, he generally complains of pain in the involved area. His hair may become loose and come out, especially when he brushes or combs it. He may develop an inflammation of his eyes. His liver and kidneys may be affected by the spirochetes. His cerebrospinal fluid and semen usually contain spirochetes. The patient with any of these symptoms is infectious and may remain so for two to three years if he is not treated effectively. Serology tests are laboratory procedures done on the blood serum to diagnose syphilis. These tests become positive during this period. The Wassermann, Kline, Kahn, and Mazzini are examples of serologic tests for syphilis.

After the early symptoms of syphilis have disappeared, the untreated or the inadequately treated patient goes through a period during which he has no symptoms. The length of this period varies. It may range from a few months to many years. The patient may have no further trouble or he may develop late syphilis. A lesion which occurs commonly in a person with late syphilis is known as a *gumma*. This lesion can be thought of as a tumor. Its center frequently is a mass of dead cells. These are usually surrounded by a capsule of hard tissue. The patient may develop a gumma in the internal organs, on the mucous membrane, or on the skin.

Since any system of the patient's body can be attacked by the spirochetes, he can have a variety of symptoms. The symptoms vary in different individuals. The two systems which are frequently affected by late syphilis are the nervous and the circulatory systems. A person with syphilis of the nervous system has *neurosyphilis*. The individual with syphilis of the circulatory system has (cardiovascular syphilis.) An example of neurosyphilis is seen in the person with (general paresis.) This patient develops mental changes, tremors, and difficulty in talking. An example of cardiovascular syphilis is seen in the person with an aneurysm of the aorta. The aorta, which is the large artery leading from the heart, may be attacked by spirochetes. When this happens, it causes the wall of the aorta to become weak. The diseased part of the aorta which becomes dilated as a result of this is known as an aneurysm. The practical nurse may find it helpful to think of an aneurysm as (resembling the bulging of a weak spot in a balloon.) The weak part of the aorta, like the weak part of a balloon, is likely to rupture.

### Treatment and Nursing Care

Penicillin is generally precribed for the patient with syphilis. The doctor may use another antibiotic especially when the patient is allergic to penicillin. The patient should be encouraged to visit his doctor regularly so that he can determine whether or not the treatment was effective. In some cases the patient may need to have the treatment repeated.

When assisting in the care of the patient with syphilis, the practical nurse should remember that the patient with an open lesion or a rash is usually infectious. If this patient is hospitalized, he is generally placed in strict isolation. Dressings soiled with body discharges from the person with an open lesion should be either disinfected or burned. Linens, dishes, and all equipment used in his care should be sterilized. Members of the nursing team usually are instructed to wear rubber gloves in addition to a protective gown when caring for this patient. They should also wash their hands thoroughly with soap under running water after caring for him.

### Gonorrhea

### Description

The patient with gonorrhea has an infection which is transmitted by direct contact. Usually this contact is by sexual intercourse. For this reason gonorrhea is known as a venereal disease. However, gonorrhea is not always transmitted by sexual intercourse. For example, a little girl may develop this condition after using a toilet seat which has recently been contaminated by a person with gonorrhea.

Gonorrhea is caused by a microorganism which is called *Neisseria gonorrhoeae.* It is commonly known as the *gonococcus.* Although this organism causes an infection which frequently involves the reproductive organs, other parts of the body such as the urethra, the urinary bladder, and the eyes can be affected.

### Symptoms

The individual develops a discharge which contains pus approximately three to five days after contact with an infected person. The female has this purulent discharge from the vagina. She may also have painful and frequent urination. The male has a discharge from the urethra. He often complains of painful and frequent urination. He generally has pus in his urine. The amount of discharge generally becomes less in two to three weeks. Recovery from the infection may take place at this time.

The patient sometimes continues to have the infection. It can spread along the reproductive tract and cause complications such as salpingitis and prostatitis. The infection may cause the fallopian tubes or the ducts from the testes to become closed. This results in sterility.

A pregnant woman with gonorrhea can infect her unborn infant as it passes through the birth canal. The eyes of the baby can be infected in this manner. An infant with a gonorrheal infection of the eyes has *ophthalmia neonatorum,* which, if untreated, usually results in blindness. The regular treatment of all newborn babies' eyes with an antiseptic, such as silver nitrate, can prevent this serious infection. This preventive measure has become a law in the majority of the states.

### Treatment and Nursing Care

The physician can confirm his diagnosis of gonorrhea by having the patient's discharge examined in the laboratory. He usually treats the patient with penicillin. Frequently he treats the patient in his office or in the clinic. The doctor generally examines the patient periodically following treatment to determine whether or not it was effective. In general, he has the patient's discharge examined in the laboratory several times to see if the gonococcus is still present. The practical nurse should remember that gonorrhea is transmitted by direct contact. She should also remember that the mucous membrane of the eyes and the genitalia are highly susceptible to infection by the gonococcus. The practical nurse should wash her hands thoroughly after caring for a patient with gonorrhea. She should keep her hands away from her face until she has washed them. Pads soiled with discharge from the part of the patient's body infected by the gonococcus should be either disinfected or burned.

*Answer for Friday*

## SUGGESTIONS FOR STUDY

1. Why is the patient with a disease of the prostate gland likely to have difficulty in emptying his bladder?
2. What special nursing care does the patient need after a prostatectomy?
3. Define the following: menopause, menorrhagia, dysmenorrhea, metrorrhagia, amenorrhea, leukorrhea, and gynecologist.
4. Why can salpingitis cause sterility?
5. Is a fibroid tumor of the uterus benign or malignant?
6. Why is it important for the woman to have an empty bladder before being transported to surgery for an operation on the reproductive tract?
7. When is a woman likely to have a prolapse of the uterus?
8. How is syphilis transmitted?
9. What kills the *Treponema pallidum?*
10. Review the common symptoms of early syphilis.
11. What special precautions should be taken by the practical nurse when helping to care for a patient with an infectious case of syphilis?
12. What complication may occur in an infant with ophthalmia neonatorum?

## REFERENCES FOR CHAPTER 20

American Cancer Society, Inc.: *A Cancer Source Book for Nurses.* The Society, New York, 1956, pp. 64-70 and 93-96.
Applebaum, Stella B., and Kavinoky, Nadina R.: "Understanding Menopause," *Practical Nurses Digest,* 4:21-22 and 31, (Jan.) 1957.

Brady, Leo; Kurtz, Ethna L.; and McLaughlin, Eileen: *Essentials of Gynecology*, 2nd ed. The Macmillan Company, New York, 1949.

Brown, Amy F.: *Medical Nursing*, 3rd ed. W. B. Saunders Co., Philadelphia, 1957, pp. 878-90.

Carter, Charles F., and Smith, Alice L.: *Principles of Microbiology*, 3rd ed. C. V. Mosby Co., St. Louis, 1957, pp. 346-52 and 492-502.

Crossen, Robert J., and Campbell, Ann J.: *Gynecologic Nursing*, 5th ed. C. V. Mosby Co., St. Louis, 1956.

Eliason, Eldridge; Ferguson, L. Kraeer; and Sholtis, Lillian A.: *Surgical Nursing*, 10th ed. J. B. Lippincott Co., Philadelphia, 1955, pp. 380-92 and 601-26.

Emerson, Charles P., Jr., and Bragdon, Jane S.: *Essentials of Medicine*, 17th ed. J. B. Lippincott Co., Philadelphia, 1955, pp. 719-25, 781-82, and 844-50.

Jensen, Julius, and Jensen, Deborah: *Nursing in Clinical Medicine*, 4th ed. The Macmillan Company, New York, 1954, pp. 783-98.

Ormsby, Hugh L.: "Prophylaxis of Ophthalmia Neonatorum," *Am. J. Nursing*, 57:1174-75, (Sept.) 1957.

Stafford, Edward S., and Diller, Doris: *Surgery and Surgical Nursing*, 3rd ed. W. B. Saunders Co., Philadelphia, 1958, pp. 415-45.

Turner, C. E.: *Personal and Community Health*, 10th ed. C. V. Mosby Co., St. Louis, 1956, pp. 328-46 and 429-34.

Van Blarcom, Carolyn C., and Ziegel, Erna: *Obstetrical Nursing*, 4th ed. The Macmillan Company, New York, 1957, pp. 1-46.

West, John P.; Keller, Manelva W.; and Harmon, Elizabeth H.: *Nursing Care of the Surgical Patient*, 6th ed. The Macmillan Company, New York, 1957, pp. 360-88.

*Nursing the Patient
with a Disease of
the Nervous System*

PART IX

Chapter 21

# THE PATIENT
# WITH A DISEASE OF
# THE NERVOUS SYSTEM

## STRUCTURE AND FUNCTION

The nervous system is composed of the brain, spinal cord, and nerves. Although this system consists of only a few organs, it plays a vital role in the functioning of the body. It helps to regulate and to coordinate the body's activities. The nervous system enables the body to function as a whole.

The central nervous system is made up of the brain and the spinal cord. Both of these are surrounded by membranes and a bony case for protection. The three membranes which cover the brain and the spinal cord are known as *meninges*. The *cranium* or *skull* is the bony case protecting the brain and its meninges. The spinal cord and its meninges are protected by bones known as *vertebrae*.

Additional protection to the central nervous system is provided by the *cerebrospinal fluid*. This is normally a clear liquid which bathes, lubricates, and protects the brain and the spinal cord. Cerebrospinal fluid also flows between the meninges.

Nerves carry messages to and from the brain and spinal cord. A *nerve* is a bundle of nerve fibers which are usually outside the central nervous system. Nerve fibers are outgrowths of the nerve cell. Gray

355

matter is made of nerve cells, and white matter is made of nerve fibers. Nerve fibers can be repaired following injury or disease, but destroyed nerve cells cannot be restored. Thus, a person is not able to use the part of his body supplied by nerve cells which have died. An individual having a disease of the nerve fibers may have a good chance of recovering the use of the affected part because the fibers can be restored or repaired.

### Brain

The brain is composed of both gray and white matter; that is, it contains nerve cells and nerve fibers. The brain is the largest mass of nervous tissue in the body. The five main parts of the brain are the cerebrum, the midbrain, the cerebellum, the pons Varolii, and the medulla oblongata. The cerebrum, which is the largest part of the brain, is located in the upper portion of the cranium. The five lobes of the cerebrum are the frontal, the parietal, the temporal, the occipital, and the insula. Mental activities, such as reason, intelligence, memory, and consciousness, are controlled by the cerebrum. The cerebrum also controls such activities as seeing, smelling, talking, and voluntary movements, such as picking up a pencil.

The cerebellum is behind and below the cerebrum. It helps to control equilibrium and muscular coordination.

The brain stem is composed of the midbrain, the pons Varolii, and the medulla. The midbrain connects the cerebrum and the cerebellum with the pons. The pons Varolii is located between the medulla oblongata and the midbrain. The pons connects the cerebrum with the medulla. The brain is connected to the spinal cord by the medulla oblongata. Many of the motor nerves (those responsible for motion) cross in the medulla. The vital centers which control automatic activities of the body, such as respiration, heartbeat, and blood pressure, are in the medulla oblongata. Such activities as sneezing and coughing are also controlled by this part of the brain. The 12 pairs of cranial nerves which originate in the brain stem control the activities of the head. These nerves serve as pathways for special senses, such as sight, smell, taste, and hearing.

### Spinal Cord

The spinal cord goes from the medulla to the lower part of the back. It contains both gray and white matter. The gray matter is

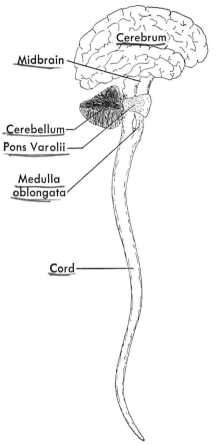

**Figure 41.** Diagram of brain and spinal cord. (Kimber, Diana C.; Gray, Carolyn E.; Stackpole, Caroline E.; and Leavell, Lutie C.: *Textbook of Anatomy and Physiology*, 13th ed. The Macmillan Company, New York, 1955.)

located in the center of the cord. Nerves going to and from the brain pass through the spinal cord. The nerves which branch off from the cord are known as *spinal nerves*. The spinal nerves connect with the peripheral nerves, which are located near the surface of the body. The spinal cord and the spinal nerves serve as pathways for the impulses between the brain and parts of the body below the head.

## ASSISTING WITH EXAMINATION

The physician performs certain procedures to aid in determining whether or not the patient has an abnormality in either the structure or the function of the nervous system. Since the practical nurse may be responsible for assisting in the care of a patient undergoing diagnostic study, she needs an understanding of these procedures.

In addition to obtaining a complete history and doing a thorough physical examination, the doctor does a neurological examination. A lumbar puncture, an x-ray examination, and an electroencephalogram may be done also to aid him in his diagnosis.

The neurological examination is a highly specialized procedure done by the doctor. A *neurologist*, who is a physician specializing in diagnosing and treating patients with disorders of the nervous system, is frequently the person responsible for this examination. The examiner tests the patient's reflexes and his special senses, such as sight, smell, and touch. He checks the patient's ability to coordinate his movements, such as those involved in walking. The physician also tests the strength of various parts of the patient's body. For example, the doctor may have the patient squeeze his hand. The neurologist also determines whether or not the patient knows the exact location and position of his extremities. For example, the patient may have to look at his feet to know where they are.

The doctor may do a *lumbar puncture*, which is known also as a *spinal tap*, to aid in diagnosis. In this procedure, he inserts a needle between the vertebrae into the spinal canal. This is known as a lumbar puncture since it is usually done in the lumbar region (lower part of the back). He usually determines the pressure of the cerebrospinal fluid when he does a lumbar puncture. He may remove some of the fluid so that it can be examined.

Air, oxygen, or a special dye which is visible by x-ray examination may be injected into the central nervous system. These substances make the outline of the soft brain and spinal cord visible by x-ray examination. A patient having *encephalography* has x-rays taken of his head after some of the cerebrospinal fluid has been replaced by air or oxygen. A patient having *ventriculography* has air placed into the ventricles (small cavities) within his brain. In order to do this examination, the neurologist makes openings in the patient's skull

*Myelogram - X-ray of cord - dye injected*

so that he can inject air or some other suitable substance into the ventricles. The patient's head is then x-rayed. This type of examination enables the physician to study the outline of the internal brain structure. The patient having an *arteriogram* has x-rays of his head made immediately after a dye has been injected into the carotid artery, which is the large artery on each side of the neck. The dye which is carried to the cerebral arteries is visible on x-ray examination. This enables the doctor to study the arteries in the brain.

An *electroencephalogram* is a tracing of the electrical waves of the brain. The brain waves of a healthy person have a definite pattern. An individual with certain brain diseases has an abnormal pattern.

*Radio isotope - determine tumor*

## TUMOR OF THE BRAIN

### Description

The patient with a *brain tumor* or an *intracranial tumor* has an abnormal growth of cells within his skull. The tumor may be *primary;* that is, it started in the brain; or it may be *secondary,* that is, the tumor started in another part of the body and spread to the brain. An intracranial tumor may be either benign or malignant.

### Symptoms

The patient's symptoms depend a great deal upon the size of the tumor, its rate of growth, its type, and its location. A large tumor which grows rapidly causes the patient's symptoms to become progressively worse. The patient with a malignant tumor which has spread from another part of his body is more likely to have an unfavorable outcome than is the patient with a malignant tumor which started in the brain and is diagnosed early.

The tumor's location within the skull is an important factor in determining the patient's symptoms. Two examples of symptoms caused by a tumor of the cerebrum are given to illustrate how the location of a tumor within one lobe of the brain can result in different symptoms. A tumor in the part of the cerebrum which controls movement may cause the patient to have weakness, convulsions, and paralysis. These symptoms occur in the part of the body which receives its nerve supply from the diseased area of the brain. If the patient's tumor is on the left side, the right side of his body is affected. A tumor in the part of the cerebrum which controls behavior may cause the patient to have personality changes. He may have sudden outbursts of crying and laughing which are unlike him. He may also become untidy or he may use vulgar language. Another example of the tumor's location affecting the patient's symptoms is seen in the patient with a tumor in the occipital lobe of his brain. This patient may have visual disturbances, such as difficulty in reading, spots before his eyes, and blindness, since the occipital lobe controls sight.

A brain tumor usually produces symptoms of increased pressure within the cranium which is known as increased intracranial pressure. Remembering that the brain is soft and is housed in a bony cage helps the practical nurse to understand the changes which take place. The soft brain yields to pressure and the hard bones of the skull do not. Thus, an abnormality such as a tumor, bleeding, and edema increases pressure within the cranium. This pressure is exerted against the soft brain rather than the hard skull. A tumor can cause the patient to have symptoms of increased intracranial pressure. These are headache, drowsiness, and visual disturbances, such as double vision and varying degrees of blindness. The pupils of his eyes become dilated if the pressure continues. Vomiting which is forceful or projectile is frequently present. The vomiting usually has no relationship to meals and may not be accompanied by nausea. As the patient's condition becomes worse, his blood pressure usually rises. Also, his pulse and respiratory rate become slower. These symptoms should be reported immediately. Muscular weakness, paralysis, loss of consciousness, and convulsions may occur. The optic nerve which is the main nerve leading to the eye, may become swollen. The doctor can see the swollen optic nerve by looking through the pupil of the eye with an ophthalmoscope. The practical nurse may hear edema (swelling) of the optic nerve referred to as papilledema or choked disk.

### Treatment and Nursing Care

The neurosurgeon removes the patient's brain tumor if possible. He may do a decompression if the patient's condition is not good enough to remove the tumor or if he cannot determine the tumor's exact location. Decompression is an operation in which the doctor removes part of the bony skull to relieve intracranial pressure. Removing part of the skull gives the brain space in which to expand. This may relieve the patient's symptoms of increased intracranial pressure. An operation to remove the tumor may be done later.

### Preoperative Care

The general principles, such as cleanliness, relief of anxiety, and adequate diet and fluids, discussed in the care of a patient before surgery in Chapter 5 apply to this patient. Care should be used to avoid nicking the skin when the patient's head is shaved. The practical nurse may be asked to give the patient a shampoo before surgery. The surgeon usually does not prescribe morphine as it depresses the patient's respiration and affects the reaction of the pupils of his eyes. The doctor may not order an enema because straining associated with a bowel movement could cause further damage by increasing intracranial pressure.

### Postoperative Care

The patient should be placed in bed gently following surgery. The neurosurgeon usually specifies the exact position for the patient. A special bed with a low headboard may be used so that it is easier for the doctor to change the patient's dressing. The bed should be ready for the patient when he is returned from surgery.

The patient's pulse, blood pressure, respiration, and temperature (rectal) should be checked frequently following surgery. Generally, the neurosurgeon leaves specific orders regarding these. Elevated temperature, and a change in the patient's pulse, respiration, and blood pressure should be reported promptly. The appearance of either fluid or blood on the bandage, paralysis, difficulty in swallowing, inability to speak, and incontinence should also be reported immediately. The nurse in attendance should be prepared to protect the patient from injury in case he has a convulsion.

In general, the doctor specifies when the nursing team should start changing the patient's position as well as the position the patient is to maintain. In helping to turn the patient, the practical nurse may be asked to turn him as one piece, or as if he were a log. This is important to prevent strain on the incision.

The neurosurgeon may prescribe a certain amount of fluid which *because of edema*

he wants the patient to receive each day. A careful record of the patient's intake and output of fluids should be kept. It is the responsibility of the nursing team to see that the patient receives the prescribed amount of fluids. When the practical nurse is feeding the patient, she should not hurry him. Nasal feedings may be necessary if the patient is drowsy or stuporous.

The unconscious patient should be kept clean and dry and should be turned frequently. The bed linen should be kept free of wrinkles to prevent pressure on the skin. Members of the nursing team responsible for the care of this unconscious patient should see that his body is kept in good alignment in order to prevent deformities. Good body alignment is of equal importance in the care of a paralyzed patient. The practical nurse should observe and report the patient's voiding and defecation. The patient should be observed frequently for symptoms of increased intracranial pressure, such as a slowing of either the pulse or respiratory rate and an increase in the blood pressure. Such observations should be reported promptly. The care of the unconscious and paralyzed patient is discussed in more detail on pages 145 to 146.

The patient's convalescence may be longer than that of a patient recovering from other types of surgery. Throughout this period he needs understanding and encouragement from all members of the health team who are caring for him. Rehabilitation plays an important role in this patient's recovery. For example, it may be necessary for him to learn to talk, or to walk, again. He may have a disability as a result of the tumor. Emphasis should be placed on his remaining capabilities rather than his disability. The aim of the health team in caring for this patient is to help him to live most happily and effectively with his disability.

## TUMOR OF THE SPINAL CORD

### Description

An individual may have a tumor on the outside of his spinal cord and develop symptoms when it presses on the cord, or he may develop a tumor within the spinal cord. The tumor may be either benign or malignant.

## Symptoms

Pain is generally an early symptom experienced by the individual with a spinal cord tumor. The pain occurs in the part of the body which receives its nerve supply from the diseased area of the spinal cord. For example, a tumor in the upper part of the spine could cause the patient to have chest pain since his chest receives its nerve supply from that part of the spinal cord. A tumor in the lower region could cause the patient to have pain in his abdomen or legs.

The patient's pain may be associated with numbness and tingling. The affected part of his body may become weak. This is usually caused by an enlargement of the tumor. The patient may lose all sensation in regions of his body which receive their nerve supply from the part of the spinal cord which is below the tumor. Paralysis may also develop. The patient has *paraplegia* when his lower limbs are paralyzed, and *quadriplegia* when all four of his extremities are paralyzed. The patient may have urinary disturbances, such as incontinence, retention, and urgency to void.

## Treatment and Nursing Care

The patient with a tumor of his spinal cord is treated by surgical removal when this is possible. The neurosurgeon reaches the tumor by doing a *laminectomy.* This is an operation in which part of the vertebrae covering the diseased cord is removed.

Remembering that the spinal cord has lost part of its protective covering helps the practical nurse to realize the importance of the patient's position after surgery. When the practical nurse is asked to assist in turning the patient, she should remember that he is to be turned as if he were a stiff board. This is important to avoid injuring the cord. Special beds are available which enable one or two nurses to turn the patient. The Foster and the Stryker frames are two examples.

This patient is particularly prone to develop decubitus ulcers. For this reason, he needs to be turned frequently. His skin should be kept clean and dry. The appearance of reddened areas should be reported promptly so that measures may be taken to prevent further irritation to the skin. The bed linen should be smooth and free of wrinkles and patches which could irritate the skin.

The patient's elimination should be checked as he is likely to become constipated and to have retention of urine. The doctor may order an enema at regular intervals to relieve constipation. He may have an indwelling catheter inserted to relieve urinary retention.

## INJURY OF THE BRAIN

### Description

Although a bony cage protects the brain, it may become injured. Damage to the brain can vary from slight bruising to severe destruction of tissue. Brain injury is known also as an *intracranial injury*.

The patient with a *concussion* of the brain loses consciousness either completely or partially. This is a minor head injury which usually follows a fall or a blow on the head. The patient's skin becomes pale and cold, and his pulse is weak. As he regains consciousness, he may vomit and complain of a headache.

A severe head injury usually causes brain tissue to be damaged and blood vessels to be torn. Blood flowing from the torn blood vessels collects within the cranial cavity and forms a clot. This condition is known as a *hematoma*. A *depressed fracture* of the skull can also cause brain damage. In this type of fracture, the bony fragments are driven inward into the brain. Blood flowing from torn blood vessels, fluid escaping from the damaged brain tissue, and a depressed fracture cause the patient to have increased intracranial pressure. The amount of damage to the brain and the location of the injury determine the seriousness of the patient's condition.

### Symptoms

The patient with an intracranial injury may have local symptoms of injury, such as a bleeding wound or a fracture. However, an external wound is not always seen. The patient may have symptoms of increased intracranial pressure, which are discussed on page 360. These are determined by the amount of brain damage. In addition to having symptoms of increased intracranial pressure, he may have bleeding from his nose, throat, or ears. The pupil of his eye on the injured side may be dilated. A severe head injury usually causes the patient to lose consciousness immediately. A deep state of unconsciousness over a period of time usually indicates an unfavorable outcome.

Inflammation of the brain, epilepsy, and paralysis may result from a brain injury. The individual's mentality is sometimes affected. Another complication is severe headaches. The patient may suffer with headaches long after his other symptoms have disappeared.

### Treatment and Nursing Care

The physician prescribes bed rest if he suspects that the patient has sustained a brain injury. The patient should be observed for symptoms of brain injury. The doctor may ask the nurse to check the patient's blood pressure, temperature, pulse, and respiration at frequent intervals. The centers which control these vital functions are located in the brain. Thus, injury of one of these centers may cause serious results. For instance, damage to the respiratory center causes the patient's respirations to become slower. A marked decrease in the respiratory rate indicates that the patient needs help in breathing. Such a symptom should be reported immediately.

Generally, the physician performs surgery on the patient with either a depressed fracture or a hematoma. The area around the wound should be cleaned and shaved before surgery. The surgeon removes damaged scalp tissue. Bone fragments may be either removed or raised from the brain. It may be necessary for the doctor to place a plate of metal or polyethylene over the opening in the scalp. The surgeon makes an opening through the scalp when it is necessary to remove a hematoma (blood clot). The patient having brain surgery because of injury needs the same type of care which was discussed in relation to the patient having surgery for a brain tumor.

## INJURY OF THE SPINAL CORD

### Description

An individual may receive an injury to his spinal cord by an object penetrating the vertebrae, such as a bullet. Also, a fracture or a dislocation may result in spinal cord injury. The cord may be completely severed or it may be partially destroyed. Bleeding and edema which follow an injury to the spinal cord may cause the patient to have paralysis which disappears when the blood and fluid are absorbed. If the patient has a complete severance of the spinal cord, he has paralysis and loss of feeling in the part of his body which received its nerve supply from the spinal cord below the injury.

### Treatment and Nursing Care

The emergency care of a patient with a spinal cord injury is directed toward preventing further injury to the cord when he is moved. He should be kept lying down until sufficient help is available to move him. Several people are needed to transfer him to a stretcher. The patient should be moved as one piece or as though he were a stiff board. His vertebrae should be kept as motionless as possible. If the person's injury is in his neck, his head and neck should be supported so that there is no movement of the cervical vertebrae.

After determining the location and the extent of the injury, the doctor tries to restore the normal contour of the spine. Traction is used frequently in treating the patient with a fracture or a dislocation of the vertebrae in the neck. This may be accomplished by the use of either tongs or a head halter. Hyperextension by the use of a special orthopedic frame is used frequently in treating the patient with a fracture or a dislocation of the lower vertebrae.

When assisting in the care of this patient, the practical nurse should remember that the patient must be turned in one piece. Skin care is of extreme importance to prevent decubitus ulcers. This patient needs an adequate intake of both food and fluids, and usually a record of his intake and output is kept. He should be checked carefully for both voiding and defecation as these are likely to be affected. Rehabilitation is an important part of this patient's treatment.

## RUPTURED INTERVERTEBRAL DISK

### Description

Vertebrae are separated by a piece of dense tissue containing cartilage. This tissue is known as an *intervertebral disk*. This serves as a cushion between the vertebrae. Each disk is surrounded by a covering. This covering may rupture and allow the inner portion of the disk to push outward. Thus, the patient has a ruptured intervertebral disk.

### Symptoms

An individual usually develops a ruptured intervertebral disk following an injury of his back, such as a strain. Frequently the patient gives a history of feeling as though something slipped in his back while bending, lifting, or reaching. The misplaced disk may press against nerve roots and cause pain or it may press against the spinal cord. The patient's pain is usually in the lower part of his back as this is the most common location of ruptured disks. However, the injury may take place in the neck vertebrae. In this case, the patient's pain would be in his neck. The patient with a ruptured disk in the lower vertebral column may have pain which goes down one leg. Exertion such as coughing, lifting, and bending increases the pain. The patient may have weakness and a loss of feeling in the part of his body supplied by the spinal nerves coming from the injured area.

### Treatment and Nursing Care

The physician may prescribe medical treatment which consists mainly of rest and traction. The purpose of these two measures is to allow the disk to return to its normal position and heal. The doctor usually recommends bed rest on a firm mattress with a fracture board beneath it. Traction may be used on both legs to obtain extension of the lower vertebrae. Head traction may be used if the ruptured disk is in the neck.

Local applications of heat may be prescribed to relieve the patient's pain. Massage may also be recommended for the same purpose.

It may be necessary for the surgeon to remove the ruptured disk. He may also do a bone graft, which strengthens the area. In this case, he removes a piece of bone from another part of the body (a long bone, such as the tibia) and places it on the vertebrae. A patient having a bone graft requires a longer period for recovery as it takes more time to heal. He has another incision which has to heal also.

The patient having surgery for a ruptured disk needs, with a few variations, the same care as other surgical patients which was discussed in Chapter 5. This patient is usually placed on a firm mattress with a fracture board beneath it. The doctor may request that the patient remain flat in bed immediately after surgery. Sometimes a body cast which reaches from the upper part of the chest to the lower part of the back is applied. The doctor may have the patient wear the cast for six to eight weeks. Some physicians allow the patient to be out of bed during this time and others do not. If the patient has had a bone graft, he may have another cast on the extremity which was used to supply the bone. The care of a patient in a cast, discussed on pages 257 to 261, applies to this patient.

The patient should be encouraged to turn himself following surgery unless otherwise ordered by the doctor. Frequently, the patient is afraid that he will injure his back by turning. In this case, he needs to be reassured that turning will not cause him to harm his back.

## EPILEPSY

### Description

An individual with epilepsy has periodic seizures. He has an abnormal discharge of energy from his brain during a seizure. This abnormal discharge of nervous energy may cause the patient to have convulsions, to lose consciousness, or to experience both.

Usually a person with epilepsy has one of the three main types of epileptic seizures. These are grand mal, petit mal, and psychomotor. The patient subject to grand mal attacks may have an aura. This is a sensation which warns him of an oncoming seizure. For example, a patient may have an aura which he describes as seeing a flash of light or feeling numb. After having the aura, he loses consciousness and has a generalized convulsion. When having a petit mal seizure, the patient loses consciousness for a few moments. This loss of consciousness generally lasts from 5 to 30 seconds. The patient may not have muscular movements or a generalized convulsion. However, he may have a jerking of small muscles rather than the generalized convulsion of grand mal attack. For instance, the patient may have a rhythmic jerking of the muscles of his face during a petit mal attack. After the seizure ends, he resumes his former activity as though nothing had happened. The patient having a psychomotor seizure has a temporary mental disturbance. He acts in a peculiar manner for a short period of time and does not remember what happened during the attack. Patients may have a variety of symptoms during a psychomotor seizure. One patient

*Jacksonian seizure - hand & foot*

may make swallowing noises, one may act dazed and mutter, and another may pull at his clothing.

## Cause

The person with epilepsy has a chronic disorder of his brain, but there is usually no organic change in his brain to account for it. However, epilepsy may occur in an individual following brain damage from a tumor, an infection, or an injury.

An individual can inherit a tendency toward developing epilepsy. A child born of parents either of whom has epilepsy or has ancestors with this disorder is more likely to develop it than is the child born into a family with no history of epilepsy. The person who has a tendency toward developing epilepsy usually starts having seizures in childhood or during adolescence.

## Treatment and Nursing Care

When the doctor suspects that a person has epilepsy, he obtains a thorough medical history from the patient and his family. In addition to doing a general physical examination, he may do a lumbar puncture so that the cerebrospinal fluid can be examined. An electroencephalogram is helpful to him in making a diagnosis. He needs an accurate description of the patient's seizures. The nurse in attendance should observe and report the patient's actions before the seizure, the time it began and ended, the part of the body affected by muscular contractions, and the presence of cyanosis. It is important to note whether the muscles relaxed during the attack. She should note whether the patient appeared unconscious and was incontinent.

The person with epilepsy needs to live as normally as possible with his disease, since no specific cure is known. He should establish a regular daily regimen which includes adequate rest. Activities which would involve a risk in case he had a seizure should be avoided. For example, he might wreck an automobile or fall into machinery during an attack.

The patient should be protected from injuring himself during a seizure. Since an epileptic is likely to have seizures at night, he should sleep with side rails on his bed. He should not sleep with removable dental appliances as these might cause him to choke during an attack. Additional measures needed by the patient having a convulsion are discussed on page 42.

Anticonvulsive drugs are helpful in controlling the convulsions of epilepsy. Phenobarbital, diphenylhydantoin (Dilantin), and trimethadione (Tridione) are three examples of drugs which may be prescribed.

## PARKINSON'S DISEASE

### Description

The patient with Parkinson's disease has a chronic disease of the nervous system. The practical nurse may hear Parkinson's disease referred to as *paralysis agitans, parkinsonism,* or *shaking palsy.*

An individual may develop Parkinson's disease at any age following encephalitis (inflammation of the brain). It may also occur in a person with cerebral arteriosclerosis. However, the cause of most cases of parkinsonism is not known. An individual is most likely to develop this disease during late middle life.

### Symptoms

During the early stages of the disease, the patient may notice weakness, trembling, and rigidity (stiffness) of the muscles in one part of his body. These symptoms gradually spread to other parts of his body. A tremor may develop while the patient is still. It usually lessens when he moves the shaking part.

The patient with a fully developed case of Parkinson's disease has an expressionless face because of the rigid muscles. His weak, rigid muscles cause his movements to be slow and stiff. When walking, he moves slowly and stiffly, does not swing his arms, and leans forward as if he were going to fall. This abnormal posture causes him to take steps which become increasingly shorter and faster. Eventually a running pace is easier for him than a walking one. Rigidity also causes the patient to have difficulty in chewing, swallowing, and talking. His speech may become weak and slurred. The tremor which developed earlier usually becomes more noticeable.

### Treatment

Unfortunately, there is no specific cure for a patient with Parkinson's disease. The physician directs his treatment toward making the patient comfortable and relieving his symptoms, such as tremors and rigidity. Drugs to relieve rigidity, rest, physical therapy, and occupational therapy may be prescribed.

## MULTIPLE SCLEROSIS

### Description

The patient with multiple sclerosis has areas of degeneration in his brain and spinal cord. These areas of degeneration occur in the myelin sheath. Nerve fibers are covered by myelin, which is a fatty sheath or covering. It may be helpful for the practical nurse to compare this sheath with the insulation on an electric wire. Electricity cannot pass through the wire if the insulation is worn away. Neither do the impulses pass through a nerve properly if the myelin sheath is diseased. When the impulses do not pass through the nerve, they do not reach the muscles. This results in either a disturbance of the function of this part of the body or in paralysis. The area has a disturbed function when it receives fewer impulses than usual. The patient is paralyzed if no impulses pass through the nerve because of the diseased myelin sheath. For example, if the patient's larynx and tongue receive fewer nerve impulses than normal, he develops speech difficulties. If his leg muscles receive fewer nerve impulses than normal, he has difficulty in walking. If his eyes receive no nerve impulses, he is unable to see.

Areas of the myelin which degenerate are replaced by scar tissue. This is known as sclerotic tissue because of its hardness. The patient develops many areas of sclerotic tissue in his brain and spinal cord. Thus, the disease is known as multiple sclerosis.

When an area of the myelin sheath begins to degenerate, it becomes edematous or swollen. The patient has symptoms of disturbed function of the part of his body supplied by that nerve. Disappearance of the edema can result in disappearance of the patient's symptoms unless the area is filled with scar tissue. This accounts for periods of time when the patient may have no symptoms; however, these reappear when the area becomes swollen again. When an area becomes sclerotic, the patient's symptoms are permanent.

The life expectancy of a patient with multiple sclerosis is usually decreased. The disease may progress either rapidly or slowly. In some cases the person lives out a normal life span and in others the patient may die in 5 to 10 years. The amount of disability from multiple sclerosis varies. Some individuals become confined to bed whereas others have only a moderate amount of disability. Infections of the lungs and urinary tract, decubitus ulcers, and malnutrition are frequent complications. The patient is more likely to develop one of these complications during the later part of his illness.

## Cause

The cause of multiple sclerosis is unknown at the present time. However, research is being done to determine its cause.

This disease usually occurs most often in individuals between 20 and 40 years of age. It seems to be more common in cold climates than in warm ones.

## Symptoms

Symptoms of multiple sclerosis vary because of the patchy distribution of the degenerating areas. The symptoms of an individual patient depend upon the location of the diseased areas and the amount of damage. In general, the patient has disturbances of motion because motor areas (those responsible for movement) are affected. The patient's voluntary muscles, (those under the control of his will) may become spastic. The muscles which receive their nerve supply from the affected part of the central nervous system may tremble. For example, the patient's hand begins to shake when he starts to pick up a glass of water. The tremor usually increases as he replaces the glass. The shaking generally disappears when he rests his hand and arm.

The patient may have difficulty in seeing. Common visual disturbances are blurred vision, difficulty in focusing the eyes, inability to control movement of the eyes, and blindness.

In addition to having difficulty with his eyes, the patient with multiple sclerosis is likely to have speech difficulties. When this happens, he may talk in a hesitant manner. His words also sound slurred.

The patient may go through periods in which he seems to be improved, only to have the symptoms return in a more exaggerated form. Intervals between the periods when the patient is not bothered with symptoms become shorter as the disease progresses. As additional areas of his central nervous system become sclerosed or hardened, the patient becomes more handicapped. He may begin to tire more easily and lose his ability to move properly. The patient may also become incontinent and paralyzed.

## Treatment and Nursing Care

Unfortunately no cure is known at the present time for the patient with multiple sclerosis. However, this does not mean that nothing can be done for him. The doctor guides the members of the health team toward rehabilitation of the patient. The aim of his rehabilitation is to help him to live as happily and effectively as possible and to remain independent for as long as possible. The patient needs to learn to live with his disability as well as to use his capabilities to the maximum. Rehabilitation is especially important during the times when the patient is not affected by the more disabling symptoms. Psychotherapy may be used to help the patient adjust to his disabling condition.

The physician may prescribe physical therapy, such as massage, warm baths, and exercise. These treatments help to strengthen the muscles, to prevent or to correct deformities, to increase muscular coordination, and to prevent atrophy (wasting away) of the muscles from lack of use. Physical therapy may be used also to relieve muscle spasm in an effort to make the patient more comfortable. The practical nurse may be asked to help the patient with prescribed exercises. The patient should avoid becoming overly tired and may need to be reminded of this. The practical nurse should encourage the patient through the long, continuous process of rehabilitation. The importance of continuing with the program under the doctor's guidance should be emphasized.

The patient may need to learn how to perform seemingly simple activities which the healthy person takes for granted. Clever devices may be purchased or made to help the person to remain independent for as long as possible. For example, the patient who has trouble in grasping objects may find it helpful to have large handles placed on objects such as his toothbrush and silverware. The bedridden patient may find the addition of a metal bar over the head of his bed of great value. This enables him to be more independent in raising himself in bed and turning. Devices to turn pages of a book can be purchased as well as equipment to project reading material on the ceiling.

Diversion plays an important part in the care of this patient. The activity selected depends upon the patient's capabilities as well as his disabilities. An example of this is seen in the patient with a visual disturbance who may not be able to read but who may be able to knit.

The physician may order certain drugs to relieve the patient of some of his symptoms. Drugs which dilate the blood vessels, such as nicotinic acid and histamine, may be prescribed. Some authorities believe that the nerve tissue has an inadequate supply of blood because the tiny arteries are smaller as a result of spasm. Thus, these drugs may be given in the hope that the blood supply can be increased by dilating the blood vessels. Drugs to relieve spastic muscles, such as neostigmine, mephenesin (Tolserol), chlorpromazine (Thorazine), zoxazolamine (Flexin), and meprobamate (Equanil), may be prescribed. The doctor may order hormones, such as cortisone and adrenocorticotropic hormone (ACTH). Vitamins, especially the B group, may be prescribed also.

The patient who is confined to bed because of his disability needs special skin care and frequent back rubs. This is important to prevent decubitus ulcers. His position should be changed frequently. The nurse should keep the patient's body in good alignment. A footboard can be used to prevent foot drop. Pillows may be used to support weak parts of the body. The incontinent patient should be kept clean and dry.

When talking with a person who has developed a speech difficulty, the practical nurse should be patient. If the person senses a feeling of impatience on the part of the listener, he is likely to have increased speech difficulty.

## MENINGITIS

### Description

The patient with meningitis has an inflammation of the meninges, the membranes which cover the brain and spinal cord. Meningitis is usually caused by pathogenic microorganisms, such as the meningococcus, the pneumococcus, the streptococcus, and the tubercle bacillus.

The invading organism usually enters the body through the nose and throat. It passes from the nose and throat into the blood stream. The organism is carried by the blood to the meninges. Remembering that the body responds to an invading organism by increasing the blood supply to the area, the practical nurse can easily understand why the cerebrospinal fluid is increased. White blood cells enter the cerebrospinal fluid in an effort to combat the infection.

## Symptoms

The patient has symptoms of an infection as well as symptoms of increased intracranial pressure when the inflammation is caused by pathogenic microorganisms. During the early part of this disease the patient usually has symptoms of an upper respiratory infection. Fever, malaise, and vomiting soon follow. The patient finds that he is more comfortable when lying on his side with his knees flexed and his head back. He complains of a headache, his neck becomes stiff, and his fever goes higher as the infection continues. The patient may develop inflamed lips, sensitiveness to light, and convulsions. He may become delirious or he may lose consciousness. Meningitis may be complicated by pneumonia and infections of the ears, sinuses, and eyes.

## Treatment and Nursing Care

The physician prescribes one of the antibiotics, such as oxytetracycline (Terramycin), or one of the sulfonamides, such as sulfadiazine, after determining which drug is effective against the invading microorganism. The principles of caring for a patient with an infection, such as rest, increased intake of fluid, diet high in calories, and good skin and mouth care apply to this patient. These are discussed in more detail in Chapter 6.

The patient should have bed rest in a quiet room. His eyes should be protected from light. This can be done by adjusting the shades and the lighting fixtures so that there is no glare or direct light shining in his eyes. The nurse in attendance should be prepared to protect the patient from injuring himself in case he has a convulsion. The patient's position should be changed frequently. It may be less painful for the patient if two people turn him.

The patient is placed in an isolation unit during the infectious stage. An individual caring for this patient should wear a gown to protect her clothing and a face mask. When assisting in the care of a person with meningitis, the practical nurse should follow the isolation procedure used in that particular hospital. In some institutions the gown is used again and in others a clean gown is worn each time a person enters the unit. The nurse should wash her hands thoroughly before and after caring for the patient. This helps to prevent carrying infection to the patient as well as away from him to others.

Meningitis is usually spread by secretions from the upper respiratory tract. Because of this, paper tissues soiled with secretions from the nose and throat should be collected in a paper bag and burned. Soiled linen should be disinfected according to the hospital procedure. For example, it may be boiled for 30 minutes or it may be soaked in a disinfectant. Equipment used for treatments as well as dishes should be boiled. The room should be cleaned thoroughly and aired for 24 hours before being used by another patient. The mattress and pillows should be placed in direct sunlight for 24 hours.

## POLIOMYELITIS

### Description

The patient with poliomyelitis has an infectious disease caused by a filtrable virus. This is a virus so small that it can pass through a fine filter, such as porcelain. After entering the body, the virus can spread to the central nervous system and affect the spinal cord and the brain. The infection frequently involves the anterior portion of the gray matter in the spinal cord. (This gray matter which is in the center of the cord is made of nerve cells). In this case, the patient has *acute anterior poliomyelitis*. The part of the brain which is more often affected is the medulla. In this case, the patient has *bulbar poliomyelitis*. The respiratory and the circulatory centers in the medulla may be involved. This can result in respiratory and circulatory failure.

The patient regains use of the affected muscles if the nerve cells are not injured too severely. Muscles supplied by nerve cells which die are paralyzed permanently. However, this does not mean that other muscles cannot be trained to take over some of the job previously performed by the paralyzed muscles.

Poliomyelitis may occur in epidemic form, especially during the summer and fall. It can affect older children and adults, but is more common in young children. The exact manner in which poliomyelitis is spread is not completely understood. However, it is thought that the virus may enter the body through either the gastrointestinal tract or the upper respiratory system.

## Symptoms

The patient frequently has symptoms of an infection, such as fever, malaise, and headache during the early stage of poliomyelitis. Symptoms of a gastrointestinal disturbance, such as vomiting and diarrhea, are common. Symptoms of an upper respiratory infection, such as a sore throat, are likely to develop during this stage. The infection may end here. This patient makes a rapid recovery and may not know that he has had poliomyelitis.

Infection which spreads to the spinal cord causes the patient to have pain in the muscles supplied by the area which is inflamed. His neck may also become stiff and sore. The affected muscles may become weak and paralyzed. They soon begin to atrophy, or become smaller. Muscles in the legs, arms, back, and shoulders are frequently affected. Muscles of the face and chest may be involved also. The patient is likely to have difficulty in talking, in swallowing, and in breathing when the medulla is affected. The location and the amount of paralysis depend upon the area of the central nervous system which is affected as well as the amount of damage. The acute symptoms of fever, malaise, and pain usually disappear in five to six weeks. The patient may be left with paralyzed muscles which can result in deformities, or he may have no paralysis.

## Prevention

A vaccine is used to prevent paralytic poliomyelitis. This vaccine, which was developed by Dr. Jonas E. Salk, is prepared from the three types of poliomyelitis viruses. Although the viruses are killed, they retain their ability to cause the human body to produce antibodies. In other words, the person who has received the poliomyelitis vaccine has antibodies in his blood which combat the poliomyelitis virus if it enters his blood stream. However, the fact that this vaccine exists does not wipe out the disease. Individuals likely to develop poliomyelitis must receive this preventive medicine if they are to benefit by it. The practical nurse is often in a position to encourage relatives or friends to consult their doctor about being given the poliomyelitis vaccine. She can also encourage them to receive the full course of treatment, which currently consists of three injections.

### Treatment and Nursing Care

Bed rest is prescribed for the patient during the acute stage of poliomyelitis. Measures to prevent deformities should be started early. The patient should be placed on a firm mattress which has a fracture board under it. A board can be placed at the foot of the bed to keep the patient's feet in a good position. The doctor usually recommends that the patient be placed in a natural position on either his back or his abdomen with his arms at his side. The nurse in attendance should keep the patient's body in good alignment. The nurse should handle the patient's affected extremities gently to avoid hurting him.

The practical nurse may be asked to make the patient's bed with blankets instead of linen. Cotton blankets are used frequently because they absorb moisture more quickly than sheets. The patient's bed should be kept dry and free of wrinkles to prevent skin irritation.

The patient with poliomyelitis should be placed in isolation during the acute stage. He may be isolated with a group of patients affected with the same disease, or he may be isolated separately. Discharges from the patient's nose, throat, and mouth should be collected in paper tissues which are placed in a paper bag and later burned. Laundry, dishes, and equipment used for treatments should be either sterilized or disinfected. It may be necessary to disinfect all waste material from the body before allowing it to enter the sewage disposal system. This is necessary because body wastes, especially from the intestines, may contain the poliomyelitis virus. Disinfecting all of the patient's waste materials may not be necessary in some localities because of an effective sewage disposal system. The nursing team should follow the rules of the local health department regarding this.

Retention of urine and constipation occur frequently during the acute stage. For this reason, the patient's elimination should be checked carefully.

The physician may prescribe a form of the Kenny method of treating the patient with poliomyelitis. This type of treatment includes warm, moist packs, and physical therapy. Moist heat to the affected area relieves muscle spasm and pain. It also stimulates circulation in the affected part.

Wool or part-wool blankets are cut the size and shape of the area being treated. The pieces may be folded or two pieces may be sewed together so that the pack is made of two thicknesses. The packs can be made hot and moist by wringing them out of boiling water with a wringer or by using a hot-pack machine. The warm moist packs are applied to the affected muscles. Care should be taken to avoid burning the patient. The warm pack is covered with waterproof material, and a piece of dry woolen material is then placed over the waterproof material. This helps to retain the heat. The doctor designates the frequency with which the nurse is to apply the packs.

Physical therapy is generally started during the early part of the paralyzed patient's illness. The program, which usually consists of rest, exercise, muscle re-education, and heat, may be continued for several years. The patient should be encouraged to continue with this plan of treatment until he has been rehabilitated to the maximum. The affected muscles can be re-educated to an amazing degree. The patient may be taught to use unaffected muscles to perform a particular function.

The physician attempts to correct any deformities which might have developed. Braces, physical therapy, and surgery may be used to accomplish this aim. Surgery may be done also to improve the function of a group of muscles. For example, a tendon in the thumb can be transplanted in order to improve the ability of the involved muscles to grasp and hold objects.

## HERPES ZOSTER

### Description

The patient with herpes zoster (shingles) has an infection of a group of nerves, which is caused by a virus. The patient develops an inflammation of either his skin or mucous membrane along the course of the nerve from the infected area. The inflammation often occurs along the course of an intercostal nerve (one between the ribs).

Generally the first symptom experienced by the patient is severe pain along the path of the nerve. This is soon followed by the formation of vesicles, which are tiny sacs containing fluid. The patient may continue to have pain after the vesicles have disappeared. Herpes zoster can be serious in either a debilitated or an elderly person.

### Treatment

The doctor directs treatment toward making the patient comfortable, since no specific therapy is known. Drugs, such as aspirin, codeine, and sometimes morphine, may be ordered to relieve the patient's pain. The physician may prescribe the application of a soothing powder or lotion.

## NEURITIS

### Description

The patient with neuritis has an inflammation of one or more nerves. Neuritis may be caused by injury of a nerve. For example, the nerve in the arm may be injured by pressure from the improper use of crutches. Infections, pressure from a growing tumor, deficiency of vitamins, metabolic disturbances such as diabetes, and poisons, such as arsenic, lead, and mercury, are some additional causes of neuritis.

The practical nurse may hear the physician speak of different types of neuritis. It should be helpful to her to know that this condition may be classified in various ways. For instance, neuritis may be classified according to its cause. Alcoholic neuritis is caused by drinking an excessive amount of alcohol. Neuritis may also be classified according to the number of nerves involved. The term multiple neuritis is used to refer to a patient having several nerves inflamed, whereas the patient with mononeuritis has one nerve inflamed. These are only a few of the different types of neuritis.

The patient with neuritis has varying degrees of pain depending upon the location and amount of inflammation. The amount of pain may range from a burning and uncomfortable sensation to severe pain. The patient may develop weakness and paralysis of the part supplied by the affected nerve or nerves.

Treatment

The physician directs treatment toward removing the underlying cause if possible. For instance, the patient with a vitamin deficiency is treated with vitamins, the patient with diabetes is treated for this disease, and the patient with an injury is treated for this.

## NEURALGIA

Description

The patient with neuralgia has pain along the course of a nerve or nerves. He has periods of severe, stabbing pain. These periods of pain usually last for a short length of time, disappear, and then return. Neuralgia may last for weeks and sometimes many months. The patient may have no inflammation to account for his pain or he may have a lesion which irritates the nerve. For example, a growing tumor may press on a nerve and cause pain.

Neuralgia is often classified according to the nerve affected. For instance, a person with intercostal neuralgia has pain radiating along the path of one or more intercostal nerves in the chest. The patient with trigeminal or facial neuralgia has pain along the pathway of the trigeminal nerve in the face.

Treatment

The physician tries to determine whether or not there is an underlying cause of the patient's neuralgia. He directs his treatment toward relieving the underlying cause if one is found. Bed rest may be recommended for the patient with an acute case of neuralgia. Salicylates, such as aspirin, are frequently prescribed to relieve pain. The local application of heat by an electric heating pad or a hot-water bottle may be ordered to relieve discomfort. The physical therapist may be asked to apply additional heat to the painful area by the use of a diathermy machine or an infrared lamp.

In some cases, the doctor blocks the nerve by injecting alcohol. This substance causes temporary paralysis which relieves pain. It may be necessary for the physician to cut the affected nerve if the patient continues to have severe pain.

## SCIATICA

### Description

An individual with sciatica has neuralgic pain along the course of the sciatic nerve. This is a large nerve which leaves the lower part of the spine and goes down the back of each leg.

A person with sciatica has pain which radiates down his thigh and the back of his leg. Exercise such as walking usually increases the pain. He may also have a feeling of numbness, tingling, and tenderness along the pathway of the sciatic nerve.

Sciatica may result from injury, inflammation of the nerve, and unknown causes. A ruptured intervertebral disk, arthritis, and sprain of the lower part of the back are examples of some of the causes of injury to the sciatic nerve. An individual may have an attack of sciatica after becoming chilled. The patient with sciatica is treated in a similar way to the one with neuralgia.

## SUGGESTIONS FOR STUDY

1. Review the functions of various parts of the brain.
2. Which nerves control the functions of your head? Your body?
3. Define the following in your own words: encephalography, ventriculography, electroencephalogram, neurologist, decompression, herpes zoster, neuralgia, and sciatica.
4. What factors determine the symptoms experienced by a patient with an intracranial tumor?
5. Review the symptoms of increased intracranial pressure.
6. Members of the nursing team should observe the patient suspected of having a brain injury for what symptoms?
7. Discuss the nursing care of a patient who has had brain surgery.
8. What could account for the disappearance of paralysis in a patient recovering from a spinal cord injury?
9. What is a ruptured intervertebral disk?
10. Review the three main types of epilepsy.
11. Does the patient with epilepsy always have convulsions?
12. Describe the symptoms usually seen in a patient with paralysis agitans.
13. Review the changes which occur in the spinal cord and brain of a person with multiple sclerosis.

14. What age group is most often affected by multiple sclerosis?
15. How does the shaking of a patient with Parkinson's disease differ from the shaking of a person with multiple sclerosis?
16. Discuss the nursing care of a patient with meningitis.
17. Review the care needed by a patient with poliomyelitis which has caused paralysis.

### REFERENCES FOR CHAPTER 21

Boyd, Theodore E.: "How the Present Poliomyelitis Vaccine Was Discovered," *Am. J. Nursing*, **57**:722-25, (June) 1957.

Brooks, Stewart M.: *Basic Facts of Medical Microbiology*. W. B. Saunders Co., Philadelphia, 1958, pp. 157-61.

Brown, Amy F., *Medical Nursing*, 3rd ed. W. B. Saunders Co., Philadelphia, 1957, pp. 494-95, 610-84, and 747-52.

Carini, Esta, and de Gutierrez-Mahoney, C. G.: "Head Injuries," *Am. J. Nursing*, **56**:54-58, (Jan.) 1956.

Carter, Charles F., and Smith, Alice L.: *Principles of Microbiology*, 3rd ed. C. V. Mosby Co., St. Louis, 1957, pp. 287-88 and 463-67.

Eliason, Eldridge; Ferguson, L. Kraeer; and Sholtis, Lillian A.: *Surgical Nursing*, 10th ed. J. B. Lippincott Co., Philadelphia, 1955, pp. 481-524.

Emerson, Charles P., Jr., and Bragdon, Jane S.: *Essentials of Medicine*, 17th ed. J. B. Lippincott Co., Philadelphia, 1955, pp. 600-672 and 824-31.

Gorson, Albert G.: "The Practical Nurse and Epilepsy," *Practical Nurses Digest*, **4**:9-10, (Mar.) 1957.

Gotten, Nicholas, and Wilson, Letitia: *Neurologic Nursing*, 3rd ed. F. A. Davis Co., Philadelphia, 1957.

Hodges, Lucien R.: "Tumors of the Brain," *Am. J. Nursing*, **58**:58-60, (Jan.) 1958.

Holcomb, Kathryn L.: "Diagnosis: Multiple Sclerosis—and Katie Fights Back," *Am. J. Nursing*, **55**:467-70, (Apr.) 1955.

Hull, Edgar, and Perrodin, Cecilia: *Medical Nursing*, 5th ed. F. A. Davis Co., Philadelphia, 1954, pp. 522-46.

Jensen, Julius, and Jensen, Deborah: *Nursing in Clinical Medicine*, 4th ed. The Macmillan Company, New York, 1954, pp. 570-634, 667-71, and 697-700.

Kimber, Diana; Gray, Carolyn E.; Stackpole, Caroline E.; and Leavell, Lutie C.: *Textbook of Anatomy and Physiology*, 13th ed. The Macmillan Company, New York, 1955, pp. 217-311.

Larson, Carroll B., and Gould, Marjorie: *Calderwood's Orthopedic*

*Nursing*, 4th ed. C. V. Mosby Co., St. Louis, 1957, pp. 371-437, 479-82, and 488-96.

Magee, Kenneth R., and Elliott, Alta: "Parkinson's Disease," *Am. J. Nursing*, 55:814-18, (July) 1955.

Martin, John, and Craig, Iris: "The Early Care of Patients with Injury of the Spinal Cord," *Am. J. Nursing*, 55:936-39, (Aug.) 1955.

Musser, Ruth D., and Bird, Joseph G.: *Modern Pharmacology and Therapeutics.* The Macmillan Company, New York, 1958, pp. 347-54.

O'Leary, James L.: "Electroencephalography," *Am. J. Nursing*, 55:1238-41, (Oct.) 1955.

Palmer, Mary E.: "Nursing the Patient with Multiple Sclerosis," *Am. J. Nursing*, 57:753-55, (June) 1957.

"Polio Is Still a Threat," *Am. J. Nursing*, 57:41, (Jan.) 1957.

Proudfit, Fairfax T., and Robinson, Corinne H.: *Nutrition and Diet Therapy*, 11th ed. The Macmillan Company, New York, 1955, pp. 450-57.

Raney, Rupert B.: "The Minor Concussion," *Am. J. Nursing*, 57:1444-45, (Nov.) 1957.

Schumacher, George A.: "Multiple Sclerosis," *Am. J. Nursing*, 57:751-53, (June) 1957.

Solomon, Charles, and Gill, Elizabeth S.: *Pharmacology and Therapeutics*, 7th ed. J. B. Lippincott Co., Philadelphia, 1956, pp. 199-203.

Stafford, Edward S., and Diller, Doris: *Surgery and Surgical Nursing*, 3rd. ed. W. B. Saunders Co., Philadelphia, 1958, pp. 348-73.

Taufic, Marjorie: "Rehabilitation after Craniotomy," *Am. J. Nursing*, 58:61-63, (Jan.) 1958.

Turner, C. E.: *Personal and Community Health*, 10th ed. C. V. Mosby Co., St. Louis, 1956, pp. 434-36.

*[Handwritten notes:]*

May 18, 1966

Practical Nursing Book
Psychiatric Nursing

Unit 12
Chapter 60 - P. 519
Chapter 62 - P. 569?

Intractable pain - drugs do not relie[ve]
Lobotomy - in brain sever nerves - no pa[in]
Cordotomy - for pelvic pain - sensory
nerves are cut

*Nursing the Patient*

*with a Disease of*

*the Eye and the Ear* & Skin

Test 6/ /66

PART X

Thu 8,441

# Chapter 22

# THE PATIENT WITH A DISEASE OF THE EYE

## STRUCTURE AND FUNCTION

Eyes are the organs of vision. Each eye is a rounded organ which is located in a bony cavity of the skull. This cavity which is cone-shaped has an opening in the back portion. The optic nerve, which is the nerve leading from the eye, and blood vessels pass through this opening into the cranial cavity. The front part of the eye is covered by eyelids which protect it. The eyelids are lined with a mucous membrane known as the conjunctiva. A thin layer of this membrane covers the front part of the eyeball. Eyebrows also help to protect the eye. Six muscles are attached to each eye for movement.

The exposed surface of the eyeball is moistened by tears. This fluid is produced by the tear glands which are called lacrimal glands. These glands are located above the eyeballs. After moistening the outer surface of the eye, the tears drain into lacrimal ducts which lead to the nose. This fluid overflows and runs down the cheek when it is not carried away fast enough.

The three coats, or layers of tissue, which make up the eyeball are the fibrous coat, the uvea or uveal tract, and the retina.

The sclera and the cornea form the outer fibrous coat. The sclera is the white, outer membrane which covers most of the eyeball. It extends from the back of the eyeball to the iris, which is the colored

387

part of the eye. The sclera joins the cornea in the front part of the eye. The _cornea_ is the transparent (clear) membrane which covers the iris and the pupil. Light enters the eye through this transparent window which is approximately 1.2 cm (½ in.) in diameter. The cornea normally has no blood vessels and it receives nourishment from lymph.

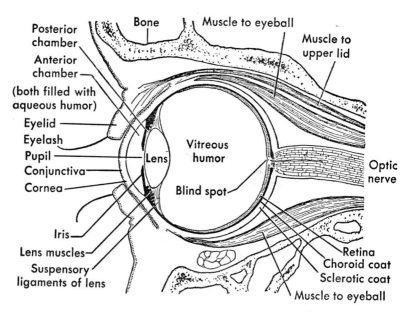

Figure 42.   Diagrammatic median section of the human eye and associated structures. (Woodruff, Lorande L., and Baitsell, George A.: _Foundations of Biology,_ 7th ed. The Macmillan Company, New York, 1951.)

The middle layer of the eyeball which is known as the _uvea_ or _uveal tract_ is made of the choroid, the ciliary body, and the iris. The _choroid_ is the structure which lines the sclera. The choroid has a rich supply of blood vessels. The _ciliary body_, which is attached to the front part of the choroid, contains blood vessels, nerves, and a muscle called the _ciliary muscle._ The third part of the uveal tract is the _iris._ This is the rounded, colored portion of the eye which is behind the cornea. The black circle in the middle of the iris is an opening known as the *pupil*. Light passes through the center of the eyeball by way of this opening. Muscles in the iris control the size of the pupil.

The *retina* is the inner coat of the eyeball. It is a sensitive membrane containing many nerve cells. Light rays are normally focused on the retina, and an image is formed.

The *crystalline lens* is a transparent body filled with a jellylike substance and is surrounded by an elastic capsule. The lens is located behind the pupil. The ciliary muscle which is attached to the side of the lens can change the shape of the lens by contracting and relaxing.

The crystalline lens divides the cavity within the eyeball into two parts. The cavity in front of the lens is filled with a clear, watery fluid known as *aqueous humor*. The cavity behind the lens is filled with fluid called the *vitreous humor*. This fluid resembles clear jelly. The vitreous humor plays an important role in helping the eye to maintain its shape.

## Vision

Perfect vision depends upon proper accommodation, refraction of the light rays, proper functioning of the pupils, teamwork between the two eyes, and transmission of nerve impulses to the brain. The ability of a person to adjust or focus his eyes on objects at varying distances is known as *accommodation*. This is made possible by a change in the shape of the crystalline lens. The ciliary muscle attached to the side of the lens contracts and relaxes. This causes the lens to change its shape so that rays of light from various distances can be focused properly on the retina. An individual loses his ability to focus his eyes properly as he grows older because the tissue involved becomes less elastic.

*Refraction* is the bending of light rays. These rays must be bent so that they are brought into focus on the retina in order for a person to see properly. The cornea, the aqueous humor, the crystalline lens, and the vitreous humor refract (bend) the light rays so that they are focused properly on the retina. The direction of a light ray is changed when it passes through a transparent substance of different density. For example, the direction of a light ray is changed when it passes at an angle from the air into water. This light ray is refracted or bent. A person has defective vision when the light rays entering his eyes are not focused properly on the retina. This type of visual defect is known as an *error of refraction.* An eye examination to determine this type of visual defect is spoken of as *refraction of the eye.* In other words the doctor measures the ability of a person's eyes to bend light rays.

The pupils must become larger and smaller in order to control the light rays entering the eye. The size of the pupil is controlled by the circular muscle in the iris. When the muscle contracts, it causes the pupil to become smaller. This reduces the amount of light entering the eye. When the muscle of the iris relaxes, it causes the pupil to become larger. This increases the amount of light entering the eye.

An individual normally has two eyes which function as a team so that he sees one object instead of two when he uses both eyes. Teamwork between the two eyes enables a person to determine distance and depth more accurately.

Nerve impulses caused by the light rays which form an image on the retina must be carried to the brain in order for a person to see. These impulses are carried by the optic nerve to the center of sight in the brain. A person is able to see when this area in the brain interprets the impulses as a sensation of color and form. An individual has good vision when (1) he has proper accommodation of the lens, (2) the clear structures within the eyeball refract the light rays so that they are focused on the retina, (3) the pupils react to light properly, (4) the two eyes work together, and (5) the nerve impulses are transmitted to the center of sight in the brain.

## HYGIENE OF THE EYES

The ability to see is a priceless gift which is made possible by the proper functioning of our eyes. In many cases these organs of sight are unknowingly subjected to harmful conditions. The public is becoming more interested in learning how to avoid these harmful conditions and to conserve sight. Many industries have active programs directed toward protecting the workers' eyesight. For example, they provide adequate lighting for their employees. They also provide protection for their workers' eyes from extreme heat and light.

Another example of the public's interest in the conservation of sight is seen in the construction of schools. Adequate lighting is considered as an essential factor when building a new school.

Eyestrain frequently results from using the eyes for close work, especially under unfavorable conditions. For example, reading in a moving car can cause eyestrain. The muscles which control the movement of the eyeball as well as those within the eye which control the entrance of light rays attempt to carry out the individual's wishes regarding his vision. The muscles become tired because of this abnormal effort to pull the eye into focus. The person's eyes become strained.

The practical nurse should be familiar with the measures which are important to eye health. Remembering that eyestrain frequently follows use of the eyes for close work, the practical nurse can easily understand the importance of good lighting for such activities. The light should come from above and behind the person engaged in close work. The individual should rest his eyes frequently by gazing into the distance. This allows the eye muscles to relax.

Glare such as that which comes from an unshaded lamp in front of a person's work should be avoided. The muscles of the iris react to glare by contracting in order to reduce the amount of light which enters the eye. This can result in eyestrain.

An individual should protect his eyes from direct rays of the sun as these may destroy parts of the retina. Sunglasses are used commonly for this purpose.

Cleanliness is an important measure in the prevention of eye infection. The skin about the eyes should be kept clean by the use of soap and water. Clean washcloths and towels should be used. Also, these should not be used by another person. The habit of rubbing one's eyes with his fingers is not safe because of the possibility of carrying an infection to them.

A foreign body in the eye, such as a particle of dust or ash, should be removed with care. When a person gets something in his eye he usually has an increased amount of tears and blinks more frequently. These natural reactions of the eye may wash the foreign body away. It may be necessary to turn the top eyelid inside out so that the object can be located. In some cases the foreign body may be removed by gently touching it with a sterile cotton applicator which has been moistened with sterile water or saline solution. The person should consult his physician if the particle is not immediately removed. He should also see the doctor when the foreign body is located in the cornea. An individual with a foreign particle embedded in his eyeball may need surgery to have it removed. The physician may remove a particle of steel with a magnet. Additional treatment may be necessary dependent upon the amount of injury to the eye.

The practical nurse should know the symptoms of eye trouble. A burning sensation, itching, inflammation, and pain in the eyes should indicate to the person that he needs to consult an eye physician. Disturbances of vision, such as spots before the eyes, having to hold reading material too close or too far from the eyes, and blurred vision, are also symptoms of eye trouble.

## COMMON VISUAL DEFECTS

### Introduction

Glasses are prescribed frequently to correct common visual defects. *Glasses* are lenses which help the crystalline lens of the eye to bring light rays into focus on the retina. In other words, glass lenses are used when a person has difficulty in focusing his eyes properly. These lenses are ground so that the person has either an artificial curvature or a lack of curvature to compensate for the eye defect.

The *ophthalmologist*, who is also called an *oculist*, is a physician specializing in the diagnosis and treatment of a person with a disease or a defect of the eye. He has been prepared to treat a person with an eye defect or disease either medically or surgically. An ophthalmologist can frequently determine whether or not the patient has a condition in his eye which is caused by a disease elsewhere in his body, such as syphilis, arteriosclerosis, diabetes, certain types of kidney disease, and a brain tumor. The ophthalmologist gives the patient a prescription for glasses when necessary. This prescription can be filled by an *optician*. He is an individual who grinds the lenses according to the doctor's recommendation. The optician can be compared with the pharmacist who fills the doctor's prescription for medicine. The optician is not licensed to examine a person's eyes or to test vision.

The *optometrist* is an individual who is licensed to measure the visual powers of a person. He can recommend glasses or exercises to correct a visual defect. Since he is not a physician, he is not allowed to use drugs to aid in the eye examination or to prescribe drugs.

## Nearsightedness

A person with nearsightedness, which is also called *myopia*, can see better when objects are close to him. Myopia occurs when an individual's eyeball is too long or the crystalline lens is too rounded. Light rays entering his eye are focused in front of the retina rather than on it. Nearsightedness can be corrected by glass lenses which cause the light rays to be focused properly on the retina.

## Farsightedness

A person with farsightedness, which is also called *hypermetropia*, can see better when objects are at a distance from him. Hypermetropia occurs when an individual's eyeball is too short or when the lens or cornea is too flat. Light rays entering the eye are focused behind the retina rather than on it. Farsightedness can be corrected by glasses which cause the light rays to be focused properly on the retina.

## Astigmatism

An individual with astigmatism has an irregular curvature of the cornea or of the crystalline lens. This prevents the light rays from focusing at one point on the retina. As a result, the image formed on the retina is blurred. Thus, the patient with astigmatism has blurred vision. This type of visual defect can also be corrected by glasses.

## Presbyopia

A person with presbyopia may see distant objects distinctly but he cannot see close objects clearly. This condition occurs with the aging process. The crystalline lenses become less elastic. This decreases the power of accomodation of the lenses. Glasses can be prescribed to improve this type of visual defect also.

## STYE

### Description

The patient with a stye has an acute inflammation on the edge of his eyelid. It is known also as a *hordeolum*. The area becomes red, swollen, and painful.

### Treatment

The doctor generally recommends the application of warm compresses. The patient's head should be turned to the side so that the solution cannot run into the unaffected eye. The hands should be washed thoroughly before and after applying the compresses to prevent spreading the infection. The application of heat usually causes the stye to drain. In some cases the doctor has to make a small incision into the infected area to allow for drainage. It usually heals after the pus has been removed.

## CONJUNCTIVITIS

### Description

A person with conjunctivitis has an inflammation of the conjunctiva. It may be caused by an infection, an allergy, or an injury.

### Symptoms

The patient usually has redness and swelling of the conjunctiva. His discomfort may range from a feeling of having grit in the affected eye to acute pain. He usually has an increased amount of tears. He may complain of burning and itching, especially when the inflammation is caused by an allergy. A discharge containing pus generally occurs when the inflammation is caused by the gonococcus. The patient with conjunctivitis may develop an infection of the cornea, if he is not treated.

### Treatment

The doctor directs his treatment toward relieving the underlying cause of the inflammation. For example, suitable drugs are prescribed to combat infection. The doctor may prescribe an antihistamine for the patient with an allergy. He may also attempt to determine and to remove the substance to which the patient is allergic. Irrigation of the affected eye and the instillation of mild antiseptic drops may be ordered.

## STRABISMUS

### Description

An individual with strabismus is unable to direct both eyes toward the same object. This is caused by a lack of coordination between the muscles which control the movement of the eyes. The person is said to be *cross-eyed* when the eye is turned toward the nose and *wall-eyed* when the eye turns outward. Strabismus is known also as *squint*.

### Cause

Squint may be congenital. This is the case commonly in children. An individual may also develop strabismus because of paralysis of the nerves which supply the eye muscles.

### Treatment

The doctor prescribes glasses and muscle exercise in some cases. However, many patients require surgery for correction. The ophthalmologist changes the position of the faulty muscles during the operation. He may have to do surgery several times in order to correct the condition. Unlike most patients following eye surgery, this patient usually is allowed to be out of bed soon after operation. Also, he generally does not have to keep his head still. The reason for this difference is that the surgeon was dealing with muscles outside the eyeball and the eye was not opened.

## ULCERATION OF THE CORNEA

### Description

An individual with an ulceration of the cornea has an open lesion of this transparent membrane. A corneal ulcer frequently follows an infection of the eye, such as conjunctivitis or an injury to the cornea.

## Symptoms

Although ulceration of the cornea may cause the patient to have no great discomfort, it can cause him to experience pain and discomfort from light. He may also have an increased amount of tears.

A scar may form in the area of the corneal ulcer during the healing progress. The practical nurse can realize the seriousness of this condition when she remembers that the cornea normally is transparent. Light rays must pass through this clear window into the eye for a person to see. If the scar is located directly over the pupil, it prevents light rays from entering the eye. Thus the person has diminished or no vision in the affected eye.

## Treatment

The physician may prescribe a medication, such as atropine, to dilate the pupil. This causes the ciliary and iris muscles to rest. Another means of resting the eye is the application of a dressing over the affected eye. An antibiotic ointment may be ordered to combat infection. The doctor may order warm compresses to the eye to relieve pain and to help the healing process.

The ophthalmologist may find it necessary to remove the diseased tissue from the cornea. Following this he may cover the area with a tiny flap of the conjunctiva. In general, this type of treatment is used when there is danger of the ulcer perforating. This could happen if the patient exerted himself suddenly, such as by sneezing or coughing. Perforation could result in loss of sight as well as loss of the eye.

An operation known as either a *corneal transplant* or as *keratoplasty* may be performed on the patient who has little or no vision because of a scarred cornea. In this procedure, the ophthalmologist removes the damaged cornea and puts in its place another piece of cornea. This tissue which is transplanted in the patient's eye was removed earlier from the eye of a deceased person. Eye banks are being established in various areas throughout the country to receive these eyes and to make the corneas available to surgeons. Some civic organizations aid in obtaining donor eyes by encouraging individuals to donate their eyes to a specific bank. The eyes are removed soon after death and shipped immediately. Such groups as local police, volunteer motor corps drivers, and airline employees work together closely to speed this delivery to the eye bank. A cornea suitable for transplantation is then made available to the surgeon. He in turn has the next patient on the list hospitalized. After removing the damaged cornea from the patient's eye and putting the donated tissue in its place, the surgeon sutures the new piece of cornea into place. This patient needs the nursing care which is discussed later in this chapter under the heading "Nursing the Patient Having Eye Surgery" (pp. 401-5). Usually his sight is slow to return following a corneal transplant. The doctor generally advises him to wear dark glasses and to avoid straining his eyes by overuse.

## CATARACT

### Description

The patient with a cataract has a clouding (opacity) of the crystalline lens. The capsule surrounding the lens may become cloudy also. Cataracts may develop in both eyes. Remembering that light rays enter the eye through the clear lens, the practical nurse can readily understand that the patient with a cataract has a decrease in vision.

### Cause

An infant may be born with cataracts. When this occurs the condition is known as *congenital cataracts*. An individual may develop a cataract later in life because of injury or a disease affecting another part of the eye, such as an inflammation of the choroid. This condition may also be associated with a disease elsewhere in the body, such as diabetes. A person is more likely to develop a cataract later in life in connection with the aging process. Thus, cataracts are more common in older people.

### Symptoms

The patient with a cataract has blurred vision. He finds it necessary to hold reading material or work closer to his eyes. He may notice that a piece appears to be missing from an object. Or he may notice that he sees black spots which move when he moves his eyes. These symptoms occur as a result of local areas of cloudiness within the crystalline lens. The patient continues to lose his vision as the clouding process continues within the lens.

### Treatment

The ophthalmologist treats the patient with a cataract by surgical removal. This offers the patient a good chance for having his sight restored. Surgery for the removal of a cataract usually is carried out under local anesthesia. This is done to prevent strain on the incision of the eye from nausea and vomiting which frequently follow general anesthesia. The nursing care of a patient having eye surgery which is discussed later in this chapter is applicable to the patient having a cataract removed.

The surgeon may not remove the cataract until it is mature. This means that all of the jellylike substance in the lens has become cloudy. Frequently the patient who has cataracts in both eyes has only one removed at a time. This is done in case the patient should have complications which would interfere with the success of the surgery.

Approximately six to seven weeks after removal of the cataract, the patient usually is tested for glasses. Properly fitted lenses should enable the patient to have vision which is almost normal. However, the practical nurse needs to understand that the patient's vision does not change to near perfect as soon as the glasses are fitted. The patient has to become adjusted to the new lenses before he can achieve the maximum amount of vision.

### GLAUCOMA

#### Description

A person with glaucoma has increased pressure within the eyeball. This is a serious eye disease which eventually results in blindness if not treated. It is one of the leading causes of blindness in the United States. Glaucoma is more common in individuals over 45 years of age.

#### Cause

The exact cause of glaucoma is unknown. However, it is generally believed to be associated with the improper drainage of a normal fluid (aqueous humor) of the eye. Also, glaucoma may follow other diseases of the eye such as an inflammation of the iris.

## Symptoms

An individual may have either acute or chronic glaucoma. In an acute case, the patient often complains of pain in the diseased eye and may have nausea and vomiting. The pupil of the affected eye is dilated. The patient also has increased tension within the eyeball. This is determined by the ophthalmologist who measures the tension within the eye with an instrument called the *tonometer*.

The person with chronic glaucoma may be only vaguely aware of gradual impairment of vision. Frequently this patient has one eye involved and then the other one. His symptoms develop slowly over a period of time. One of the main symptoms noticed by the patient is that his side vision is not as good as it used to be. He may also have difficulty in adjusting his eyes to darkened rooms.

## Treatment

The ophthalmologist directs his treatment of the patient with glaucoma toward reducing the tension within the eyeball. He may prescribe drugs to contract the pupil, perform surgery to improve drainage of aqueous humor, or both. If the patient has surgery, he needs the nursing care which is discussed later in this chapter under the heading "Nursing the Patient Having Eye Surgery." At the present time, sight which the person has lost because of this condition cannot be restored. However, the above treatment can be used successfully in many cases of early glaucoma to prevent further loss of vision. For this reason, a person with symptoms of glaucoma should be encouraged to consult a competent physician. Individuals over 40 years of age should have an eye examination by an ophthalmologist at least once every two years.

After the patient has used drugs to contract his pupil, he generally has to continue their use. These should be used regularly as prescribed by the doctor. Surgery may have to be repeated in an effort to maintain proper drainage of the eye fluid. The patient with glaucoma should avoid strenuous physical exercise, such as lifting heavy objects, because of its affect on the tension within the eye. Emotional upsets, such as worry and excitement, should be avoided for the same reason. The patient should be encouraged to continue his regular visits to the doctor as he needs continuous treatment to prevent further loss of vision.

## DETACHMENT OF THE RETINA

### Description

Normally the retina fits against the choroid. An individual has a detachment of the retina when this membrane becomes separated from the choroid. The separation may be either partial or complete. The practical nurse may find it helpful to think of a detached retina as being similar to wallpaper which has become loose from the wall. The retina has become loose from the choroid layer of the eyeball.

### Cause

Detachment of the retina may be caused by such factors as a tumor of the eye, an eye injury, or an accident which causes the person to be shaken up although he may have no direct injury to the eye. An individual with a severe case of myopia may develop this condition. An older person may have a detached retina because of degenerative changes in the eye associated with the aging process. It can also occur for no apparent reason.

### Symptoms

Recalling that light rays must be focused properly on the sensitive retina in order for a person to see helps the practical nurse to remember that a detached retina causes a loss of vision. This loss of vision may be either partial or complete depending upon the location and amount of retinal detachment.

### Treatment

The physician generally prescribes complete bed rest for the patient with a detachment of the retina. The practical nurse can expect the doctor to order a bandage, an eye mask, or pinhole glasses for both eyes. *Pinhole glasses* are dark glasses with a tiny opening in the center of each lens. The patient can see straight ahead through these small openings. Pinhole glasses help the patient to avoid moving his eyes excessively. Occasionally, bed rest with a fixed head position and covering the eyes cause the retina to fall back into its normal position resulting in a return of vision. However, surgery is usually necessary in order to ensure the permanent return of the retina to its proper place. The patient needs the nursing care included in the following discussion which deals with the nursing care of a patient before and after having eye surgery.

## NURSING THE PATIENT HAVING EYE SURGERY

The patient with a foreign body in his eye, ulceration of the cornea, a cataract, glaucoma, detachment of the retina, an eye injury, or a tumor of the eye may be treated by surgery. Since the practical nurse frequently is responsible for assisting in the care of a patient having eye surgery she needs an understanding of the basic principles involved.

### Preoperative Care

The preoperative care of a particular patient varies with the ophthalmologist, the institution, and the specific type of surgery to be performed. In addition to the care of a patient before surgery which was discussed in Chapter 5, this patient has a special need for being oriented to his new surroundings. For example, the thoughtful nurse shows him the physical setup of his unit and how to call the nurse. She should also introduce him to the other patients in the nursing unit or room with him. Meeting members of the nursing team who will be caring for him after his eyes are bandaged helps him to feel more confident.

In addition to the anxieties and fears often experienced by individuals before surgery, this patient usually has great concern over his vision. He may be afraid that he will be either partially or completely blind.

Local preparation of the eyes prior to surgery varies with different surgeons and hospitals. The practical nurse should receive specific directions from her team leader or head nurse when asked to assist with this. She should remember to wash her hands thoroughly before and after helping to care for the patient's eye.

A woman's hair should be combed and arranged so that it will stay in place after surgery. This is necessary because the physician may not allow the patient's hair to be combed for several days following the operation. If her hair is long it can be plaited into two braids.

### Postoperative Care

Eye surgery is frequently performed under local anesthesia. This is done to prevent nausea and vomiting which often occur after general anesthesia. The strain associated with vomiting could have a harmful effect upon the newly operated eye. Another advantage of local anesthesia is that the patient is awake and can cooperate with those caring for him. For example, he can maintain the fixed head position recommended by the doctor. Also, the conscious patient is less likely to bother the eye dressing.

### *Position*

The patient should be placed gently on his bed after surgery. The physician usually specifies the position in which the patient is to remain for a certain length of time. This is important to prevent the escape of vitreous humor through the incision. Movement not allowed by the doctor may ruin the effect of surgery.

In general, the patient is placed flat in bed on his back. Sandbags may be placed on either side of his head to remind him to keep it in the position ordered by the doctor. Side rails can be placed on his bed to remind him that he is to stay in bed.

Members of the nursing team share the responsibility of helping the patient to remain in the position specified by the doctor. When assigned to care for this patient, the practical nurse should receive specific instructions regarding his position and amount of movement permitted. The signal cord should be placed within easy reach. The patient who is not allowed to move should be encouraged to ring for the nurse when necessary rather than to move in an attempt to care for himself. The practical nurse should try to anticipate the needs of this patient in an effort to prevent him from moving unnecessarily. As the patient is permitted more freedom of movement, he needs to have articles, such as a radio and water, placed in a convenient position on the bedside stand.

### *Attitude of the Practical Nurse*

The practical nurse needs to understand that the patient recuperating from eye surgery may become extremely fearful of losing his vision. He may also be unable to care for himself because of his bandaged eyes and enforced rest. These factors call for a patient, calm, and understanding nurse.

Both eyes are often bandaged following an eye operation. This reduces movement of the treated eye. When both eyes are covered with a dressing or a mask, the patient loses one means of contact with the world around him. In other words, he kept in touch with his surroundings by seeing, hearing, touching, smelling, talking, and tasting. Now his ability to see is absent. Although he may be able to see later, he cannot keep in touch with those around him by sight at the present time. The ability to hear and to talk frequently becomes more important to this patient.

When entering the patient's room, the practical nurse should speak to him in a pleasant manner to avoid startling him. This could cause him to jump and to jar his eye unnecessarily. Loud, unexpected noises should be avoided for the same reason. The practical nurse should tell the patient who she is until he has learned to recognize her voice. She should also tell the patient what she is going to do before beginning to care for him. The thoughtful practical nurse tells the patient when she is leaving the room.

Members of the nursing team can help the patient with bandaged eyes by stopping in frequently to speak to him. This simple, kindly act can be of much value to the patient. It often helps him to feel that someone is interested in him and that he is not alone. This friendly word in passing helps to divert the patient's thoughts from the fears which keep entering his mind. It also helps him to keep in contact with those around him. Frequent chats with others can help to prevent the patient from becoming mentally confused. Knowing that an older person is more likely to become confused, the practical nurse can readily understand the importance of not leaving the elderly patient alone for long periods of time.

### Activities

The practical nurse recalls that it was stated earlier in this discussion that the nursing team should keep the patient in the position prescribed by the doctor. In addition to this, the nursing team shares the responsibility of helping the patient to limit his activities according to the doctor's plan. Generally the patient is to lie quietly in bed for a short while after surgery. The doctor increases the amount of activity gradually.

The patient usually is instructed by the doctor to avoid coughing and sneezing. If he has to cough, he should do so gently. He can avoid sneezing by pressing his upper lip.

During the time that the patient has to lie quietly on his back, he may complain of backache. The nurse can rub the lower part of his back by slipping her hand gently under his back. Another measure to relieve this discomfort resulting from inactivity is to place a small pillow under the lower part of his back. The patient's back should be rubbed after his doctor allows him to turn.

The patient may not be allowed to do various daily activities or to have them done for him for varying lengths of time after surgery. For example, combing the hair, brushing the teeth, and shaving may not be allowed for a day or two after surgery. The practical nurse should seek specific instructions from the head nurse or team leader before doing these activities or allowing the patient to do them. The practical nurse may be asked to give the patient a partial bath instead of a complete one. She may be told to let the patient use mouthwash instead of brushing his teeth during the first day or two after surgery.

As his condition improves, the patient is allowed to increase his activities. Members of the nursing team as well as the patient need to know which activities are allowed by the doctor.

If the patient who has both eyes bandaged or has lost his vision is allowed to walk, he needs the help of a nurse. She should have the patient take her arm. Walking a short distance ahead of the patient serves as a guide for him. The patient should be told approximately how far they plan to walk. He should be helped to locate both the arms and the back of the chair before sitting down.

The doctor usually instructs the patient to avoid bending forward, lifting heavy objects, and exercising strenuously for several months after eye surgery. The patient should be encouraged to follow the doctor's instructions after being discharged. He may also need to be encouraged to keep appointments for care after leaving the hospital.

### Diversions

Having visitors to talk with him as well as members of the nursing team helps the patient to occupy himself while his eyes are bandaged. Listening to the radio and having someone read to him frequently are enjoyable diversions for this patient. These activities also help the patient to keep in contact with those around him.

### Diet

The physician may order a liquid diet at first to prevent chewing which could jar the affected eye. The patient is allowed to have other foods as ordered by the doctor. The patient with both eyes covered needs to be fed. When feeding the patient, the practical nurse should tell him what he has on his tray. His clothing should be protected with a napkin. She should follow the patient's preferences as to what he would like to eat next. When a patient is learning to feed himself, he needs to be told what he has on his tray and the location of the food. Placing the food on his plate according to the hands of a clock is frequently helpful. For example, the meat can be placed at 6 o'clock.

### Dressings

The practical nurse may be assigned to assist the doctor in changing the dressings. She should arrange the lighting so that it does not shine into the patient's eyes when the dressing is removed. She should have all equipment which the doctor needs.

The patient should avoid rubbing his eye after he is allowed to go without a dressing. The doctor may recommend that the patient wear a stiff, double eye mask while sleeping. The purpose of this is to prevent the patient from rubbing his eyes while asleep or just after awakening.

## REHABILITATION OF THE BLIND PERSON

Members of the nursing team share the responsibility of helping the patient who is losing his sight, or has lost his sight, to live a satisfying life. He needs to learn to be as independent as possible. The individual faced with permanent blindness needs specialized help in adjusting to his loss of sight. He may be taught by specialists in this field or by other individuals who are blind.

After losing his vision, the person has the problem of accepting this fact. He frequently goes through a period of depression after becoming blind. He may also feel isolated. Since his sense of sight is gone, he depends upon other senses, such as feeling and hearing, to keep him in touch with his surroundings. Because of this, he should be spoken to frequently by those who are around him.

Vocational rehabilitation programs throughout the United States are rendering an invaluable service in the rehabilitation of blind citizens. Many individuals learn to live a satisfying life because of these programs. In many cases the person is taught a new vocation. The older individual can learn to be independent in the activities of daily living, such as eating, dressing, and walking. Learning to take care of his daily needs helps the person to regain and to maintain his self-respect. Carving, knitting, crocheting, and other diversional activities play an important part in the total rehabilitation program.

Individuals inexperienced in rehabilitation of the blind frequently are overprotective. This attitude does not encourage the person to become as independent as possible. Another error of inexperienced people in dealing with a blind person is to talk too loudly. Although the person is blind, he is not necessarily deaf.

Objects which are likely to cause the sightless person to have an accident should be removed from his surroundings. For example, scatter rugs, a misplaced toy, and water on the floor may cause him to fall. Furniture should be left in the same place so that he can learn to move about as freely as possible. Doors should be kept either closed or opened completely. This prevents his walking into a door which is partially open.

SUGGESTIONS FOR STUDY

1. What factors are necessary in order for a person to have perfect vision?
2. Discuss the main functions of an ophthalmologist, an optician, and an optometrist.
3. In what ways can you improve the hygiene of your own eyes?
4. What visual defects can be corrected with glasses?
5. How does the ophthalmologist usually treat a person with strabismus?
6. Why would an ulceration of the cornea be considered serious?
7. In what type of eye disease would the ophthalmologist be likely to do a keratoplasty?
8. What are the causes of a cataract?

9. Why would a person with cataract have loss of vision? What can be done to correct this?

10. What are the symptoms of glaucoma?

11. How is a person with glaucoma generally treated?

12. How does the nursing care of a patient having a squint corrected by surgery differ from the care of most patients having eye surgery? What is the reason for your answer?

13. Discuss the postoperative care of a patient having eye surgery in regards to position, activities, diet, diversions, and the practical nurse's attitude.

14. Is there a vocational rehabilitation center for the blind citizens of your state? A visit to such a center would be beneficial to the practical nurse. Ask your instructor if this center is close enough for a visit to be arranged.

## REFERENCES FOR CHAPTER 22

Bindt, Juliet: A Handbook for the Blind. The Macmillan Company, New York, 1952.

Clark, Graham, and Shaw, Cora L.: "The Patient with Retinal Detachment," Am. J. Nursing, 57:868-71, (July) 1957.

Eliason, Eldridge; Ferguson, L. Kraeer; and Sholtis, Lillian A.: Surgical Nursing, 10th ed. J. B. Lippincott Co., Philadelphia, 1955, pp. 431-56.

Esau, Margaret; Fallon, Barbara R.; Frentzos, Kathryn G.; Phillips, Elisabeth C.; and Tourtillott, Eleanor A.: Practical Nursing Today, Attitudes–Knowledge–Skills. G. P. Putnam's Sons, New York, 1957, pp. 78-79 and 286-90.

Gamble, Richard C.: "The Medical Eye Examination," Am. J. Nursing, 57:1590-92, (Dec.) 1957.

Gill, Helen Z. (ed.): Basic Nursing, 4th ed. The Macmillan Company, New York, 1955, pp. 119-21 and 580-84.

Harman, Palmer: "The Truth about Eyestrain," Practical Nurses Digest, 4:10-11, (Nov.) 1957.

Kimber, Diana; Gray, Carolyn E.; Stackpole, Caroline E.; and Leavell, Lutie C.: Textbook of Anatomy and Physiology, 13th ed. The Macmillan Company, New York, 1955, pp. 719-34.

Manhattan Eye, Ear, and Throat Hospital: Nursing in Diseases of the Eye, Ear, Nose and Throat, 10th ed. W. B. Saunders Co., Philadelphia, 1958, pp. 3-119.

Newton, Kathleen: Geriatric Nursing. C. V. Mosby Co., St. Louis, 1950, pp. 290-310.

"One Blinding Flash," Am. J. Nursing, 56:621, (May) 1956.

Shepard, Mary E.: *Nursing Care of Patients with Eye, Ear, Nose, and Throat Disorders.* The Macmillan Company, New York, 1958, pp. 3-95.

Stafford, Edward S., and Diller, Doris: *Surgery and Surgical Nursing,* 3rd. ed. W. B. Saunders Co., Philadelphia, 1958, pp. 374-95.

Terry, Florence J.; Benz, Gladys S.; Mereness, Dorothy; and Kleffner, Frank R.: *Principles and Technics of Rehabilitation Nursing.* C. V. Mosby Co., St. Louis, 1957, pp. 194-96.

Turner, C. E.: *Personal and Community Health,* 10th ed. C. V. Mosby Co., St. Louis, 1956, pp. 199-210.

West, John P.; Keller, Manelva W.; and Harmon, Elizabeth H.: *Nursing Care of the Surgical Patient,* 6th ed. The Macmillan Company, New York, 1957, pp. 529-57.

# THE PATIENT
# WITH A DISEASE OF
# THE EAR

## STRUCTURE AND FUNCTION

Hearing is made possible by normal functioning of the two ears and the auditory (acoustic) nerves which lead to the centers of hearing in the brain. Each ear is composed of the external ear, the middle ear, and the internal ear.

The external ear consists of the part which protrudes from the side of the head and the external auditory canal. The part which projects from the side of the head is known as the *pinna*. It is composed mainly of cartilage, fatty tissue, muscles, and skin. The pinna helps to funnel sound waves into the *external auditory canal* which leads inward. This tubelike passage is approximately 2.5 cm (1 in.) in length. The external auditory canal is lined with skin which contains a few hairs near the external opening. The inner part of the canal has glands which secrete the yellowish, pasty earwax known as *cerumen*. The hair and the cerumen help to prevent foreign substances from entering the ear. The external auditory canal is separated from the middle ear by a membrane known as the *tympanic membrane* or the *eardrum*.

The middle ear is a small bony cavity located in the temporal bone of the skull. This cavity contains three small movable bones which connect the tympanic membrane with the internal ear. These three bones are the *malleus*, which is similar in appearance to a hammer; the *incus*, which resembles an anvil; and the *stapes*, which is similar to a stirrup. The malleus connects the tympanic membrane

*409*

with the incus, and the incus is connected with the stapes. Part of the stapes fits into the small oval window of the thin bony wall which separates the middle ear from the internal ear. The oval window is known also as the *fenestra vestibuli.*

The middle ear has five openings. There is one opening between the external auditory canal and the middle ear. It was stated earlier in this discussion that this opening normally is covered by the tympanic membrane. Two small openings are situated in the thin bony wall which separates the middle ear from the internal ear. The small tube which leads from the middle ear to the pharynx (throat) is known as the *eustachian* or *auditory tube.* Normally, air enters the middle ear from the throat through the eustachian tube. This helps to equalize the pressure of air on both sides of the eardrum. Another small opening in the middle ear leads to the mastoid cells. The part of the temporal bone which projects downward behind the ear is known as the *mastoid.* This contains spaces filled with air which are known as *mastoid cells.*

The internal ear is located beyond the middle ear in the temporal bone. The internal ear is also called the *labyrinth* because it contains an intricate system of connecting canals and cavities. The cochlea, the semicircular canals, and the vestibule are three of the main structures which are included in this discussion. The *cochlea,* which is similar in appearance to a snail shell, contains fluid and branches of the auditory nerve. The three small *semicircular canals,* which help to control equilibrium, contain fluid and nerve endings. The *vestibule,* which is the cavity between the cochlea and the semicircular canals, also contains fluid. It is connected with the middle ear by the small oval window.

Objects or bodies which produce sound vibrate to produce waves. These travel through air, enter the external auditory canal, and cause the stretched tympanic membrane to vibrate. These vibrations rapidly pass through the three small movable bones in the middle ear to the fluid of the inner ear. Movement of this liquid stimulates the endings of the auditory nerve. The impulses are then carried to the centers of hearing in the brain and interpreted as sound.

## ASSISTING WITH EXAMINATION

The practical nurse is often asked to assist the physician in examining the patient's ear. This may be done as part of a general physical examination or it may be done as a single procedure. In either case, the practical nurse should provide adequate lighting, a head mirror, ear specula (plural for speculum) of different sizes, an otoscope, and cotton-tipped applicators. A movable lamp placed behind the patient can be adjusted so that its light is reflected from the doctor's head mirror into the ear. The *ear speculum* is a small, hollow instrument which is similar to a funnel in shape. The physician inserts it into the external auditory canal so that he can see its walls

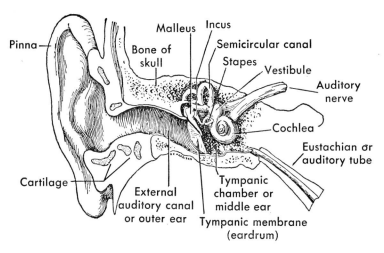

**Figure 43.**   Front view of a median section of the human ear, right side. Note the transmitting mechanism of tympanum (eardrum) and three bones: malleus, incus, and stapes. Somewhat idealized. (Woodruff, Lorande L., and Baitsell, George A.: *Foundations of Biology,* 7th ed. The Macmillan Company, New York, 1951.)

as well as the tympanic membrane. Several ear specula are needed so that the doctor can select the proper size for a particular patient. The *otoscope* is another instrument used for examination of the external auditory canal and the tympanic membrane. It contains a light which can be directed through an attached speculum. A small magnifying lens in the otoscope enables the doctor to see the tympanic membrane better. The physician may need the cotton-tipped applicators to remove wax and other secretions from the external auditory canal which interfere with examination.

The practical nurse may be asked to have the patient either lying down or seated in a chair for an ear examination. She may be responsible for holding the patient's head when a special chair with a head support is not used. A special chair such as this is usually found in the clinic and in the doctor's office. The physician is not able to do a complete examination if the patient's head is not still. Sudden movement of the head may also cause injury from the speculum. When the patient is unable to hold his head still or if he is too young to cooperate, the assistant is responsible for holding the head still.

The physician sometimes has to irrigate the external auditory canal before he can complete his examination. This may be done to remove substances, such as a mass of earwax or drainage. Unless it is otherwise specified by the doctor, the practical nurse should have the temperature of the solution near that of the body as the use of warmer or colder solution can cause the patient to have an earache. Nausea and dizziness may also occur. The doctor may order the instillation of a small amount of warmed substance, such as sweet oil or hydrogen peroxide, before doing an irrigation. This is done to soften the plug of earwax.

A variety of tests can be used to determine the person's ability to hear. In general, the ear not being tested is closed. Rough estimates of the patient's hearing can be made by the use of either a ticking watch or a tuning fork. The examiner may also whisper to the patient for this purpose.

An *audiometer* is used for more specific information. This is an instrument used to measure an individual's ability to hear. The *otologist,* a physician who specializes in conditions of the ear, can determine more definitely the exact amount of hearing loss. He can also determine the amount of sound conducted through the air by way of the external auditory canal as well as the amount conducted through the mastoid. Knowing whether sound is conducted through either the air or the bone and the amount of hearing loss guide the otologist in his diagnosis and treatment.

## FOREIGN BODIES

The individual with a foreign body in his ear should be advised to see his doctor. Since there is danger of injuring the tympanic membrane and the external auditory canal, an inexperienced person should not attempt to remove the foreign body.

The physician may irrigate the external auditory canal to remove the foreign body. However, peas, beans, and similar objects are likely to swell when moistened; in this case, the otologist uses alcohol instead of water for the irrigation. An insect can be killed by the instillation of a few drops of either oil or alcohol which has been warmed. After removing the foreign body and drying the ear, the doctor frequently places dry cotton in the opening. This is done to prevent chilling and an earache.

## OTITIS MEDIA

### Cause

The patient with otitis media has an inflammation of the middle ear. The infection may follow such diseases as the common cold, a sore throat, tonsillitis, scarlet fever, and measles. If the practical nurse recalls that the middle ear is connected to the throat by the eustachian tube, she can readily understand that an infection can spread from the nose and throat to the middle ear.

### Symptoms

The patient may complain that the affected ear feels full and stuffy, and aches. *Tinnitus*, which is a sensation of ringing, may be present in one ear or in both ears. Upon examining the ear, the physician may find a reddened and bulging eardrum. The patient may also have general symptoms of an inflammation, such as malaise and fever.

If the patient is not treated or if he does not respond to treatment, his symptoms may become more severe. The inflammation can cause fluid to form in the middle ear and result in a temporary loss of hearing. Pressure from the fluid can cause the eardrum to rupture. In this case, the patient has a discharge from his ear. The infection can spread from the middle ear to the mastoid cells by way of the opening between the two structures. A patient sometimes develops chronic otitis media. This may result in a discharge from the involved ear for months. A permanent loss of hearing can result from otitis media.

## Treatment and Nursing Care

The physician directs his treatment toward relieving the cause of otitis media as well as relieving the inflammation. For example, he would treat the patient with tonsillitis complicated by otitis media for both conditions. A suitable drug to combat the infection, such as an antibiotic or one of the sulfonamides, is almost always prescribed.

The physician may on occasion do a *myringotomy*. This is a surgical procedure in which he makes an opening into the tympanic membrane. A myringotomy is not done very frequently now as many infections of the middle ear respond to drug therapy. A general anesthetic is often used for a myringotomy since it is quite painful. After the operation, the doctor may place sterile cotton in the external auditory canal. The nurse in attendance should observe and report the type and amount of drainage. A change in the drainage should also be reported.

Other treatments which the doctor may sometimes order are irrigation of the ear and the instillation of drops of medication into the external auditory canal. If a member of the nursing team is responsible for irrigating the external auditory canal, she should remember that the solution should enter the canal with low force. This is especially important when the eardrum is ruptured or when it has been incised. The ear of an adult should be lifted upward and backward in a gentle manner to straighten the canal. The external auditory canal of a child can be straightened by drawing the ear downward and backward gently. When ordering the instillation of a drug into the external auditory canal, the doctor usually specifies the number of drops to be used. The prescribed drug should be warmed to body temperature unless otherwise ordered. The patient should be lying down with the ear to receive the drops upward. After straightening the external auditory canal, the nurse drops the prescribed number of drops into the canal. The patient should remain in this position for at least five minutes after the drops have been instilled to permit adequate absorption of the drug. The nurse may be requested by the doctor to place a piece of cotton into the ear opening.

## MASTOIDITIS

### Description

The patient with mastoiditis has an inflammation of the mastoid, generally caused by the spread of an infection from the middle ear.

Although mastoiditis is not very common now since sulfonamides and antibiotics are used, it can be a serious disease. A thin piece of bone separates the tiny air cells of the mastoid from the membranes which cover the brain. Remembering this, the practical nurse can readily understand how the infection can spread to the brain.

### Symptoms

The patient usually complains of pain around and behind his ear and of headache on the affected side. The tip of the mastoid is tender. He may have an increased amount of drainage from his ear and a greater loss of hearing. Such general symptoms of infection as malaise and fever are also present.

### Treatment and Nursing Care

The physician directs his treatment toward relieving the otitis media as well as the mastoiditis. He nearly always prescribes a suitable drug, such as an antibiotic or a sulfonamide, to combat the infection. Measures, such as bed rest, an increased intake of fluids, and a nourishing diet, generally recommended for the patient with an infection, are also important in the care of this patient.

Surgery may be indicated when the patient does not respond favorably to the medical treatment. A *simple mastoidectomy*, which is removal of the infected part of the mastoid, is usually done. Sometimes a radical mastoidectomy may be necessary. This is especially true in a chronic case of long standing which did not respond to other treatment. In a *radical mastoidectomy*, the surgeon removes the tympanic membrane and nearly all of the contents of the middle ear as well as the infected portion of the mastoid. Following a radical mastoidectomy, the patient continues to have a loss of hearing in the affected ear, but further loss is generally prevented.

The nursing care of a patient before surgery, discussed on pages 46 to 53, is applicable to this patient. If the practical nurse is asked to shave the part, she should learn which side of the head is to be prepared. In general, an area of approximately 5 cm (2 in.) around the affected ear should be shaved.

In addition to the nursing care needed by most patients following surgery, discussed on pages 53 to 56, this patient should be encouraged to move his head frequently. Such movement helps to prevent and to relieve the painful, stiff neck which often follows a fixed position of the head and neck during surgery.

## OTOSCLEROSIS

### Description

An individual with otosclerosis has a growth of new bone which is usually around the oval window. It was stated earlier in this chapter that sound vibrations were carried through the middle ear to the inner ear by the chain of three movable bones in the middle ear. Part of one of these bones, the stapes, fits into the oval window of the thin bony wall which separates the middle ear from the inner ear. Sound vibrations reaching the stapes cause it to move. Movement of the part which fits into the oval window causes the fluid in the inner ear to move. An abnormal growth of bone around the oval window prevents the stapes from moving. Thus, the sound waves do not reach the inner ear. This results in a progressive loss of hearing as the new bone continues to develop. Deafness caused by otosclerosis is known as conductive deafness because the sound waves are not transmitted or conducted properly.

### Treatment and Nursing Care

The otologist may create a new pathway for the sound waves so that they can reach the inner ear. In other words, a detour is made around the obstruction. This surgical procedure is known as a fenestration. The surgeon creates a new opening or window in the bone covering the inner ear and places the tympanic membrane over the new window. This permits the sound waves to be transmitted from the tympanic membrane to the inner ear.

Dizziness and nausea are frequent discomforts following fenestration. This is caused by a disturbance of the equilibrium apparatus in the inner ear. The doctor generally asks the nursing team to keep the patient flat in bed for the first day or two postoperatively. In helping the patient to change his position, the practical nurse should encourage him to move slowly and with as little help from her as possible. If the patient has nausea and vomiting, he should be told to lie quietly and to avoid moving his head. A drug, such as dimenhydrinate (Dramamine), used for motion sickness, may be prescribed. The physician allows the patient to increase his activities as the nausea and dizziness disappear.

Special instructions to the patient before leaving the hospital usually include information about dizziness because this may continue for several weeks. The otologist recommends to the patient that he take tub baths, rather than showers, during the healing period and explains that this prevents water getting into the ear. The patient should be encouraged to continue his follow-up visits to the doctor until he is discharged, at which time the doctor will advise the patient whether it is safe for him to take showers and to go swimming. If the patient's hearing is not improved by the fenestration, he may be advised by his physician to get a hearing aid.

## DEAFNESS

### Cause

The person handicapped by deafness has either a complete loss or a partial loss of hearing. It may be caused by poor conduction of sound waves or by inadequate perception. Two types of deafness are conductive and perceptive.

*Conductive deafness* occurs when the sound waves do not reach the inner ear properly. Since the waves must pass through the external auditory canal and the middle ear to reach the inner ear, an abnormal condition of these structures can cause a loss of hearing. A plug of earwax or a foreign body in the external auditory canal, perforation of the eardrum, and otitis media can cause conductive deafness. Chronic otitis media may result in either impairment or destruction of the bones in the middle ear. Thus, sound is not conducted properly to the inner ear. Otosclerosis, which was discussed earlier in this chapter, is another cause of conductive deafness. Also, a person may be born with a defect in the part of the ear responsible for the conduction of sound.

*Perceptive deafness* occurs when the sound waves go through the middle ear but are not received properly by the brain. This is caused by damage to the auditory nerve or to its sensitive branches in the inner ear. An individual may be born with a defect in the part of the ear responsible for the perception of sound. Injury of the auditory nerve may cause perceptive deafness. For example, a brain tumor pressing on this nerve, a skull fracture, and prolonged exposure to loud noises may result in deafness. Toxins associated with certain diseases, such as syphilis, mumps, and measles, can damage the auditory nerve. It can also be injured by an infection of the middle ear.

### Prevention

Either a partial or a complete loss of hearing causes limitations to the individual. Because of this, measures to prevent the loss of hearing are important. Periodic examinations of children in an effort to discover conditions which could result in deafness are helpful. An individual with the common cold or other upper respiratory infections may develop complications which could result in deafness. The proper care of an individual with such infections helps to prevent complications involving the ears. The person with symptoms associated with an ear infection or with a loss of hearing should be encouraged to consult his physician.

The habit of putting nothing into the external auditory canal is a safe one. Hard objects, such as a hairpin or a match stick, are likely to scratch the delicate tissue. A tiny splinter from the match stick may become embedded in the earwax and cause a plug to form. The use of a washcloth, soap, and water should be all that is needed to keep the canal from becoming blocked. If an individual does have a collection of wax in his ear, he should consult his doctor, who may remove the plug of earwax by irrigating the canal.

Many industries have active programs to conserve the hearing of their employees. This is especially important when the workers are exposed to loud noises over a long period of time. Reduction of noise in the vicinity of the employee, the use of material on the walls, ceilings, and floors to absorb sound, the use of ear protectors, and periodic testing of the employees' hearing are examples of measures used to aid in the prevention of deafness.

## Treatment

The otologist attempts to relieve the underlying cause of deafness in order to prevent further loss of hearing and to improve the patient's hearing when possible. For example, the patient with chronic otitis media is treated for this condition or the patient with otosclerosis may have a fenestration done.

If the physician is unable to improve the patient's hearing, he may recommend a *hearing aid*, an instrument that amplifies the vibrations. Various types are available to suit the needs of different individuals. Usually a small inconspicuous part of the hearing aid is inserted in the ear or pressed over the mastoid behind the ear. The rest of the apparatus may be worn in the earpiece of eyeglasses or in the person's clothing. Other types of hearing aids are attached to the seats in public places, such as churches and theaters.

When the physician finds that a hearing aid does not help the patient, he may direct him to a lipreading class. The child with a marked loss of hearing should receive special instruction in lipreading as well as in speaking.

## Nursing Care

The practical nurse is responsible for nursing many patients with varying degrees of deafness. Often this handicap is not the condition for which the patient is being treated. An example of this is seen in the deaf boy who was hospitalized for pneumonia. Although he was being treated for pneumonia, his deafness influenced the practical nurse's approach to him. She needed to know how to care for the person with a loss of hearing as well as one with pneumonia.

In talking with the person who has a loss of hearing, the practical nurse should stand facing the patient so that he can see her expression as well as her lips. She should speak clearly, a little louder, and somewhat slower than usual. Pausing occasionally may also be helpful. After learning whether the patient has a better ear, she should direct her voice to that side.

The practical nurse should determine whether the patient understands what she is saying to him. This is especially important when she is explaining a treatment or a procedure to be followed. A person with defective hearing is likely to agree with what is said to him by saying "yes" when he does not understand. Knowing this the practical nurse can often avoid a misunderstanding by talking further with the patient when he does say "yes" to a question. For example, the practical nurse may be asked by the head nurse to tell the patient not to eat anything and not to drink any fluids after midnight in preparation for an x-ray the next morning. In order to determine whether the patient understood the procedure to be followed, she asked him if he had been prepared in this manner before for an x-ray. After being told "yes" by the patient, she asked him when this was done. He replied that he had been given similar instructions several years ago when his stomach was x-rayed. By spending a few extra minutes in talking with this patient, the practical nurse felt assured that the patient understood what she was saying to him. The practical nurse should repeat the statement without impatience when she finds that the patient does not comprehend what she is saying. She may find it helpful to use other words in repeating the instructions.

Remembering that a hearing aid is important to the patient as well as expensive, the practical nurse is careful when handling it. The thoughtful nurse remembers to give the patient his hearing aid. Of course, she should put it on for the patient when he is unable to do so. The hearing aid should be attached securely. The type which is attached to the clothing can be pinned in the patient's pocket. The hearing aid which is a part of the eyeglasses should be placed comfortably and securely on the patient's face. The practical nurse can usually find out from the patient or from some member of his family how to turn the hearing aid on and how to adjust the volume when he is unable to do this. Since water can harm a hearing aid, it should not come in contact with the instrument. It should be turned off and put in a safe place at night.

An individual handicapped with deafness may have difficulty in expressing himself in addition to hearing. This is especially true when the impaired hearing either prevents or complicates the process of learning to talk. For example, a person who is deaf at birth or becomes so in early childhood needs special instruction in order to speak and to lipread. His speech may be difficult to understand because he does not hear the voices of other people to use for comparison. If the patient is totally deaf and has not learned to talk he may have to communicate with others by writing. Then the practical nurse must write messages to the patient when he is unable to understand speech by watching the talker's lips.

When talking with the person who lipreads, the practical nurse should stand in front of him. The light should shine on her face so that the patient can see her lips. Speaking slowly and distinctly and pausing occasionally help the lipreader in understanding the speaker.

The practical nurse should pay full attention to the person who has difficulty in talking. In addition to listening to him she should look at him. The practical nurse should try to catch the main meaning of his speech rather than the details. When she does not understand what the patient is saying, she should not try to give the patient the impression that she does. Having the patient write the message and then to speak what he has written help the listener to become accustomed to his speech.

## SUGGESTIONS FOR STUDY

1. Why is it important for the patient's head to be still while the doctor examines the ear?

2. Why should the temperature of solution to be put in the ear be near that of the body?

3. What is an otoscope? An audiometer?

4. Why is the person with an infection of the nose and throat likely to develop otitis media?

5. What is otosclerosis? How does it cause deafness?

6. Review the nursing care of a patient following a fenestration.

7. Discuss measures which can be used to help in the prevention of deafness.

8. How can the practical nurse determine whether a deaf patient understands what she says to him?

9. Discuss the care of a hearing aid.

10. Review the factors to be remembered when talking with a person handicapped by deafness.

REFERENCES FOR CHAPTER 23

Davidson, Louise E., "A Hearing Conservation Program," *Am. J. Nursing*, **55**:582-83, (May) 1955.
Eliason, Eldridge; Ferguson, L. Kraeer; and Sholtis, Lillian A.: *Surgical Nursing*, 10th ed. J. B. Lippincott Co., Philadelphia, 1955, pp. 457-64.
Freeland, Lorraine S.: "The Practical Nurse and the Hard-of-Hearing Patient," *Practical Nurses Digest*, **5**:9-10 and 30, (May) 1958.
Gill, Helen Z. (ed.): *Basic Nursing*, 4th ed. The Macmillan Company, New York, 1955, pp. 121-23 and 584-87.
Harmer, Bertha, and Henderson, Virginia: *Textbook of the Principles and Practice of Nursing*, 5th ed. The Macmillan Company, New York, 1955, pp. 558-59, 819-21, 911-16, and 1164-66.
Kimber, Diana; Gray, Carolyn E.; Stackpole, Caroline E.; and Leavell, Lutie C.: *Textbook of Anatomy and Physiology*, 13th ed. The Macmillan Company, New York, 1955, pp. 709-19.
Manhattan Eye, Ear, and Throat Hospital: *Nursing in Diseases of the Eye, Ear, Nose and Throat*, 10th ed. W. B. Saunders Co., Philadelphia, 1958, pp. 123-71.
Rapier, Dorothy K.; Koch, Marianna J.; Moran, Lois P.; Fleming, Viola L.; Cady, Elwyn L.; and Jensen, Deborah: *Practical Nursing, A Textbook for Students and Graduates*. C. V. Mosby Co., St. Louis, 1958, pp. 244-47.
Seitock, Bertha B., "The Deaf Child," *Am. J. Nursing*, **56**:594-96, (May) 1956.
Shepard, Mary E.: *Nursing Care of Patients with Eye, Ear, Nose, and Throat Disorders*. The Macmillan Company, New York, 1958, pp. 99-156.
Stafford, Edward S., and Diller, Doris: *Surgery and Surgical Nursing*, 3rd. ed. W. B. Saunders Co., Philadelphia, 1958, pp. 411-15.
Terry, Florence J.; Benz, Gladys S.; Mereness, Dorothy; and Kleffner, Frank R.: *Principles and Technics of Rehabilitation Nursing*. C. V. Mosby Co., St. Louis, 1957, pp. 197 and 309-11.
Turner, C. E.: *Personal and Community Health*, 10th ed. C. V. Mosby Co., St. Louis, 1956, pp. 194-99 and 522-24.
Warfield, Frances: *Keep Listening*. The Viking Press, New York, 1957.
West, John P.; Keller, Manelva W.; and Harmon, Elizabeth H.: *Nursing Care of the Surgical Patient*, 6th ed. The Macmillan Company, New York, 1957, pp. 557-72.

*Nursing the Patient with a Disease of the Skin*

PART XI

# Chapter 24

# THE PATIENT
# WITH A DISEASE OF
# THE SKIN

## STRUCTURE AND FUNCTION

The body is covered by skin. Some of its many functions include protection of the body from infection, injury, and loss of fluid. The skin helps to regulate body heat because of its rich blood supply and sweat glands. Water and certain salts are eliminated through the skin. A person keeps in touch with his immediate surroundings through the many nerve endings in the skin. For example, he can feel the touch of an object on his skin. He can also tell whether or not the object is hot or cold or if it causes pain.

The two main layers of skin are the epidermis and the dermis. The outer layer of the skin, which is the *epidermis*, has no blood vessels. It is composed mainly of flattened, dead cells. The epidermis serves as a protective covering for the living cells beneath it. This dead layer of cells is continuously receiving additional cells from the tissue below it and having cells removed from its top portion.

The layer of tissue below the epidermis is the *dermis*. It contains small blood vessels, lymph vessels, nerves, hair follicles, sebaceous glands, and sweat glands. The *sebaceous glands* secrete an oily substance which protects, moistens, and softens the skin. The *sweat*

425

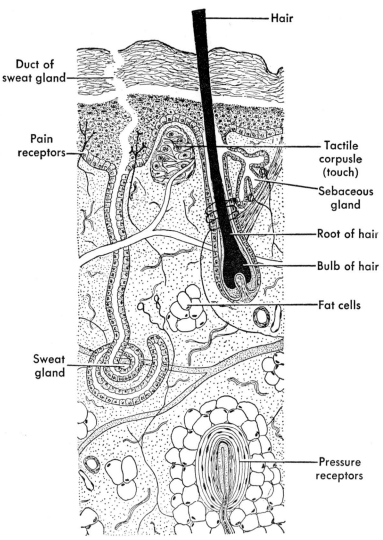

Labels on figure:
Hair
Duct of sweat gland
Pain receptors
Tactile corpusle (touch)
Sebaceous gland
Root of hair
Bulb of hair
Fat cells
Sweat gland
Pressure receptors

**Figure 44.** Diagram of skin showing glands and other structures. (Stackpole, Caroline E., and Leavell, Lutie C.: *Textbook of Physiology,* The Macmillan Company, New York, 1953.)

426

*glands* secrete perspiration. Evaporation of this fluid helps to control body heat.

## SOME DERMATOLOGIC CONDITIONS

Dermatologic conditions, which are skin disorders, are common. *Dermatology* is the branch of medicine which deals with the structure and function of the skin, its diseases, and the treatment of persons with these diseases. The *dermatologist* is a physician specializing in this branch of medicine.

Although the care of a person with a dermatologic condition is considered a specialty, the practical nurse needs an understanding of the main principles which are generally accepted in the care of this patient. Only a few of the more common skin disorders are discussed briefly in this chapter.

### Acne Vulgaris

#### Description

Acne vulgaris, which is known as pimples, occurs commonly during adolescence. Although it appears most often on the face, it can develop on the back, chest, and other parts of the body. Acne vulgaris is associated with overactivity and inflammation of the **sebaceous glands. This results in** formation of blackheads; *papules*, which are small, rounded, raised areas; and *pustules*, which are blisters filled with pus.

#### Treatment

Measures to improve the general health of the individual are important. These include adequate rest, outdoor activities, regular hours, cleanliness, and a well-balanced diet. The doctor may recommend that the patient avoid certain foods, such as chocolates and nuts.

Specific instructions regarding the care of the skin should be obtained from a doctor. In general, he recommends meticulous cleanliness of the skin by washing it frequently with soap and water. The patient is usually advised not to squeeze the blackheads or the pimples because of the danger of injuring the tissue. The doctor sometimes prescribes medication to be applied to the area. Severe cases may be treated with x-ray therapy.

## Athlete's Foot

### Description

Athlete's foot is caused by fungi, which are low forms of plant life. Since fungi grow in moist surroundings, they are frequently found in and around showers and swimming pools.

Tiny blisters filled with fluid (vesicles) may form on and between the toes. The area appears red and may become cracked and scaly. The person frequently experiences local stinging and itching. The infection can spread to other parts of his feet and body. Bacteria may invade the cracked skin and cause a secondary infection.

### Treatment

Keeping the feet dry and clean helps to get rid of the infection. Exposing the affected part to air and sun is beneficial when this is possible. Medication in the form of an ointment and a powder may be prescribed to combat the infection. The person is generally directed to apply the ointment at night and to remove it in the morning. The powder is then dusted on his feet. He may be advised to sprinkle powder into his shoes. The patient may be told to wear clean, white hose or socks while being treated. The doctor may advise the person to boil the hose or socks to prevent reinfection. He may also recommend that the patient place his shoes in a closed box containing a jar of formalin for a specific length of time to kill the fungi in them. The shoes should be exposed to air for approximately two days before being worn again. This is necessary to prevent irritation from the fumes of the formalin.

## Dermatitis

Dermatitis is a general term used to indicate an inflammation of the skin. A person can have an acute or chronic case. Some individuals develop dermatitis in infancy and continue to have recurrences throughout their life. There are many types of dermatitis which can be classified in various ways. For example, it may be classified according to its cause. Some of the many causes of dermatitis are infection, injury, cold weather, drugs, allergy, and exposure to the sun, radium, or x-ray. An example of an inflammatory skin condition caused by an allergy is seen in the person with *contact dermatitis*. After coming in contact with the irritating substance, his skin becomes inflamed. He may have a combination of localized symptoms, such as redness, macules, papules, vesicles, and pustules. *Macules* are discolored, unelevated spots, and *papules* are small rounded, raised areas. The size of the papules may range from that of a pin point to that of a split pea. *Vesicles*, which are blisters filled with fluid, as well as pustules may develop in the inflamed area. *Pustules* are small rounded, raised areas containing pus. Oozing, scaling, crusting, and leathery thickening may occur.

An example of contact dermatitis is seen in the person with an allergy to poison ivy (oak). After coming in contact with this plant, he develops a rash and other local symptoms of inflammation. The individual can sometimes prevent this reaction by washing the area thoroughly with warm water and soap promptly after coming in contact with the poison ivy.

### Herpes Simplex

An individual with herpes simplex (fever blisters) has patches of tiny blisters, usually about the lips. Herpes simplex is believed to be caused by a virus. This is not a serious condition and generally disappears without treatment. The local application of spirit of camphor may be used to hasten the disappearance of the blisters.

### Impetigo Contagiosa

#### *Description*

Impetigo contagiosa is an infectious disease of the skin. It may may be caused by streptococci or staphylococci. Although impetigo contagiosa occurs most often in infants and children, it can affect persons of any age. The infection spreads rapidly in infants and can be dangerous.

A small blister which contains watery fluid forms at first, and then pus. In other words, the patient has vesicles which become pustules. The tiny bleb ruptures, and the fluid which escapes carries bacteria to other parts of the skin. This results in the formation of new vesicles. A yellowish crust forms over the site of the ruptured blister.

### Treatment

The patient with impetigo contagiosa should be isolated since this is an infectious disease. It can be transmitted by direct contact and by the articles which have become contaminated by the fluid or the crust from the infected area.

The physician may request the nurse to rupture the blisters. This should be done in such a manner that the fluid does not come in contact with the skin around the infected area. He may prescribe the application of an ointment, such as ammoniated mercury, to the ruptured blister. The nurse should wash her hands thoroughly with soap and running water before and after carrying out this treatment.

### Nursing Care

The practical nurse should receive definite instructions from her team leader or head nurse when asked to assist in caring for the patient with a dermatologic disorder. She can expect this patient to need special skin care. The practical nurse should not use soap and water on the patient unless they are ordered by the doctor. Instead of using regular toilet soap which can have an irritating effect on the skin, she may be told to use a specially prescribed soap.

The physician frequently orders variations in the bath. He may ask the nurse to have the temperature of the water similar to that of the body. This is done to prevent dilating the blood vessels of the skin with heat. The type of soap, if any, should be indicated. The nurse should pat the patient's skin dry instead of rubbing it. The doctor may leave an order for the nurse to clean the patient's skin with an oil, such as olive oil or mineral oil, or a specially prescribed solution.

An emollient bath may be ordered for the patient with a generalized inflammation of the skin. This type of bath has a soothing effect on the skin. Oatmeal or a mixture of cornstarch and baking soda are examples of substances which may be prescribed. The bath is prepared according to the hospital procedure and the doctor's orders. In general, the temperature of the solution should be between 33.9° to 35.6° C (93° to 96° F).

The physician prescribes suitable ointments, pastes, medicated solutions, lotions, and dusting power when necessary. Either hot or cold applications may be ordered in the form of compresses, dressings, and soaks.

## BREAST CONDITIONS

### Structure and Function

The breasts are known as *mammary glands*. Their function is to secrete milk to nourish the newborn. Both sexes have these glands. However, the breasts normally develop and function only in the female. The mammary glands of a young girl become larger during puberty because of the action of hormones. Some women notice temporary changes which are associated with the menstrual period. The breasts frequently become smaller after menopause.

Each breast is made of connective tissue, fatty tissue, and 15 to 20 lobes. These lobes contain glandular tissue. A duct leads from each lobe to an opening in the nipple. The nipple is surrounded by dark- or pink-colored skin which is called the *areola*. The remaining portion of the skin which covers each mammary gland has a color similar to that which covers most of the body.

Glandular tissue of the breasts becomes active during pregnancy. This causes the breasts to increase in size and the areola to become larger and darker. A yellowish fluid called *colostrum* is secreted by the glands within the breasts during the later part of pregnancy. An increased amount of colostrum is secreted for the first few days after delivery. This secretion is then replaced by milk.

### Mastitis

#### Description

The woman with mastitis has an infection of the breast. The infection may involve the entire mammary gland or a part of it. Although mastitis occurs most often in a woman who has recently delivered, it can occur at other times. Bacteria usually enter through a crack in the nipple and spread to other parts of the breast.

#### Symptoms

The infected breast is swollen and painful, and may appear inflamed. The patient usually has general symptoms of an infection, such as fever and malaise. Mastitis can be complicated by a breast abscess.

### Treatment

The doctor may order either cold or hot applications to the inflamed breast to relieve discomfort. The nurse may be responsible for emptying the breast of the new mother with a breast pump. An appropriate antibiotic is almost always prescribed.

## Chronic Cystic Mastitis

### Description

The woman with chronic cystic mastitis has an irregular, excessive growth of certain tissues in the breast. In other words, some of the breast tissue grows abnormally fast for varying lengths of time. This excessive growth of tissue results in the blockage of ducts and the development of *cysts*, which are sacs containing fluid. Many cysts may form. Both breasts are often affected.

### Symptoms

The patient may consult the doctor because she notices small lumps in the breasts. Tenderness and pain are common complaints of the woman with chronic cystic mastitis.

### Treatment

The common treatment for this condition is surgical removal of the cyst. However, the physician may keep the patient under close observation for a while before deciding whether or not to do surgery. If the cyst is removed, it is examined by the pathologist for malignancy. Sometimes an entire breast is removed although the growths are benign. Removal of a breast is known as a mastectomy.

## Benign Tumor

A benign tumor of the breast usually is freely movable and grows slowly. However, if the doctor finds that a woman has a breast tumor, he generally removes tissue from it or the entire tumor for examination. A definite diagnosis can be made only after the tumor has been removed by the surgeon and examined microscopically by the pathologist.

## Cancer

### Description

The breasts are frequently affected by cancer. Although it is more common in women between the ages of 40 and 60, cancer of the breast can develop at any age. It may also occur in men.

Cancer of the breast can be cured if it is diagnosed and treated early. Because of this, women are encouraged to examine their breasts monthly following the menstrual period. This is especially important for those over 35 years of age. The woman can examine her breasts for dimpling, swelling, a depressed area, and retraction of the nipple by looking in the mirror. She should then lie upon her back and examine each breast systematically for lumps. If she finds a lump, she should consult her physician without delay. In addition to self-examination, she should have regular physical examinations.

### Symptoms

The woman with early cancer of the breast usually has a small, firm lump which does not cause pain. Pain is a later symptom. The tumor is usually not freely movable since it is growing into other tissues of the breast. As the growth enlarges, it can cause the breast to change in shape. Skin over the area does not move easily and may appear to have small dimples in it like an orange peel. The nipple may appear either higher or lower than the one of the unaffected breast. The nipple may be drawn inward and bleed as the malignant growth becomes larger. Cells from the malignant tumor can spread to the lymph nodes in the axilla. They may also spread to the chest, the bones, and other parts of the body. If the abnormal growth continues, it can affect the skin of the breast and cause it to become ulcerated. The open lesion is subject to infection.

### Treatment and Nursing Care

If the surgeon suspects that the patient has a malignancy, he usually removes some of the tissue from the tumor and has it examined by the pathologist. The tissue is frequently examined while the surgeon and the patient wait in the operating room so that, in case of malignancy, he can do an immediate mastectomy. If he learns definitely that the growth is malignant, he generally does a *radical mastectomy*. In this operation, he removes the entire breast, muscles of the chest wall, and lymph nodes in the axilla. X-ray therapy may be used before or after surgery.

The nursing care of the patient before surgery, discussed on pages 46 to 53, is applicable to this patient. However, the practical nurse needs to understand that the woman who is scheduled for this type of surgery is likely to have many fears. For example, she may be afraid of not being cured or of being unattractive because of losing one breast. She needs understanding from members of the nursing team who care for her.

Postoperatively, this patient needs care similar to that discussed on pages 53 to 56. She should be observed closely for bleeding and symptoms of shock. Remembering that the breasts have many large blood vessels which were cut during surgery helps the practical nurse to remember the importance of checking the dressing frequently for blood. Shock is a complication which may follow a long and extensive operation. Thus, it is important for the nurse who is caring for this patient to check the blood pressure, pulse, and respiration at frequent intervals. Of course, she should report symptoms of shock immediately.

Some surgeons request the nurse to elevate the patient's arm on the operative side by placing it on pillows. This is done to prevent edema of the arm.

After the patient has reacted from the anesthetic, she should be encouraged to breathe deeply at frequent intervals, to aid in the prevention of pulmonary complications.

The practical nurse may be asked to move the patient's arm on the affected side during the early postoperative period. She should have definite directions regarding this. As the patient improves, she should be encouraged to use her arm as much as possible. These exercises are important in helping the patient to regain full use of her arm.

Prosthetic forms can be purchased which match the size and shape of the breast removed. The patient should not wear this until the wound has healed, and she has the doctor's approval. Some surgeons prefer to recommend the type of prosthetic appliance to be used.

## BURN

### Description

Injury to the body caused by heat, electricity, x-ray, radium, and chemicals is known as a burn. Although a burn can and does affect other parts of the body, it almost always involves the skin. Heat is one of the more common causes of burns.

Burns are classified according to the amount of tissue which is either damaged or destroyed. The three-degree classification is frequently used. The person with a *first-degree* burn has a reddened skin. The one with a *second-degree* burn has blisters; whereas the person with a *third-degree* burn has an actual destruction of skin. Tissues below the skin, such as fat, muscles, and bone, may also be destroyed in varying amounts. An individual may have all three degrees of burn. However, a burned area usually has two degrees. For example, a burned person may have a reddened skin as well as blisters.

### First Aid

A clean, soothing substance such as petrolatum or a paste of baking soda can be applied to a first-degree burn. A second-degree burn may be cared for in the same manner if the injured area is not large. The person giving first aid should avoid breaking the blisters. A small, third-degree burn can be cared for by applying a soothing substance and then covering it with a dressing. The person should be treated by the doctor if much of the skin is burned. The area can be protected with a clean towel or a sheet until the doctor sees the patient.

An individual with a severe burn should be carried to the hospital. Remembering that one of the complications of a severe burn is shock helps the practical nurse to understand the importance of early measures to prevent this. The patient should be kept lying down and warm. The burned area should be covered with a freshly laundered towel or sheet. No attempt should be made to remove particles of clothing which stick to the burned region or to apply an ointment or any other substance. After draping the burned region, the person giving first aid should cover the patient with blankets in an effort to keep him warm. The patient may be given fluids to drink if his condition permits and if there is delay in transferring him to the hospital.

## Treatment and Nursing Care

Since the practical nurse may be responsible for assisting in the care of a severely burned patient, she needs to be familiar with the usual methods of treatment and nursing care. Understanding the purposes and importance of these measures enables her to be a more valuable member of the health team.

The physician usually plans his treatment of the patient who has an extensive burn with certain objectives in mind. These are: (1) prevention of, or controlling, shock, (2) relieving pain, (3) preventing infection, (4) controlling the loss of body fluids, (5) promoting healing, (6) preventing deformities, and (7) rehabilitation. Throughout the course of treatment he guides other members of the health team in helping the patient to avoid or to overcome emotional difficulties which are often associated with a severe burn.

### Prevention of, or Controlling, Shock

The doctor directs his early treatment of this patient toward preventing or controlling shock. The practical nurse recalls that this was an important factor in the first-aid care of a severely burned person. Keeping the patient warm by placing him in a comfortably warm room and by covering him adequately helps to prevent shock. The foot of the bed may be elevated. Intravenous fluids, such as glucose, saline, plasma, or blood, are generally administered to help replace fluids being lost, and to control shock. As the patient's condition improves, he is given liquids by mouth.

### Relieving Pain

Suitable drugs are ordered to relieve the severe pain which is often associated with an extensive burn. Since pain may influence the state of shock, relief of pain can help to prevent or to control shock. Morphine is a medication which is frequently selected by the physician for this purpose. A large dose may be prescribed in an effort to relieve the patient's pain. For example, 15 to 30 mg (¼ to ½ gr) may be ordered.

After the burned areas have been treated by the doctor, the patient needs rest. This is an important factor in the care of a burned patient because rest helps to prevent further shock and to promote healing. Knowing that the relief of pain is necessary for a person to rest, the practical nurse can understand why the doctor usually orders a drug for this purpose. The nursing team plays an important role in making the patient comfortable so that he can rest. Nursing measures, such as a comfortable position and a soothing backrub, when the patient's back is not burned, also help him to rest.

### Preventing Infection

Sterile technique is necessary in the care of a burn in order to aid in preventing infection. For this reason, the patient may be taken to the operating room. The physician generally cleans the injured area before treating it. It may be necessary for him to remove pieces of clothing which cling to the burned area by moistening the area with a sterile solution, such as normal saline.

The doctor may use either the closed method of treating the patient's burns or the open method. In the *closed method* of treatment, the physician covers the injured portion with sterile dressings. This helps to prevent further loss of fluid through the burned surface and to prevent infection. He frequently applies a sterile ointment, such as petrolatum or gauze containing petrolatum, to the burned tissue before bandaging it. The use of a lubricating substance helps to prevent the dressing from sticking to the raw surface. This helps to reduce pain associated with later dressings. Approximately one week may elapse before the doctor changes the dressing.

Members of the nursing team responsible for the care of a patient with bandaged extremities should observe his toes or fingers for symptoms of poor circulation. Swelling, numbness, coldness, cyanosis, and the absence of a pulse should be reported promptly to her team leader or head nurse.

The patient with bandages on his chest should be encouraged to take deep breaths frequently. He should have his position changed often or be reminded to turn himself. Sometimes a Balkan frame with a hand trapeze is placed on the patient's bed to aid him in turning himself. These measures are important in preventing pneumonia.

In the *open* or *exposure method* of treatment, the physician cleans the wound if necessary but does not apply a dressing. The burned area is exposed to air so that a protective crust can form. This may take several days or longer. After the crust has formed, it prevents further loss of vital body fluids. The burned area must be kept as clean as possible. For this reason, the patient is placed on sterile bed linen. Gowns and face masks are worn by those who care for him. A bed cradle is often placed over the patient to prevent linen from sticking to the burned surfaces and to keep him warm. Additional heat is sometimes obtained by the use of light bulbs in the bed cradle which are placed at a safe distance from the patient.

When caring for a burned patient, the practical nurse should observe him for symptoms of infection. She should report an elevated temperature, an increased respiratory or pulse rate, restlessness, pain, and a foul odor from the burned tissue to her team leader or head nurse.

Another important measure in the prevention of infection is cleanliness. The part of the patient's body which is not burned should be kept clean and dry. In addition to helping to prevent infection, cleanliness makes the patient more comfortable, aids in the removal of waste from the unburned skin, and helps to control offensive odors. Another measure to relieve the foul odor which comes from burned tissue is proper ventilation. Deodorants and commercial products which absorb odors may also be used for this purpose.

Tetanus antitoxin and antibiotics may be prescribed to prevent and to control infection. *Tetanus antitoxin* is a drug given to prevent an infection known as *tetanus*. The practical nurse may have heard this disease referred to as *lockjaw*. This drug usually is given to the patient soon after he has been burned. Penicillin is an example of an antibiotic which may be prescribed to control infection.

### Controlling the Loss of Body Fluids

The person who has a large amount of skin destroyed by a burn loses much of his body fluid. This results in a reduction of the fluids which are normally circulating in the body. The patient's blood may become concentrated because of this decreased amount of fluid. He may develop shock and die if these fluids are not replaced. In addition to shock, he may have kidney damage as a result of excess fluid loss.

Realizing the dangers of excess loss of body fluids should help the practical nurse to understand the importance of replacing them. It was stated earlier in this discussion that the patient is usually given intravenous fluids until he is able to take an adequate amount by mouth.

Laboratory procedures to determine the patient's hemoglobin and hematocrit (proportion of red cells to a specific amount of blood) are often ordered. These blood tests help the physician in determining the amount of blood concentration caused by the fluid loss. Knowing the patient's hemoglobin and hematocrit reading helps him plan the amount of fluids needed by the patient.

The physician may request the insertion of an indwelling catheter. The amount of urine drained through the catheter should be measured frequently and reported by the nurse. A urinalysis is generally ordered. This request may be repeated at periodic intervals. Knowing the amount of urine draining from the catheter and having a report of the urinalysis help the doctor to adjust the fluid therapy to the patient's needs.

Members of the nursing team who care for this patient should keep an accurate record of his intake and output. If the practical nurse notices that the patient is passing a smaller amount of urine or none at all, she should report this immediately to her team leader or head nurse. Urine which seems to have blood in it should be saved in case the doctor wants it sent to the laboratory.

### Promoting Healing

Measures to improve the patient's general condition, such as adequate rest, ample fluids, and cleanliness, are important factors in helping the burned area to heal. The prevention of infection, which has already been discussed, also aids the healing process.

The doctor may order a diet high in proteins, vitamins, and calories. This is done in order to meet the increased nutritional demands of the body during the healing process. The patient may need to be encouraged to eat because he has a loss of appetite. The practical nurse may want to review the care of a patient with anorexia (loss of appetite), which is discussed on page 27.

Grafting may be necessary to hasten healing. In doing a graft, the surgeon takes skin from another part of the patient's body and places it on the raw area. Skin grows from the small islands of transplanted tissue to cover the wound.

### Preventing Deformities

Abnormal contractures of damaged tissue can result in deformity. If the doctor uses a dressing on the extremity, he places the limb in good position before applying the bandage. In an attempt to prevent deformity, sometimes a leg or an arm is splinted after being bandaged. The patient treated by the exposure method should be kept in good body alignment also.

Members of the nursing team are responsible for helping the severely burned patient to keep his body in good alignment. Weakened muscles may be supported by the use of pillows, sandbags, rolled towels, and a footboard. A bed cradle may be used to keep the bedclothes from pressing on the affected part. The patient should be encouraged to move as his condition improves. The doctor may ask the physical therapist to give special care, such as massage and exercise, to aid in preventing or correcting deformities.

### Rehabilitation

The person who is handicapped because of a severe burn needs help in achieving the maximum amount of use of the affected part of his body. The specialized service of other members of the health team, such as the physical therapist and the occupational therapist, are beneficial in helping the patient to return to a satisfying and useful way of life. Plastic surgery is necessary for the correction of deformities in some cases.

The occupational therapist may be asked to plan suitable diversions for the patient during his long period of hospitalization. This valuable member of the health team can select and guide the patient in activities which help to prevent or to correct deformities in addition to occupying his mind. The occupational therapist can also be helpful to the patient in planning for a future job.

## CANCER

### Description

The skin is the part of the body which is most often affected by cancer. It is more common in elderly people. Cancer of the skin can be frequently cured because it is usually recognized early and is easy to reach for treatment. The malignancy may spread to another part of the body or it may remain localized.

A sore that does not heal, an abnormal growth, scaly patches which persist, or any change in a wart or a mole may be a symptom of skin cancer.

## Treatment

The usual treatment of a patient with skin cancer is surgery, radiation therapy, or a combination of both. Plastic surgery may be necessary to repair a defect resulting from the treatment. The patient sometimes needs a dressing over the area for a long period of time until repair to the wound is complete. The skin around the area should be kept clean. Scotch tape may be used instead of adhesive for the patient with sensitive skin, and especially in those requiring a dressing for a long period of time.

## SUGGESTIONS FOR STUDY

1. Review the functions of the skin.
2. Why is it advisable for a person not to squeeze pimples?
3. Why should a person with athlete's foot keep his feet clean and dry?
4. Describe a macule, a papule, a vesicle, and a pustule.
5. What can a person do in an effort to prevent contact dermatitis after he has handled poison ivy?
6. Describe the skin changes in an individual with impetigo contagiosa.
7. What adaptations of the daily bath might be necessary in caring for the patient with a dermatologic condition?
8. At what age is a woman most likely to develop cancer of the breast?
9. Discuss the nursing care of a patient recuperating from a radical mastectomy.
10. Describe a first-degree burn. A second-degree burn. A third-degree burn.
11. What first-aid care should be given to a person with a severe burn before being transferred to the hospital?
12. What are the main objectives in caring for the patient with a severe burn? Discuss ways in which the practical nurse can help to accomplish these objectives.

13. What are the two main methods commonly used in treating a patient's burn? Which method have you seen used?

14. Why is the rate of cure high in patients with skin cancer?

## REFERENCES FOR CHAPTER 24

Alexander, Sarah E.: "Nursing Care of a Patient after Breast Surgery," *Am. J. Nursing*, 57:1571-72, (Dec.) 1957.

American Cancer Society, Inc.: *A Cancer Source Book for Nurses*. The Society, New York, 1956, pp. 56-63.

Brown, Amy F.: *Medical Nursing*, 3rd ed. W. B. Saunders Co., Philadelphia, 1957, pp. 471-523.

Eliason, Eldridge; Ferguson, L. Kraeer; and Sholtis, Lillian A.: *Surgical Nursing*, 10th ed. J. B. Lippincott Co., Philadelphia, 1955, pp. 397-430.

Emerson, Charles P., Jr. and Bragdon, Jane S.: *Essentials of Medicine*, 17th ed. J. B. Lippincott Co., Philadelphia, 1955, pp. 445-504.

Gill, Helen Z. (ed.): *Basic Nursing*, 4th ed. The Macmillan Company, New York, 1955, pp. 46-49 and 515-22.

Goldman, Leon: "Parasitic Diseases of the Skin," *Am. J. Nursing*, 56: 1570-72, (Dec.) 1956.

Hackett, Angela M.: "The Care of a Patient with Contact Dermatitis," *Am. J. Nursing*, 58:84-86, (Jan.) 1958.

Harmer, Bertha, and Henderson, Virginia: *Textbook of the Principles and Practice of Nursing*, 5th ed. The Macmillan Company, New York, 1955, pp. 1175-81.

Higginbotham, Sarah: "Arm Exercises after Mastectomy," *Am. J. Nursing*, 57:1573-74, (Dec.) 1957.

Jensen, Julius, and Jensen, Deborah: *Nursing in Clinical Medicine*, 4th ed. The Macmillan Company, New York, 1954, pp. 813-39.

Kimber, Diana; Gray, Carolyn E.; Stackpole, Caroline E.; and Leavell, Lutie C.: *Textbook of Anatomy and Physiology* 13th ed. The Macmillan Company, New York, 1955, pp. 670-94, and 766-69.

Knapp, Margaret F.: *Cancer Nursing: A Manual for Public Health Nurses*. National Cancer Institute, Public Health Service, Department of Health, Education, and Welfare, Washington, D. C., and the New York State Department of Health, Albany, 1955, pp. 48-51 and 55.

Lea, Walker A.: "Rouges and Rashes," *Am. J. Nursing*, 58:82-84, (Jan.) 1958.

Popma, Alfred M.: "Cancer of the Breast," *Am. J. Nursing*, 57:1570-71, (Dec.) 1957.

Proudfit, Fairfax T., and Robinson, Corinne H.: *Nutrition and Diet Therapy*, 11 ed. The Macmillan Company, New York, 1955, pp. 506-15.

West, John P.; Keller, Manelva W.; and Harmon, Elizabeth H.: *Nursing Care of the Surgical Patient*, 6th ed. The Macmillan Company, New York, 1957, pp. 187-93 and 504-27.

# GLOSSARY

**abdominal paracentesis.** Withdrawal of fluid from the peritoneal cavity by the use of a hollow needle or a trocar.

**abdominoperineal operation.** Surgical removal of the rectum, anus, and part of the colon through abdominal and perineal incisions.

**abscess.** A collection of pus.

    **stitch abscess.** That which occurs around a skin suture.

**accommodation.** The adjustment of an organ, an organism, or a part of the body; especially the ability of the eye to focus on objects at varying distances.

**acne vulgaris.** An inflammatory condition often affecting the face and characterized by the formation of blackheads, papules, and postules; also known as pimples.

**adhesion.** An abnormal union of surfaces which are normally separate.

**albuminuria.** The presence of albumin in the urine.

**allergen.** A substance which causes an allergic reaction.

**allergy.** An abnormal reaction to certain substances which ordinarily have no effect on other individuals.

**amenorrhea.** A condition in which a woman has an absence of menstruation.

**amino acids.** Chemical compounds obtained from proteins.

**ampulla of Vater.** A short, dilated tube formed by the common bile duct and pancreatic duct as they enter the duodenum.

**anal fissure.** An ulcerating crack or crevice in the mucous membrane of the anus.

**anaphylactic shock.** A state of shock which may follow the injection of a substance to which the person is allergic; anaphylaxis.

**anemia.** A decrease in the number of red blood cells, or in the amount of hemoglobin; both may be reduced.

**anesthetic.** A drug which causes a loss of feeling.

**aneurysm.** A dilatation of the wall of an artery, such as a dilatation of the aorta caused by syphilis.

**angina pectoris.** A condition in which a person has attacks of chest pain caused by an insufficient blood supply to the heart muscle.

**angioneurotic edema.** Localized, swollen areas of the skin or the mucous membrane sometimes caused by a food allergy; giant urticaria.

**ankylosis.** Stiffness of a joint; union of the bones in a joint.

**anorexia.** Loss of appetite.

**antacid.** A drug which neutralizes acids.

**antibiotic.** A substance made from certain microorganisms which either checks the growth or kills other microorganisms.

**anticoagulant.** A drug used to prevent the clotting of blood.

**antispasmodic.** A substance which relieves convulsions or spasmodic pains.

**anuria.** Lack of urinary output caused by failure of the kidneys to excrete urine or by an obstruction in the urinary tract.

**anus.** External opening of the colon.

**aphasia.** Either the loss of speech or an impairment of speech.

**aphonia.** Inability to speak; loss of the voice.

**apnea.** A temporary absence of breathing.

**appendectomy.** Surgical removal of the vermiform appendix.

**appendicitis.** An inflammation involving the vermiform appendix.

**arteriogram.** X-ray examination of an artery after the injection of a suitable dye; for example, the arteries in the brain may be examined in this manner.

**arteriosclerosis.** A condition of the arteries in which soft, fatty substances are deposited on the inside of the vessels causing the walls to become thicker. As calcium is deposited in these areas, it causes the artery to become rigid, hard, brittle, and less elastic. Hardening of the arteries.

**arteriosclerotic heart disease.** An abnormal heart condition caused by hardening of the coronary arteries.

**arthritis.** An inflammatory condition of one or more joints.

> **degenerative joint disease.** A chronic condition of the joints which is less likely to cause deformity than rheumatoid arthritis. Generally progresses slowly. The patient may have an increase in the size of the bones of the affected joints and spur formation. The inflamed joints are usually painful, stiff, and enlarged. The joint changes are not as marked as those associated with rheumatoid arthritis. It is more common in late middle life. Also known as hypertrophic arthritis and osteoarthritis.

> **rheumatoid arthritis.** A chronic condition which can affect many joints. The patient usually has general symptoms of inflammation such as fever and malaise. The inflamed joints generally are painful, swollen, and have a decreased ability to move. Ankylosis and deformity may occur. It is more common between 20 and 50 years of age.

**artificial pneumothorax.** The injection of air or gas into the pleural cavity to cause the lung to collapse; used in the treatment of pulmonary tuberculosis.

**ascites.** An abnormal collection of fluid in the peritoneal cavity.

**asthma.** A condition in which the patient has attacks of dyspnea. Frequently refers to bronchial asthma.

> **bronchial asthma.** That caused by an allergy. Allergic asthma.

> **cardiac asthma.** That caused by failure of the left ventricle which results in congestion of the lungs.

**astigmatism.** Impaired vision resulting from an irregular curvature of either the cornea or the crystalline lens of the eye.

**atherosclerosis.** A form of arteriosclerosis in which deposits of fat are made in the innermost wall of an artery.

**athlete's foot.** An inflammation of the feet and sometimes the hands caused by fungi. Tiny blisters filled with fluid form on the affected areas.

**audiometer.** An instrument used to measure a person's hearing ability.

**aura.** A sensation which warns a person of an oncoming convulsion.

**bacteria.** Microorganisms belonging to the plant kingdom. Some cause infectious disease such as tuberculosis and typhoid fever.

**bile.** A fluid secreted by the liver which aids in the digestion and absorption of fats.

**biopsy.** Removal of tissue from the body for microscopic examination; often used to determine presence of cancer.

**bradycardia.** Slow heart action. The pulse rate is usually below 60.

**bronchogram.** X-ray examination of the bronchial tree after an iodized oil has been injected into the bronchi.

**bronchopneumonia.** An inflammation of the lungs distributed around the bronchi.

**bronchoscope.** An instrument which can be inserted through the mouth, throat, and trachea into the bronchi. It enables the doctor to examine the bronchial walls; sometimes used in treatment.

**bronchoscopy.** An examination of the bronchial walls with a bronchoscope.

**bursa.** A small sac containing fluid; located so as to prevent friction between surfaces which move upon one another.

**bursitis.** An inflammatory condition of a bursa.

**calcification.** The deposit of lime salts in the body's tissues.

**calculus.** A hard body formed in a cavity or elsewhere in the body; stone.

  **renal calculus.** One located in the kidney; kidney stone; nephrolithiasis.

**callus.** A gluey substance which forms around the fractured ends of a bone. Lime salts and bone cells are deposited in the callus and cause it to harden.

**cancer.** A malignant tumor or one which threatens an individual's life.

**carcinoma.** A malignant tumor of epithelial tissue.

**cardiac cycle.** The regular series of changes which occur in the heart with each heartbeat. Systole, diastole, and the rest period are the three phases which make up this series of changes.

**cardiac orifice.** The opening between the esophagus and stomach.

**caseation.** Death of a group of cells which results in the formation of a cheese-like substance; occurs frequently in tuberculous infections.

**cast.** 1. A substance which has assumed the shape of a cavity in which it was molded. A common example is seen in the casts found in urine. These casts are formed when a substance hardens in the tubule of the kidney and is later washed out by the flow of urine.
  2. A mixture which becomes hardened as it dries, such as plaster of

Paris. This is used to immobilize parts of the body. Crinoline containing plaster of Paris is moistened and molded over the affected area. As the plaster dries, it becomes hardened.

**catamenia.** Menstruation.

**cataract.** Clouding of the crystalline lens of the eye.

**cauterization.** The destruction of tissue by the use of a chemical or by using electricity which is passed through a thin blade or a wire loop.

**cecostomy.** An operation in which an artificial opening is made into the cecum through the abdominal wall.

**cecum.** The large pouch at the beginning of the large intestine.

**cerebral hemorrhage.** Ruptured blood vessel in the brain; stroke.

**cerebral vascular accident.** A disease of the arteries in the brain resulting in an inadequate blood supply; apoplexy; stroke; cerebral accident. It may be caused by hemorrhage, a thrombus, or an embolus.

**cerumen.** Earwax.

**chancre.** A lesion which develops in an area through which invading microorganisms have entered the body. The term usually refers to the area through which spirochetes enter the body and cause syphilis.

**cholangitis.** An inflammation of the bile ducts.

**cholecystectomy.** Surgical removal of the gallbladder.

**cholecystitis.** An abnormal condition in which the gallbladder is inflamed.

**cholecystostomy.** An operation in which an opening is made into the gallbladder, usually to allow its contents to drain.

**choledochostomy.** An operation in which an opening is made into the common bile duct.

**cholelithiasis.** The presence of gallstones in the gallbladder or in one of the bile ducts.

**cilia.** Hairlike projections of mucous membrane in various parts of the body.

**circulation.** Movement from place to place in a set course, such as the flow of blood in the body's blood vessels.

    **pulmonary circulation.** The flow of blood from the right side of the heart through the lungs, to the left side of the heart.

    **systemic circulation.** The flow of blood from the left ventricle, through the blood vessels of the body and back to the heart again; general circulation.

**climacteric.** Menopause.

**colic.** Abdominal pain caused by muscle spasm.

**colitis.** An inflammation of the colon.

    **mucous colitis.** That characterized by the passage of mucus.

    **ulcerative colitis.** That characterized by ulceration of the mucous membrane.

**collapse therapy.** A method of treating pulmonary tuberculosis in which the lung is collapsed.

**colostomy.** An operation in which an opening is made through the abdominal wall into the colon and an artificial anus is formed.

**colporrhaphy.** An operation in which the vagina is repaired by suture.

  **anterior colporrhaphy.** One in which a cystocele is repaired.

  **posterior colporrhaphy.** One in which a rectocele is repaired.

**coma.** A state of unconsciousness from which the person cannot be aroused.

**commissurotomy.** An operation in which a stenosed heart valve is made larger.

**common bile duct.** The tube which is formed by the hepatic and cystic ducts and leads to the duodenum.

**concussion.** Pertains to a severe shaking or jarring of a part of the body; often used in referring to the condition which follows a fall or a blow on the head resulting in either partial or complete loss of consciousness.

**congenital defect.** Abnormal developmental condition present at birth.

**congestion.** An abnormal amount of blood in a part of the body.

**congestive heart failure.** A condition in which the heart is unable to pump blood properly. This results in an abnormal collection of fluid in various parts of the body. Cardiac failure; cardiac decompensation.

**conization.** Removal of tissue by the use of electricity, especially of the cervix.

**conjunctiva.** The mucous membrane which lines the eyelids and covers the front part of the eyeball.

**conjunctivitis.** An inflammatory condition of the conjunctiva.

**constipation.** A condition in which the person has fewer stools than usual. There is a longer period of time between bowel movements.

  **atonic constipation.** Type associated with decreased muscle tone of the colon.

  **spastic constipation.** Type associated with increased muscle tone of the colon.

**convulsion.** Involuntary contractions of the muscles.

**coronary arteries.** The blood vessels which supply the heart with blood.

**coronary occlusion.** A heart attack caused by closure of a coronary artery which nourishes the heart; coronary thrombosis; myocardial infarction; "a coronary."

**cough.** A violent, involuntary exhalation of air following a deep inspiration.

**cranium.** The bony case which protects the brain and its meninges; skull.

**cretinism.** Hypothyroidism which started during fetal life or early infancy.

**culture.** Pertaining to the growth of microorganisms on an artificial nutrient substance, such as bouillon, agar, gelatin, or blood serum. Microorganisms from the throat, blood, urine, and other parts or secretions of the body are grown frequently in the laboratory to determine the cause of illness.

**cyanosis.** A bluish color of the skin and mucous membranes caused by an inadequate amount of oxygen in the hemoglobin of the blood.

**cyst.** An abnormal sac which contains liquid or semifluid material.

**cystectomy.** 1. The surgical removal of the urinary bladder, or the gallbladder.

2. The surgical removal of a cyst.

**cystic duct.** The tube leading from the gallbladder.

**cystitis.** An inflammation of the urinary bladder.

**cystocele.** A condition in which the urinary bladder has prolapsed into the vagina.

**cystoscope.** An instrument used by the doctor to examine and to treat conditions of the urinary bladder, ureters, and kidneys.

**cystotomy.** An operation in which an incision is made into the bladder.


**deafness.** A loss of hearing which may be either partial or complete.

    **conductive deafness.** That which occurs when the sound waves do not reach the inner ear properly.

    **perceptive deafness.** That which occurs when the sound waves go through the middle ear properly but are not received properly by the brain.

**decompression.** The removal of pressure; especially the surgical relief of intracranial pressure.

**defecation.** Evacuation or emptying the contents of the rectum.

**deformity.** An abnormal size or shape of the body or a part of the body.

**degeneration.** Progressive deterioration of the body's cells often associated with the aging process. It results in a loss of the cells' ability to function effectively.

**dehydration.** An abnormal loss of water from the body's tissues.

**dermatitis.** A general term used to indicate an inflammation of the skin.

**dermatologist.** A physician specializing in dermatology.

**dermatology.** The branch of medicine dealing with the structure and function of the skin, its diseases, and the treatment of persons with these diseases.

**dermoid cyst.** A sac containing different kinds of tissues, such as teeth and hair; teratoma.

**desensitization.** Method of treating a patient with an allergy. An extract of the allergen is given to the patient in an effort to help him to build up a tolerance to that substance, or to become less sensitive to it. It is known also as hyposensitization.

**diathermy.** The use of a machine which sends an electric current into the tissues below the skin to produce local heat.

**dilatation and curettage.** An operation in which the cervix is dilated and the lining of the uterus is scraped with a curette; D and C.

**diplococci.** Oval-shaped bacteria which grow in pairs.

**diuretic.** A substance which increases the output of urine.

**diverticulitis.** An inflammation of a diverticulum.

**diverticulum.** A pouch or sac branching off from a structure; for example, a diverticulum may be located in the esophagus, the stomach, or the intestine.

**duodenum.** The upper part of the small intestine, beginning at the stomach.

**dyspepsia.** Indigestion.

**dysphagia.** Difficult swallowing, or an inability to swallow.

**dyspnea.** Difficult breathing, or shortness of breath.

**edema.** Collection of fluid in the tissues; dropsy.

**electroencephalogram.** A tracing or graphic record of the electrical waves of the brain.

**embolism.** The obstruction of a blood vessel by an abnormal particle which has been circulating in the blood stream.

  **cerebral embolism.** That which occurs in a blood vessel of the brain.

  **pulmonary embolism.** That which occurs in a blood vessel in the lungs.

**embolus.** An abnormal particle, such as a blood clot or clumps of bacteria, which circulates in the blood stream until it lodges in a blood vessel and causes embolism.

**emotions.** A person's feelings, such as love, hate, fear, anxiety, worry, anger, jealousy, disgust, depression, and joy.

**empyema.** A collection of pus in an organ, a cavity, or a hollow space; for example, pus may form in the pleural cavity or the gallbladder.

**encephalography.** X-ray examination of the brain after some of the cerebrospinal fluid has been replaced by air or oxygen.

**endocarditis.** An inflammatory condition of the endocardium.

  **bacterial endocarditis.** That caused by bacteria.

**endocardium.** The membrane lining the inside of the heart.

**endocervicitis.** An inflammation of the membrane lining the cervix; cervicitis.

**endometrium.** The mucous membrane which lines the inside of the uterus.

**endotoxin.** A poisonous substance stored within a living microorganism and given off after this organism dies.

**enterostomy.** An operation in which an artificial opening is made into the intestine through the abdominal wall.

**epilepsy.** An abnormal condition in which the person has an increased discharge of energy from the brain at various times. This abnormal discharge of energy may cause loss of consciousness, convulsions, or both.

**epistaxis.** Nosebleed.

**eructation.** Burping or belching.

**esophageal speech.** A method of speaking by swallowing air and producing sounds when the air is forced back from the stomach. It is used by a patient who has had a laryngectomy.

**estrogenic hormone.** A substance produced mainly by an ovarian follicle and causing changes in the uterine mucosa. Follicular hormone; estrone; theelin.

**exotoxin.** A poisonous substance which is excreted by a living micro-organism.

**expiration.** Act of forcing air out of the lungs; exhalation.

**extensor.** A muscle used to straighten a part of the body.

**farsightedness.** *See* hypermetropia.

**fenestration.** An operation in which an opening is made in the bone covering the inner ear. This opening is covered by tympanic membrane. Sound waves are then transmitted from the tympanic membrane to the inner ear.

**fever.** A rise in the body's temperature above normal.

**fever blisters.** *See* herpes simplex.

**fibrinogen.** A substance in the blood necessary for clotting.

**fibromyoma.** A tumor of a muscle in which muscle tissue and white fibers are intermingled; frequently found in the uterus.

**flatulence.** The presence of gas in the gastrointestinal tract.

**flexor.** A muscle used to bend a part of the body.

**follicle-stimulating hormone.** A substance secreted by the anterior part of the pituitary gland; this hormone stimulates follicles to grow in the female and aids in the development of mature germ cells in the male.

**foot drop.** A condition in which the foot falls; the foot is bent downward in an abnormal position.

**fracture.** A broken bone.

**fulguration.** The destruction of tissue by the use of electric sparks.

**gallbladder.** A pear-shaped organ located under the liver for the storage of bile.

**gangrene.** Death of a portion of the body.

**gastrectomy.** An operation in which part or all of the stomach is removed; frequently called partial or subtotal gastrectomy when part of the stomach is removed.

**gastric gavage.** A method of giving liquid nourishment by means of a tube which has been inserted through the throat and esophagus into the stomach. The tube may be passed through either the nose or the mouth to the throat.

**gastric lavage.** Washing out or irrigation of the stomach.

**gastroscope.** An instrument used to examine the inside of the stomach.

**gastrostomy.** A permanent, artificial opening into the stomach.

**glaucoma.** An eye disease in which the pressure within the eyeball is increased.

**glomerulonephritis.** An inflammation of the kidneys which involves the glomeruli.

**glycosuria.** A condition in which sugar is present in the urine.

**goiter.** An enlarged thyroid gland.

**graafian follicle.** A small sac containing an ovum in the ovary; a mature ovarian follicle.

**grand mal seizure.** An attack of epilepsy characterized by loss of consciousness and a generalized convulsion.

**gumma.** A lesion which develops in a person with late syphilis.

**gynecologist.** A physician specializing in gynecology.

**gynecology.** A branch of medical science which deals with diseases of women, especially those of the reproductive organs.


**hematemesis.** Vomiting of blood.

**hematoma.** A collection of clotted blood which readily becomes enclosed in a capsule.

**hematuria.** The presence of blood in the urine.

**hemiplegia.** Paralysis affecting one side of the body.

**hemoglobin.** The coloring matter in red blood cells; it has the vital function of picking up oxygen and releasing it to the body's cells.

**hemophilia.** A disease characterized by a prolonged time for the blood to clot. This is a rare hereditary disease which occurs only in males but is transmitted only through females.

**hemoptysis.** The expectoration of blood from the respiratory tract.

**hemorrhoidectomy.** Surgical removal of hemorrhoids.

**hemorrhoids.** Varicose veins of the anal canal and lower part of the rectum.

    **external hemorrhoids.** Those located around the anal orifice.

    **internal hemorrhoids.** Those located in the area of the junction of the anal canal and the rectum.

**hepatic duct.** The tube through which bile leaves the liver.

**hepatitis.** An abnormal condition in which the liver is inflamed.

**hernia.** An abnormal protrusion of part of the contents of a cavity through its wall; rupture.

    **congenital hernia.** One which is present at birth.

    **incisional hernia.** One which develops in an operative scar; ventral hernia.

    **inguinal hernia.** A protrusion of part of the abdominal contents through the inguinal canal in the groin.

    **irreducible hernia.** One which cannot be forced back into the cavity by gentle pressure.

    **reducible hernia.** One which can be forced back into the cavity by gentle pressure.

    **umbilical hernia.** An abnormal protrusion of part of the abdominal contents through the umbilicus.

**herniorrhaphy.** An operation in which a hernia is repaired.

**herpes.** A condition in which either the skin or mucous membrane is inflamed and tiny blisters filled with fluid form.

**herpes simplex.** That which is believed to be caused by a virus and occurs frequently about the lips; also called fever blisters.

**herpes zoster.** That which occurs along the course of a nerve and is associated with neuralgic pain; also called shingles.

**Hodgkin's disease.** An abnormal condition of the lymph nodes.

**hordeolum.** A stye.

**hormone.** A substance produced by an organ or a certain group of cells and carried by the blood to another part of the body where it has a specific effect. For example, one hormone produced by the pituitary gland in the head is carried by the blood to the ovaries where it stimulates a follicle to develop. Another example is seen in the thyroid gland in the neck which secretes thyroxin. This hormone is carried by the blood to the body's cells to control their metabolism.

**hydrocele.** An abnormal accumulation of fluid in a sac within the scrotum.

**hydronephrosis.** An abnormal collection of urine in the pelvis of the kidney because of an obstruction in the urinary tract.

**hydrotherapy.** The use of water in the treatment of a patient.

**hyperglycemia.** An increased amount of sugar in the blood.

**hypermetropia.** A condition characterized by the ability to see objects better when they are at a distance; farsightedness.

**hypertension.** High blood pressure.

    **essential hypertension.** That occurring without a known cause; also called primary hypertension.

    **malignant essential hypertension.** A severe case occurring without a known cause.

**hypertensive heart disease.** Disease of the heart resulting from high blood pressure.

**hyperthyroidism.** An abnormal condition in which the thyroid gland is overactive; toxic goiter.

**hypertrophy.** An abnormal increase in the size of an organ or a part.

**hypodermoclysis.** The injection of a large amount of fluid into the tissue beneath the skin; subcutaneous infusion.

**hypoglycemia.** A decreased amount of sugar in the blood.

**hypothyroidism.** An abnormal condition in which the thyroid gland is underactive.

**hypoxia.** Oxygen deficiency.

**hysterectomy.** Surgical removal of all or part of the uterus.

    **abdominal hysterectomy.** Removal is done through an incision in the abdomen.

    **vaginal hysterectomy.** Removal is done through the vagina.


**ileocecal valve.** A muscular structure located between the small and large intestine to prevent material from returning to the small intestine.

**ileostomy.** An operation in which an artificial opening is made into the ileum through the abdominal wall.

**ileum.** The lower part of the small intestine leading from the jejunum to the large intestine.

**ilium.** The broad upper part of the hipbone.

**impetigo contagiosa.** An infectious disease of the skin which may be caused by streptococci and staphylococci. Vesicles, pustules, and crusts form on the affected area.

**incontinence.** Loss of the control of natural evacuations, especially involuntary micturition and/or defecation.

**indwelling catheter.** A hollow tube left in the patient's bladder for drainage of urine; retention catheter.

**infection.** Inflammatory process caused by a pathogen.

**inflammation.** A defensive reaction of the body to any injury.

**injury.** Damage or harm to the body produced by such factors as a blow, a foreign body, a chemical, electricity, heat, cold, or a pathogen.

**inspiration.** Act of taking air into the lungs; inhalation.

**intestinal obstruction.** An abnormal condition in which there is a hindrance to the normal flow of contents within the intestines.

**intestinal resection.** Surgical removal of part of the intestine.

**intravenous.** Within the veins.

**intussusception.** The slipping of one part into another; especially the slipping of one portion of the intestine into another.

**ischiorectal abscess.** An abscess in the soft tissue near the anus or the rectum.

**isolation.** Separation of a patient from other persons because of a contagious disease.

**jejunum.** The middle part of the small intestine, beginning at the duodenum and ending at the ileum.

**jaundice.** Yellowness of the skin, eyes, mucous membranes, and body secretions caused by bile pigments in the blood.

    **hemolytic jaundice.** That which occurs when the destruction of red blood cells is abnormally fast.

    **nonobstructive jaundice.** That which occurs when the liver cells are damaged and are unable to eliminate bile pigments properly.

    **obstructive jaundice.** That which occurs when the flow of bile through either the common bile duct or the hepatic duct is blocked.

**keratoplasty.** Plastic surgery of the cornea; especially a corneal transplant.

**lacrimal gland.** A gland which is located above the eye and produces tears; tear gland.

**laminectomy.** An operation in which part of the vertebrae covering the spinal cord is removed.

**laparotomy.** An operation in which an incision is made through the abdominal wall.

  **exploratory laparotomy.** That which is done to allow the surgeon to search for the diseased area.

**leukemia.** A group of diseases in which there is an abnormal increase of white blood cells.

**leukocytosis.** An abnormal increase in the number of white blood cells.

**leukopenia.** An abnormal decrease in the number of white blood cells.

**leukorrhea.** A vaginal discharge.

**lobectomy.** Removal of a lobe of an organ. The term is often used in referring to removal of a lobe of the lung.

**locomotor system.** Parts of the body concerned with motion, especially bones, muscles, and joints; the muscular and skeletal systems.

**lumbar puncture.** A procedure in which the physician inserts a needle between two of the lumbar vertebrae into the spinal canal to remove cerebrospinal fluid, in order to determine the pressure of the fluid, or to inject medication; also called spinal tap or spinal puncture.

**luteinizing hormone.** A substance produced by the anterior part of the pituitary gland. This hormone stimulates the corpus luteum to develop and to produce progesterone in the female. It also stimulates the testis in the male to produce testicular hormones.

**macule.** A discolored, unelevated spot on the skin.

**malaise.** A general and indefinite feeling of discomfort or illness.

**malignancy.** Threatening to a person's life, such as cancer.

**mastectomy.** Surgical removal of the breast.

**mastitis.** An inflammatory condition of the breast.

**mastoidectomy.** The surgical removal of part or all of the mastoid air cells.

**mastoiditis.** An inflammation of the air cells in the portion of the temporal bone behind the ear which is known as the mastoid.

**meatus urethrae.** The opening of the urethra.

**meninges.** The membranes covering the brain and spinal cord.

**meningitis.** An inflammatory condition of the membranes covering the brain, the spinal cord, or both.

**menopause.** The period in a woman's life when menstruation stops; climacteric.

**menstruation.** The normal, periodic discharge of bloody fluid from the uterus; catamenia.

**metabolism.** Process by which foodstuffs are used to produce energy, changed into tissue elements, and stored in the body's cells; changes which occur to food from the time it is digested until it is eliminated.

**metastasis.** Transfer of disease from one area of the body to another.

**metrorrhagia.** Uterine bleeding between menstrual periods.

**microorganism.** A tiny living body visible only through a microscope.

**micturition.** The act of discharging urine from the bladder; urination; voiding.

**milk leg.** Thrombophlebitis.

**multiple sclerosis.** An abnormal condition in which the person has areas of degeneration in the brain and spinal cord. These areas are replaced by scar tissue. Parts of the body receiving their nerve supply from the diseased areas have disturbed function.

**murmur.** An abnormal heart sound heard by the doctor with a stethoscope.

**myelin.** The fatty substance which forms a sheath or covering around nerve fibers.

**myocardium.** Muscle tissue of the heart.

**myopia.** A condition characterized by the ability to see objects better at close range; nearsightedness.

**myringotomy.** An operation in which an opening is made into the tympanic membrane.

**myxedema.** An advanced form of hypothyroidism in adults.

**nausea.** A feeling of discomfort in the region of the stomach and a tendency to vomit.

**nearsightedness.** *See* myopia.

**neoplasm.** A new growth or an abnormal growth of cells; tumor.

**nephrectomy.** The surgical removal of a kidney.

**nephritis.** An inflammatory condition of the kidneys.

**nephrolithotomy.** The surgical removal of a stone from the kidney through an incision into that organ.

**nephrotomy.** An operation in which an incision is made into the kidney.

**neuralgia.** Pain along the course of one or more nerves.

**neuritis.** An inflammatory condition of one or more nerves.

**neurologist.** A physician specializing in neurology.

**neurology.** The branch of medicine dealing with the structure and function of the nervous system, its diseases, and the treatment of persons with these diseases.

**oliguria.** Decrease in the amount of urine produced.

**oophorectomy.** Surgical removal of an ovary.

**oophoritis.** An inflammation of either one or both ovaries.

**ophthalmia neonatorum.** A gonorrheal infection of a newborn baby's eyes.

**ophthalmologist.** A physician specializing in ophthalmology; oculist.

**ophthalmology.** The branch of medicine dealing with the structure and function of the eye, its diseases, and the treatment of persons with these diseases.

**ophthalmoscope.** An instrument used to examine the inside of the eye.

**optician.** An individual who makes lenses according to the doctor's recommendation.

**optometrist.** An individual licensed to measure the visual powers of a person without the use of drugs.

**orthopedics.** The branch of surgery concerned with the treatment of a patient with a deformity, a disease, or an ailment of the locomotor system.

**orthopedist.** A physician specializing in orthopedics.

**orthopnea.** A condition in which the patient feels that he must sit up in order to breathe.

**osteomyelitis.** An inflammation of the bone which frequently involves the marrow.

**otitis media.** An inflammatory process of the middle ear.

**otologist.** A physician specializing in otology.

**otology.** The branch of medicine dealing with the structure and function of the ear, its diseases, and the treatment of persons with these diseases.

**otosclerosis.** An abnormal growth of new bone usually around the oval window between the middle ear and inner ear. This results in progressive loss of hearing.

**otoscope.** An instrument used to examine the external auditory canal and the tympanic membrane.

**pain, referred.** The presence of pain in an area of the body which is not the diseased place.

**palpitation.** An awareness of heart action which may appear to be fast or fluttering.

**pancreatitis.** An inflammatory condition of the pancreas.

**panhysterectomy.** Removal of the entire uterus.

**Papanicolaou smear.** Microscopic examination of the body's secretions to determine presence of malignant cells; cytologic test for cancer.

**papilledema.** An abnormal condition in which the optic nerve becomes edematous; choked disk.

**papule.** A small, rounded, raised area on the skin.

**paraffin-dip treatment.** The use of melted paraffin for the application of heat.

**paralysis.** Loss of muscle function often caused by injury to the nervous system.

**paralysis agitans.** A chronic disease of the nervous system. Parkinson's disease; shaking palsy; parkinsonism.

**paralytic ileus.** Loss of muscle function of the intestines; adynamic ileus.

**paraplegia.** Paralysis of the legs.

**paresis.** A slight loss of muscle function.

    **general paresis.** A late form of syphilis in which the nervous system is affected. The patient has mental changes, tremors, and difficulty in talking.

**pathogen.** An agent which causes disease, usually a microorganism.

**pedicle.** A slender projection which acts as a stem.

**pericardial tap.** Withdrawal of fluid from the pericardium with a needle; paracentesis of the pericardium.

**pericardium.** Membranous sac covering the heart.

**perineorrhaphy.** An operation in which the perineum is repaired by suture.

**perineum.** 1. The part of the body between the pubic arch in the front and the coccyx in the back.
2. The portion of the body between the vulva and the anus in the female and between the scrotum and the anus in the male.

**periosteum.** A membrane which covers most of the surface of a bone.

**peristalsis.** Wormlike wave of contraction in hollow, muscular tubes, such as the intestine. This motion forces the contents of the tube toward its opening.

**peritoneal cavity.** The space between the two layers of the peritoneum which may become a cavity.

**peritoneum.** Serous membrane covering the abdominal organs.

**peritonitis.** An inflammation of the peritoneum.

**pessary.** An appliance which is fitted into the vagina.

**petit mal seizure.** An attack of epilepsy characterized mainly by a loss of consciousness for a short period of time.

**phlebitis.** A condition in which a vein is inflamed.

**physical therapy.** Treatment of a patient by use of physical agents and special procedures, such as massage and exercise. Heat, cold, and electricity are examples of physical agents.

**pleura.** Serous membrane covering the lungs.

**pleurisy.** An inflammation of the pleura. It is called "pleurisy with effusion" when fluid collects in the pleural cavity.

**pneumonectomy.** Removal of an entire lung.

**pneumonia.** An infection of the lungs causing the spongy lung tissue to become more solid.

  **bacterial pneumonia.** That caused by bacteria.

  **bronchial pneumonia.** See bronchopneumonia.

  **hypostatic pneumonia.** That caused by staying in one position too long.

  **lobar pneumonia.** An acute illness in which one or more lobes are involved.

  **primary atypical pneumonia.** Virus pneumonia.

  **virus pneumonia.** That caused by a virus.

**pneumoperitoneum.** 1. The injection of air into the peritoneal cavity for examination of the abdomen by x-ray or to push the diaphragm upward into the chest cavity causing the lung to collapse.
2. A collection of gas in the peritoneal cavity.

**poliomyelitis.** An infectious disease caused by a filtrable virus.

  **acute anterior poliomyelitis.** A form in which the anterior portion of the gray matter in the spinal cord is affected. Muscles receiving their nerve supply from the diseased area may become weak and paralyzed.

  **bulbar poliomyelitis.** A type in which the medulla of the brain is affected. The respiratory and circulatory centers may be involved.

**polydipsia.** Extreme thirst.

**polyp.** An abnormal growth of tissue which appears to be growing on a stalk.

**polyuria.** An excessive output of urine.

**presbyopia.** Faulty vision in which the person can see distant objects better than close objects; occurs with the aging process.

**progesterone.** A substance produced by the corpus luteum; it causes changes in the uterine mucosa in preparation for the fertilized ovum.

**prognosis.** Prediction of the length, course, and outcome of a disease.

**prostatectomy.** The surgical removal of part or all of the prostate gland.

> **perineal prostatectomy.** Removal of the prostate through an incision in the perineum.
>
> **retropubic prostatectomy.** Removal of the prostate through an opening in the lower part of the abdomen. The surgeon reaches the gland by going behind the bladder.
>
> **suprapubic prostatectomy.** Removal of the prostate through an incision in the bladder above the pubic region.
>
> **transurethral prostatectomy.** Removal of the prostate through a special cystocope which has been inserted into the urethra.

**protozoa.** Microorganisms belonging to the animal kingdom.

**pruritis.** Itching.

**psychiatrist.** A physician specializing in psychiatry.

**psychiatry.** A branch of medicine dealing with the treatment of patients with mental disorders.

**psychomotor seizure.** An attack of epilepsy characterized by temporary mental disturbances.

**psychosomatic medicine.** A special branch of medicine which emphasizes the close relationship between the mind and the body of an individual.

**psychotherapy.** Treatment of an individual's mind.

**purulent.** Made of pus.

**pus.** A collection of dead tissue cells, bacteria, and dead white blood cells.

**pustule.** A small, rounded, raised area on the skin containing pus.

**pyelitis.** An inflammation in the pelvis of either one or both kidneys.

**pyelogram.** An x-ray examination of the kidneys and ureters.

> **intravenous pyelogram.** That following the intravenous injection of a special dye. X-ray films are taken as the dye is removed from the blood by the kidneys.
>
> **retrograde pyelogram.** That following the injection of a special dye into the pelvis of the kidney through a ureteral catheter. X-ray films are taken while the dye is in the pelvis of the kidney and while it is being excreted through the ureters.

**pyelonephritis.** An inflammation involving the entire substance of either one or both kidneys.

**pyloric orifice.** The opening between the stomach and small intestine.

**pyloric stenosis.** An obstruction in the pyloric opening of the stomach.

**pylorus.** The lower end of the stomach.

**pyuria.** A condition in which pus is present in the urine.

**quadriplegia.** Paralysis of all four extremities.

**radiation sickness.** Illness following radiotherapy. It may also follow exposure to radiant energy, such as that associated with explosion of an atomic bomb.

**radiotherapy.** Treatment of disease by the use of rays, such as x-ray and radium; radiation therapy.

**radium.** Metallic element which gives off rays. For this reason, it is referred to as radioactive.

**radon.** A gas given off by radium.

**radon seed.** Tiny tube filled with the gas given off by radium; radon implants. These tubes may be placed in the body tissue as a treatment for cancer and other diseases.

**rale.** Abnormal sound in air passages in the thoracic cavity.

**rectocele.** A condition in which the rectum has prolapsed into the vagina.

**rectum.** Lower portion of the large intestine, leading from the sigmoid colon to the anal canal.

**reduction.** The replacement of a broken bone or a dislocated joint to its normal position.

  **closed reduction.** That which is done by external manipulation.

  **open reduction.** That which is done through a surgical incision.

**refraction.** 1. The bending of rays.

  2. The bending of light rays as they pass through substances which have different densities. Light rays are bent as they pass through the eye so that they will be focused properly on the retina.

**rehabilitation.** Assistance given to help a person in regaining the greatest amount of usefulness and maximum degree of health which are possible with his handicap.

**resection.** An operation in which a section or segment of an organ is removed.

**residual urine.** An abnormal amount of urine left in the bladder after urination.

**respiration.** Process by which the living exchange gases with their environment; breathing.

  **Cheyne-Stokes respiration.** A type of breathing in which the respirations show a gradual increase in depth and rate, followed by a gradual decrease in depth and rate, and then apnea. The cycle starts again after the apnea. This type of respiration may also be described as periods of deep snoring respirations interrupted by periods of apnea.

**salpingectomy.** Surgical removal of a fallopian tube.

**salpingitis.** An inflammation of the fallopian tubes.

**salpingo-oophorectomy.** Surgical removal of either one or both fallopian tubes and ovaries.

**sarcoma.** Malignant tumor of connective tissue, such as bone, cartilage, fat, and tendons.

**sciatica.** A condition in which the patient has pain along the course of the sciatic nerve.

**sclerosis.** A hardening of certain body tissues, such as the arteries and nervous system.

**shingles.** *See* herpes zoster.

**shock.** A condition in which the patient has an insufficient amount of blood circulating in the body, especially the vessels in the outer part of the body. It may be caused by a marked dilation of the blood vessels or by an actual loss of blood.

**spore.** A microorganism covered with a tough membrane which causes it to be more difficult to kill.

**spur.** An outgrowth of tissue.

**staphylococci.** Oval-shaped bacteria which grow in grapelike clusters.

**stenosis.** A narrowing of a portion of the body such as a cavity or a tube.

**stomatitis.** An inflammation of the mouth.

**strabismus.** An abnormal condition of the eyes in which the person is unable to direct both eyes toward the same object. It is caused by a lack of coordination between the muscles controlling eye movement; also called squint.

**strangulation.** 1. Constriction of an area which checks the normal flow of blood, such as strangulation of an obstructed part of the intestine.

2. An obstruction of the air passages resulting in an oxygen deficiency, such as choking a person by pressing on the trachea.

**streptococci.** Oval-shaped bacteria which grow in chain formation.

**stye.** An acute inflammation on the edge of the eyelid; also called hordeolum.

**subcutaneous.** Under the skin; hypodermic.

**suppuration.** Process of pus formation.

**sympathectomy.** Surgical removal of a part of the sympathetic nervous system.

**symptom.** A change in the body or functioning of the body which indicates disease or a change in the disease.

  **objective symptom.** That which is seen, felt, heard, smelled, or determined by others.

  **subjective symptoms.** That which is felt by the patient.

**synovia.** Clear fluid found in various joints and bursae; also known as synovial fluid.

**synovial membrane.** Tissue lining the capsule which protects freely movable joints.

**tachycardia.** Rapid heart action.

**paroxysmal tachycardia.** That which occurs periodically.

**teamwork.** Sharing and working together for a common goal.

**tenesmus.** Painful straining without having a bowel movement.

**test(s).** A special procedure or method of examination.

    **concentration test.** A type of kidney function test used to determine whether the kidneys are concentrating the urine properly.

    **elimination diet test.** Diet used as an aid in determining specific foods to which a person is allergic.

    **intradermal test.** A type of skin test in which substances are injected between the skin layers to determine specific causes of allergy.

    **kidney function test.** Various types of tests designed to determine whether the kidneys are removing the proper amount of waste materials from the blood in the proper length of time.

    **ophthalmic test.** Procedure to determine substances to which a person is allergic. An allergen is dropped into the conjunctival sac. Redness and swelling of the membrane indicate that the patient is allergic to that substance.

    **phenolsulfonphthalein test.** A type of kidney function test in which phenolsulfonphthalein, a harmless red dye, is injected intravenously or intramuscularly. This dye, which is removed mainly by the kidneys, colors the urine. Urine specimens are collected at specific times after the dye is injected. The amount of dye in the urine is determined in the laboratory. Also called P.S.P. test.

    **scratch test.** A type of skin test to determine substances to which a person is allergic. Known allergens are dropped into scratches on either the back or arm.

    **sensitivity test.** A laboratory procedure used to determine which antibiotics will be effective against microorganisms growing in a certain part of the patient's body.

    **serology test.** Laboratory examination of blood serum to diagnose syphilis.

    **skin test.** Procedure to determine the reaction of skin, especially to an allergen. It is useful in determining substances to which a person is allergic. The known allergens may be injected between the skin layers, dropped into scratched areas, or placed on the skin.

    **test dose.** Administration of a small amount of a drug which is likely to cause an allergic reaction before giving the full dose.

    **tuberculin test.** A test to determine whether a person has or has had a tuberculosis infection.

**tetanus.** 1. State of continuous muscular contractions.

    2. An infectious disease caused by the bacillus, *Clostridium tetani*, which grows only in the absence of oxygen. Bacilli enter the body through a puncture or penetrating wound. This infection causes the patient to have almost continuous muscle spasms and is often fatal. Frequently called lockjaw.

**tetany.** A condition in which a decreased amount of calcium in the blood results in muscular spasms.

**thoracentesis.** The withdrawal of fluid from the chest cavity; chest aspiration.

**thoracoplasty.** An operation in which portions of the ribs are removed to reduce the size of the chest wall; used in the treatment of pulmonary tuberculosis.

**thoracotomy.** An operation in which an incision is made into the thoracic cavity.

**thromboangiitis obliterans.** A chronic disease of the blood vessels, especially in the legs of young men; Buerger's disease.

**thrombophlebitis.** A condition in which a vein is inflamed and a thrombus is formed; milk leg.

**thrombosis.** The formation of a blood clot in the heart or a blood vessel.
  **cerebral thrombosis.** That which occurs in a blood vessel in the brain.

**thrombus.** A blood clot which has been formed within a blood vessel or the heart.

**thyroid crisis.** An acute condition which may follow removal of the thyroid gland; characterized by fever, restlessness, profuse perspiration, and a rapid pulse.

**tinnitus.** A sensation of ringing in either one or both ears.

**tonometer.** An instrument used to measure tension or pressure, such as the tension within the eyeball.

**tracheostomy.** An operation in which a permanent opening is made into the trachea. The edges of the opening are sutured to the skin of the neck.

**tracheotomy.** An operation in which an opening is made into the trachea.

**traction.** Drawing or pulling, especially by the use of weights, cords, pulleys, and other special equipment.

**trauma.** Injury.

**trocar.** A surgical instrument used to puncture a cavity for the drainage of fluid.

**truss.** An apparatus sometimes worn over a reduced hernia to keep it from slipping out again.

**tubercle.** A small rounded growth; frequently used in referring to the lesion caused by tubercle bacilli.

**tumor.** An abnormal growth of the body's cells; neoplasm.
  **benign tumor.** One that grows slowly, does not spread, and is surrounded by a capsule.
  **malignant tumor.** One that grows rapidly, spreads, and is not surrounded by a capsule. Cancer; malignancy.
  **Wilms' tumor.** One of the kidneys which occurs usually in infants and young children.

**ulcer.** An abnormal break in the continuity of a surface; an open lesion.

**umbilicus.** The navel.

**uremia.** Failure of the kidneys to remove urinary constitutents from the blood; kidney failure.

**uremic frost.** A white, powdery substance on the skin of a patient with uremia.

**ureter.** A long small tube which carries urine from the pelvis of the kidney to the urinary bladder.

**ureterolithotomy.** The surgical removal of a stone from the ureter through an incision into this tube.

**urethra.** A small tube which carries urine from the urinary bladder to the external opening.

**urinary stasis.** A slackening or a stoppage of the normal flow of urine through the urinary tract.

**urticaria.** A skin condition in which the patient develops itching wheals. Hives; nettle rash.

**vaginitis.** An inflammatory condition of the vagina.

**varicocele.** Varicose veins of the spermatic cord.

**varicose vein.** A dilated and tortuous vein.

**vegetation.** An outgrowth of tissue which is similar to a plant in outline.

**vein ligation.** An operation in which the upper end of a vein is tied.

**vein stripping.** An operation in which a portion of a vein is removed by pulling it from its bed beneath the skin.

**ventriculography.** X-ray examination of the ventricles of the brain after air or some other suitable substance has been injected into the small cavities in the brain.

**vermiform appendix.** Wormlike projection attached to the cecum.

**vertebrae.** The bones which protect the spinal cord and its meninges; they form the vertebral column.

**vesicle.** A small sac or blister containing fluid.

**virus.** A small microorganism seen by a high-powered electron microscope and capable of reproduction only within another living cell.

**vomit.** Ejection of contents of the stomach through the mouth.

**vovulus.** A twisting of the intestine.

**wheal.** A raised, swollen area of the skin which usually itches, tingles, or burns. This lesion often appears and disappears quickly in the patient with urticaria. It may also occur after an insect or an animal bite.

# INDEX

anemia due to increased destruction of, 156
and liver, 237, 240
and malaria, 160, 161
sulfonamides, and destruction of, 156
and red bone marrow, 251
white, 154
increased in, Hodgkin's disease, 159
leukemia, 157
*See also* Leukocytes
Blood cell count, red, 154
white, 154
differential, 154
Blood clot. *See* Hematoma; Thrombus
Blood clot formation. *See* Thrombosis
Blood clotting, and fibrinogen, 153
in hemophilia, 159
and platelets, 154
Blood clotting time, determined before tonsillectomy, 171-72
and jaundice, 240
prolonged, and epistaxis, 39
*See also* Hemophilia
Blood formation, substances necessary for, 155
Blood loss, as cause of anemia, 156
Blood pressure, elevated, in nephritis, 313, 314
*See also* Hypertension
Blood serum, action of, after injury or in infection, 70
Blood sugar, affected by exercise, 293
increased. *See* Hyperglycemia
low. *See* Hypoglycemia
normal, 288
test for, in diabetes mellitus, 290
Blood test(s), and patient with, extensive burn, 439
protein-bound iodine, for toxic goiter, 281
*See also* Test(s)
Blood transfusions, in treatment of, anemia, 156-57, 158, 159
hemophilia, 159
Blood vessel(s), chronic inflammation of. *See* Thromboangiitis obliterans
diseases of. *See* Disease(s), of blood vessels

Blueness of skin. *See* Cyanosis
B.M.R. *See* Basal metabolic rate (B.M.R.)
Body, defenses of, against disease, 69-72
functioning of, and role of central nervous system, 355-57
Body fluids, controlling loss of, in severe burn, 438-39
*See also* Dehydration
Boil. *See* Abscess
Bone, broken. *See* Fracture
inflammation of. *See* Osteomyelitis
Bone graft, in treatment of, ruptured intervertebral disk, 367, 368
Bone marrow, formation of blood cells in, 251
involvement of, in osteomyelitis, 266
Bovine tuberculosis, 190
Brace, and clubfoot, 253
Bradycardia, 40
Brain, injury of, 364-65
description, 364
symptoms, 364-65
treatment and nursing care, 365
structure and function, 356
tumor of, 359-62
description, 359
symptoms, 359-60
treatment and nursing care, 360-62
postoperative care, 361-62
preoperative care, 361
Brain stem, 356
origin of cranial nerves, 356
Breast(s), conditions of, 431-34
benign tumor, 432
cancer, 433-34
mastitis, 431-32
chronic cystic, 432
monthly examination of, 433
structure and function, 431
Breathing. *See* Respiration
difficult, eased by oxygen therapy, 128. *See also* Dyspnea
Breathing exercises, after surgery, 59
Bronchial asthma, 98-99
Bronchial tree, 180
and bronchiectasis, 183
x-ray of, 184

Industries, and programs for, conservation of eyesight, 390
  conservation of hearing, 418
Indwelling catheter, care of, after surgery, 54
  and neurosurgical patient, 364
  and urinary retention, 43
  use of, after abdominoperineal operation, 232
    after cerebral vascular accident, 146
    after cystocele repair, 343
    and patient with extensive burn, 439
    and prostatic hypertrophy, 328, 329
Infants, bronchopneumonia, 181
  congenital cataracts, 397
  cretinism, 286, 287
  dermatitis, 428
  diarrhea, 29, 30
  gonorrheal infection of eyes. *See* Ophthalmia neonatorum
  impetigo contagiosa, 429
Infection, bladder, 318-19
  description, 318
  symptoms, 318
  treatment and nursing care, 318-19
  of blood stream, and destruction of red blood cells, 156
  of breast. *See* Mastitis
  as cause of disease, 18
  definition, 67
  and diabetic patient, 289, 300
  drugs to combat, 79
  eye, prevention of, 391
  kidney, 317-18
    cause, 317
    description, 317
    symptoms, 317
    treatment and nursing care, 318
  prevention of, in severe burn, 437-38
  and white blood cells, 154
  wound, postoperative, 62
Inflammation, definition, 67
  patient with, 67-79
    body's defenses, 69-72
    introduction, 67
    and microorganisms, 68-69
    nursing care, 73-79
      general, 78-79

      local, 73-78
    symptoms, 72-73
      general, 72-73
      local, 72
Infrared lamp, use of, for patient with neuralgia, 381
Injection, subcutaneous, of insulin, 295-96
Injection sites, for insulin, 296
  rotation of, 296
Injury(ies), of brain, 364-65
  as cause of disease, 19
  causes of, 67
  prevention of, and elderly patient after prostatectomy, 329, 330
  of spinal cord, 365-66
Inspiration, 165
Instillation of drops, in ear, 412, 413, 414
Insulin, 293-96
  administration of, by subcutaneous injection, 295-96
  injection sites, 296
  and islands of Langerhans, 239
  made from pancreas of animals, 293
  manufactured by pancreas, 280, 281
  storage of, 295
  strengths of, 293
  types of, 293-95
  and utilization of glucose by body, 288
Insulin shock, 299
  emergency treatment of, 299
  relationship to diet, 291, 292
  symptoms of, 299
Insulin syringe, 295-96
Intake of fluids, for patient with cancer, 91
Intake and output, 32
  for cardiac patient, 119-20, 121
  for dehydrated patient, 34
  for edematous patient, 35
  extensive burn, 439
  gastrointestinal suction, 223
  in infection, 78-79
  nephritis, acute, 313-14
  after neurosurgery, 362, 366
  postoperatively, 55, 62
  prostatic hypertrophy, 328, 329
Internist, definition, 300

Liver [cont.]
  hepatic duct of, 238
  structure and function, 237
Liver extract, in treatment of, pernicious
    anemia, 155, 156
Lobar pneumonia, 186
Lobectomy, 198, 200
  definition, 185
Local preparation, before surgery, 51
  on eye, 401
  on head, 361, 364
  mastoidectomy, 416
Lockjaw. See Tetanus
Locomotor system, 251
Lower gastrointestinal tract, diseases of,
    See Disease(s), of lower gastro-
    intestinal tract
  structure and function, 207-8
Lower respiratory system, diseases of.
    See Disease(s), of lower respira-
    tory system
  structure and function, 180
Lumbar puncture, 358, 369
Lung(s), cancer of, 199-200
  circulation of blood through, 108
Lye, swallowing of, as cause of esopha-
    geal stricture, 208
Lymph nodes, enlargement of, Hodg-
    kin's disease, 158
  leukemia, 157
Lymph-vascular system, after injury or
    in infection, 70, 72

Macules, 429
Magnet, use of, to remove particle of
    steel from eyeball, 392
Malaise, definition, 73
Malaria, 160-61
  description, 160
  symptoms, 160-61
  treatment and nursing care, 161
  types of, 160
Malarial parasite, 160, 161
Malignancy, common sites of, 83. See
    also Cancer
Malleus, 409
Mammary glands. See Breast(s)
Mastectomy, definition, 432
  radical, definition, 434
Mastitis, 431-32
  chronic cystic, description, 432

  symptoms, 432
  treatment, 432
  description, 431
  symptoms, 431-32
  treatment, 432
Mastoid, 410
Mastoidectomy, radical, 415
  simple, 415
Mastoiditis, 415-16
  description, 415
  symptoms, 415
  treatment and nursing care, 415-16
Mattress, firm, 258
Mazzini test, and syphilis, 348
Meatus urethrae, 308
Medicine, historical development of,
    3-5
  psychosomatic. See Psychosomatic
    medicine
Medicines, administration of. See
    Drugs; Drug therapy
Membrane, synovial, 251
Men, and common sites of cancer, 83
Meninges, 355, 374, 375
Meningitis, 374-76
  description, 374-75
  symptoms, 375
  treatment and nursing care, 375-76
Menopause, 335
  and amenorrhea, 337
  artificial, 335, 339, 341
  senile vaginitis after, 345
  and uterine cancer, 346
Menorrhagia, 336-37
  cause, 336
  description, 336
  treatment and nursing care, 337
Menstrual disorders, 335-38
  amenorrhea, 337-38
  dysmenorrhea, 335-36
  menorrhagia, 336-37
  metrorrhagia, 337
Menstrual period(s), bleeding between.
    See Cancer, uterus, symptoms;
    Metrorrhagia
Menstruation, 334-35
  cessation of. See Amenorrhea
  excessive. See Menorrhagia
  irregular, due to ovarian cyst, 338
  painful. See Dysmenorrhea

Religion. *See* Spiritual needs
Remedies, self-prescribed, avoid, in appendicitis, 219
Renal calculus(i). *See* Nephrolithiasis
Renal colic, 319
Reproductive system, diseases of. *See* Disease(s), of female reproductive system; Disease(s), of male reproductive system
  structure and function, female, 331-34
    male, 325-26
Resection, intestinal, 224
  and treatment of, tuberculous patient, 197-98
Respiration, Cheyne-Stokes, 39
  definition, 165
Respiratory center, cerebral, 165
Respiratory complications, postoperative, 58-61
  causes of, 54
  bronchitis, 59-60
  pneumonia, 60
  prevention, 58-59
  pulmonary embolism, 60-61
Respiratory system, definition, 165
  lower. *See* Lower respiratory system
  upper. *See* Upper respiratory system
Rest, for patient with, arthritis, 269, 274
  brain injury, 365
  bronchitis, acute, 182
  burn, extensive, 437, 439
  cardiac conditions, 112, 114, 115, 117, 118-19
  dysmenorrhea, 336
  epilepsy, 369
  having eye surgery, 402
  hemophilia, 150
  hemoptysis, 37
  hepatitis, acute, 241
  in infection, 78
  kidney infection, acute, 318
  mastoiditis, 415
  meningitis, 375
  menorrhagia, 337
  nephritis, acute, 313
  neuralgia, acute, 381
  osteomyelitis, 266
  pancreatitis, acute, 246
  peptic ulcer, 212-13

  peritonitis, 226
  pharyngitis, acute, 170
  pleurisy and empyema, 188
  pneumonia, 187, 188
  poliomyelitis, 378
  prostatic hypertrophy, benign, 328
  pulmonary tuberculosis, 195
  retinal detachment, 400
  ruptured intervertebral disk, 367
  salpingitis, acute, 340
  thrombophlebitis, 149
  toxic goiter, 284, 286
Rest period, of cardiac cycle, 108
Retention, urinary. *See* Urinary retention
Retention catheter. *See* Indwelling catheter
Retina, 389
  detachment of, 400-401
    cause, 400
    description, 400
    symptoms, 400
    treatment, 400-401
Retroflexion, of uterus. *See* Retroversion, of uterus
Retroversion, of uterus, description, 342
  sterility caused by, 342
  symptoms, 342
  treatment, 342
Rheumatic fever, 116
Rheumatic heart disease, 116-17
  description, 116
  symptoms and complications, 116-17
  treatment, 117
Rheumatoid arthritis, 267-73
  cause, 268
  description, 267-68
  symptoms, 268
  treatment and nursing care, 268-73
    attitude, of practical nurse, 272-73
    drugs, 271-72
    exercise, 270
    heat, 269-70
    occupational therapy, 270-71
    rest and prevention of deformity, 269
    skin care, 271
Rice diet, Kempner, 141
Rigidity, of muscles. *See* Parkinson's disease
Ruptured intervertebral disk, 366-68

blood, extensive burn, 439
blood sugar, 290
concentration, of urine, 311
cytologic, for cancer, 86
to determine an allergy, 95-97
  elimination diet, 96
  ophthalmic, 96
  skin, 96
    intradermal, 96
    scratch, 96
to determine hearing, 412
diabetic. *See* Diabetes mellitus, diagnosis
Kahn, and syphilis, 348
kidney function, 311-12
Kline, and syphilis, 348
Mazzini, and syphilis, 348
metabolic, 281
phenolsulfonphthalein (P.S.P.), 312
protein-bound iodine, 281
radioactive iodine uptake study, 282
sensitivity, and urine culture, 310
serology, to diagnose syphilis, 348
sugar (glucose) tolerance, 290
and toxic goiter, 281-82
tuberculin, 193, 194
  intradermal or Mantoux, 194
  Vollmer patch, 194
urine, acetone, 290
  sugar, 290
  24-hour specimen, 290
Wassermann, and syphilis, 348
Test dose of a drug, to prevent anaphylactic shock, 100
Tetanus, 438
antitoxin, 438
Tetany, after thyroid surgery, 286
Therapy, diet, 21
drug, 21-22
fluid, in severe burn, 438-39. *See also* Dehydration
physical, 22-23
radiation. *See* Radiation therapy; Radiotherapy
x-ray. *See* X-ray therapy
*See also* Disease(s), methods of treatment
Thermometer, use of, in heat cradle, 76
  to test water for hot-water bottle, 75
Thirst, excessive. *See* Polydipsia

Thoracentesis, 189
Thoracoplasty, 197
Thoracotomy, 190
Throat, cancer of, 214-15
Thromboangiitis obliterans, 150
Thrombophlebitis, 149-50
  postoperative, 61
Thrombosis, 150
  cerebral, 138, 142, 143
  coronary, 138
Thrombus, 138, 149
  as cause of, cerebral vascular accident, 142
  coronary occlusion, 112
Thrush, 208
Thymus, 279
Thyroid crisis, 286
Thyroidectomy, 284-86
  postoperative care, 285-86
  preoperative care, 285
Thyroid gland, 279
  regulator of body metabolism, 283
  storage of iodine in, 279, 282, 284
Thyroxin, hormone, 279
Tinnitus, 413
Tissue damage, from cold, danger signals of, 78
Tobacco, use of. *See* Smoking
Toenails, care of, orthopedic patient, 259, 262
  cutting of, diabetic patient, 296
Tonometer, 399
Tonsillectomy, 171-73
  postoperative care, 172-73
  preoperative care, 171-72
Tonsillitis, 171-73
  description, 171
  treatment and nursing care, 171-73
Toxic conditions, due to gold therapy in arthritis, 272
Toxic goiter, 283-86
  cause, 283
  description, 283
  symptoms, 283-84
  treatment and nursing care, 284-86
    postoperative, 285-86
    preoperative, 285
Toxic reaction, due to hormone therapy in arthritis, 272
Toxin(s) in infection, 70, 73, 79

Vitreous humor, 389
  after eye surgery, 402
Vocal folds, paralysis of, after thyroid
    surgery, 285
Voiding, frequent, in bladder infection,
    318
  and bladder tumor, 322
  and gonorrhea, 350
  in kidney infection, 317
  and pressure on urethra, 330
  *See also* Urination
Volvulus, as cause of intestinal obstruc-
    tion, 221
Vomiting, of blood. *See* Hematemesis
  definition, 28
  projectile, 29
    caused by pressure from brain
      tumor, 360
  *See also* Nausea and vomiting
Vomitus, 28, 29
  with fecal odor, in intestinal obstruc-
    tion, 222
  in lungs, as cause of postoperative
    complication, 49

Wall-eyed. *See* Strabismus
"Wangensteen suction," 214
Wart(s), 81, 85
  symptom of, skin cancer, 441
Wassermann test, and syphilis, 348
Waste products, removal of, by kidneys,
    109
Water balance, in body, disturbed. *See*
    Dehydration
W.B.C. *See* Blood cell(s), white;
    Leukocytes
Weight check, of acutely ill cardiac
    patient, 120
  of mildly ill cardiac patient, 121
Weight loss, in diabetes mellitus, 289
Weight record, daily, for edematous
    patient, 35
    for patient with acute nephritis,
      314

Wheals, definition, 99
White blood cells. *See* Blood cell(s),
    white; Leukocytes
White matter. *See* Nerve fibers
Wilms' tumor, 321
Women, and common sites of cancer,
    83
World War II, rapid growth of prac-
    tical nursing schools following,
    6
  and shortage of professional nurses, 6
Wound infection, postoperative, 62

X-ray(s), 87, 88
  chest, 85, 86
    bronchiectasis, 184
    lung cancer, 199
    preoperatively, 48
    tuberculosis, 193, 194
  to diagnose fracture, 256
  gallbladder, 243, 244
  gastrointestinal, and diagnosis of
    peptic ulcer, 211
  of kidney, to locate stones, 320. *See
    also* Pyelogram
X-ray examination, nervous system,
    358-59
X-ray therapy, and acne vulgaris, severe
    cases of, 427
  bladder tumor, 322
  breast cancer, 434
  for bursitis, 275
  cancer of larynx, 177
  kidney tumor, 322
  lung cancer, 200
  portal of entry marks, 89
  skin cancer, 441
  *See also* Radiation therapy; Radio-
    therapy

Yeast, 68